Diagnosis of Lower Genital Tract Disease

Diagnosis of Lower Genital Tract Disease

Editors

Fabio Bottari
Anna Daniela Iacobone

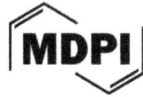

Basel • Beijing • Wuhan • Barcelona • Belgrade • Novi Sad • Cluj • Manchester

Editors

Fabio Bottari
Division of Laboratory
Medicine
European Institute
of Oncology IRCCS
Milan
Italy

Anna Daniela Iacobone
Preventive Gynecology Unit
European Institute
of Oncology IRCCS
Milan
Italy

Editorial Office
MDPI
St. Alban-Anlage 66
4052 Basel, Switzerland

This is a reprint of articles from the Special Issue published online in the open access journal *Diagnostics* (ISSN 2075-4418) (available at: www.mdpi.com/journal/diagnostics/special_issues/Lower_Genital_Tract_Disease).

For citation purposes, cite each article independently as indicated on the article page online and as indicated below:

Lastname, A.A.; Lastname, B.B. Article Title. *Journal Name* **Year**, *Volume Number*, Page Range.

ISBN 978-3-0365-9297-8 (Hbk)
ISBN 978-3-0365-9296-1 (PDF)
doi.org/10.3390/books978-3-0365-9296-1

© 2023 by the authors. Articles in this book are Open Access and distributed under the Creative Commons Attribution (CC BY) license. The book as a whole is distributed by MDPI under the terms and conditions of the Creative Commons Attribution-NonCommercial-NoDerivs (CC BY-NC-ND) license.

Contents

Preface vii

Fabio Bottari and Anna Daniela Iacobone
The Editorial of the Special Issue "Diagnosis of Lower Genital Tract Disease"
Reprinted from: *Diagnostics* 2023, 13, 2515, doi:10.3390/diagnostics13152515 1

Dana Gabrieli, Yael Suissa-Cohen, Sireen Jaber and Ahinoam Lev-Sagie
"Modified Schirmer Test" as an Objective Measurement for Vaginal Dryness: A Prospective Cohort Study
Reprinted from: *Diagnostics* 2022, 12, 574, doi:10.3390/diagnostics12030574 4

Marianna Martinelli, Chiara Giubbi, Illari Sechi, Fabio Bottari, Anna Daniela Iacobone and Rosario Musumeci et al.
Evaluation of BD Onclarity™ HPV Assay on Self-Collected Vaginal and First-Void Urine Samples as Compared to Clinician-Collected Cervical Samples: A Pilot Study
Reprinted from: *Diagnostics* 2022, 12, 3075, doi:10.3390/diagnostics12123075 12

Natasa Nikolic, Branka Basica, Aljosa Mandic, Nela Surla, Vera Gusman and Deana Medic et al.
E6/E7 mRNA Expression of the Most Prevalent High-Risk HPV Genotypes in Cervical Samples from Serbian Women
Reprinted from: *Diagnostics* 2023, 13, 917, doi:10.3390/diagnostics13050917 23

Fabio Bottari, Anna Daniela Iacobone, Davide Radice, Eleonora Petra Preti, Mario Preti and Dorella Franchi et al.
HPV Tests Comparison in the Detection and Follow-Up after Surgical Treatment of CIN2+ Lesions
Reprinted from: *Diagnostics* 2022, 12, 2359, doi:10.3390/diagnostics12102359 45

Ailyn M. Vidal Urbinati, Ida Pino, Anna D. Iacobone, Davide Radice, Giulia Azzalini and Maria E. Guerrieri et al.
Vaginosonography versus MRI in Pre-Treatment Evaluation of Early-Stage Cervical Cancer: An Old Tool for a New Precision Approach?
Reprinted from: *Diagnostics* 2022, 12, 2904, doi:10.3390/diagnostics12122904 54

Luca Pace, Silvia Actis, Matteo Mancarella, Lorenzo Novara, Luca Mariani and Gaetano Perrini et al.
Clinical, Sonographic, and Hysteroscopic Features of Endometrial Carcinoma Diagnosed after Hysterectomy in Patients with a Preoperative Diagnosis of Atypical Hyperplasia: A Single-Center Retrospective Study
Reprinted from: *Diagnostics* 2022, 12, 3029, doi:10.3390/diagnostics12123029 65

Anna Daniela Iacobone, Davide Radice, Maria Elena Guerrieri, Noemi Spolti, Barbara Grossi and Fabio Bottari et al.
Which Risk Factors and Colposcopic Patterns Are Predictive for High-Grade VAIN? A Retrospective Analysis
Reprinted from: *Diagnostics* 2023, 13, 176, doi:10.3390/diagnostics13020176 77

Anna Daniela Iacobone, Maria Elena Guerrieri, Eleonora Petra Preti, Noemi Spolti, Gianluigi Radici and Giulia Peveri et al.
Tips and Tricks for Early Diagnosis of Cervico-Vaginal Involvement from Extramammary Paget's Disease of the Vulva: A Referral Center Experience
Reprinted from: *Diagnostics* 2023, 13, 464, doi:10.3390/diagnostics13030464 91

Daniel Guerendiain, Laila Sara Arroyo Mühr, Raluca Grigorescu, Matthew T. G. Holden and Kate Cuschieri
Mapping HPV 16 Sub-Lineages in Anal Cancer and Implications for Disease Outcomes
Reprinted from: *Diagnostics* **2022**, *12*, 3222, doi:10.3390/diagnostics12123222 103

Narcisa Muresu, Biagio Di Lorenzo, Laura Saderi, Illari Sechi, Arcadia Del Rio and Andrea Piana et al.
Prevalence of Human Papilloma Virus Infection in Bladder Cancer: A Systematic Review
Reprinted from: *Diagnostics* **2022**, *12*, 1759, doi:10.3390/diagnostics12071759 115

Massimo Origoni, Francesco Cantatore, Francesco Sopracordevole, Nicolò Clemente, Arsenio Spinillo and Barbara Gardella et al.
Colposcopy Accuracy and Diagnostic Performance: A Quality Control and Quality Assurance Survey in Italian Tertiary-Level Teaching and Academic Institutions—The Italian Society of Colposcopy and Cervico-Vaginal Pathology (SICPCV)
Reprinted from: *Diagnostics* **2023**, *13*, 1906, doi:10.3390/diagnostics13111906 132

Preface

Lower genital tract diseases include vulvovaginal and HPV-related diseases, ranging from benign to pre-neoplastic and neoplastic lesions. Nowadays, there has been increasing interest in innovative methods to diagnose and prevent cervical cancer through HPV primary screening programs. However, other lower genital tract diseases are unrelated to HPV infection; hence, cytology, colposcopy, and sonography might play a crucial role in assessment and management. This Special Issue aims to address current and emerging issues in the field of the diagnosis, assessment, staging, and management of HPV-related and not-related pathology of the lower female anogenital tract. These may include new advancements in HPV testing and laboratory biomarkers, investigations on the actual role of cytology and implementation of diagnostic tools to implement differential diagnosis, and the current clinical management of lower genital tract diseases.

Fabio Bottari and Anna Daniela Iacobone
Editors

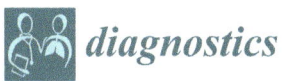

Editorial

The Editorial of the Special Issue "Diagnosis of Lower Genital Tract Disease"

Fabio Bottari [1,*] and Anna Daniela Iacobone [2]

1. Division of Laboratory Medicine, Istituto Europeo di Oncologia IRCCS, 20145 Milan, Italy
2. Preventive Gynecology Unit, Istituto Europeo di Oncologia IRCCS, 20145 Milan, Italy; annadaniela.iacobone@ieo.it
* Correspondence: fabio.bottari@ieo.it

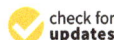

Citation: Bottari, F.; Iacobone, A.D. The Editorial of the Special Issue "Diagnosis of Lower Genital Tract Disease". Diagnostics 2023, 13, 2515. https://doi.org/10.3390/diagnostics13152515

Received: 18 July 2023
Revised: 24 July 2023
Accepted: 27 July 2023
Published: 28 July 2023

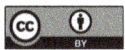

Copyright: © 2023 by the authors. Licensee MDPI, Basel, Switzerland. This article is an open access article distributed under the terms and conditions of the Creative Commons Attribution (CC BY) license (https://creativecommons.org/licenses/by/4.0/).

A range of conditions involving the vulvovaginal and anal area, and those associated with human papillomavirus (HPV) infection, which can manifest as benign, pre-neoplastic, or neoplastic lesions, can be grouped into lower genital tract diseases. Currently, there is growing interest in innovative approaches for diagnosing and preventing cervical cancer through primary human papillomavirus (HPV) screening programs. However, it is important to note that other lower genital tract diseases are not related to HPV infection. Consequently, cytology, colposcopy, and sonography might play a crucial role in their assessment and management.

The objective of this Special Issue is to address current and emerging issues in the field of the diagnosis, assessment, staging, and management of both HPV-related and unrelated pathologies of the lower ano-genital tract. Topics of interest include advancements in HPV testing and laboratory biomarkers, investigations into the actual utility of cytology, the implementation of diagnostic tools to facilitate differential diagnosis, and the current clinical management of lower genital tract diseases.

This Special Issue has had the pleasure of receiving articles that cover all the requested fields of lower ano-genital tract disease. In total, ten original articles and one systematic review have been presented.

The first article submitted to the Special Issue demonstrates how a diagnostic tool commonly used in the field of ophthalmology can be adapted to effectively evaluate vaginal dryness. Gabrieli et al. [1] presented their findings on the "modified Schirmer test," which serves as an objective scale for assessing vaginal moisture levels. This study highlights the test's potential to manage women who experience vaginal dryness.

Furthermore, in line with the theme of the Special Issue, several articles focused on HPV tests have been included. These articles explore diagnostic innovations such as self-sampling [2] and mRNA-based HPV tests [3]. Additionally, there is an article investigating the usefulness of HPV testing as a test-of-cure in post-treatment follow-up [4].

Martinelli et al. published an article presenting promising results from their pilot study on the use of the Onclarity HPV assay on vaginal samples and first-void urine samples. The accuracy of HPV testing on self-collected samples was found to be nearly equivalent to clinician-collected cervical samples. This finding represents the basis on which several studies have been conducted to validate HPV tests on self-sampling as a diagnostic tool to expand cervical cancer screening coverage [2].

Nikolic et al. showed that mRNA testing may be more relevant than HPV DNA testing for the assessment of lesion grade and in the diagnosis and monitoring of women at risk of progressive cervical disease. The HPV mRNA test shows great potential as both a screening test and a triage test for HPV DNA-positive women due to its higher specificity (detecting active infections) and greater objectivity compared to cytology. Employing the mRNA test for the improved risk stratification of HPV infection could help reduce unnecessary examinations, lower costs, and alleviate patient anxiety [3].

Bottari et al. provided evidence that the HPV test serves as a valid option for test-of-cure monitoring in patients treated for CIN2+ lesions during follow-up. Their article also emphasizes the importance of using validated HPV DNA or RNA tests, as they consistently produce comparable results. Non-validated tests do not share the same assurance, emphasizing the strong recommendation to utilize validated HPV tests exclusively in both screening and test-of-cure settings [4].

Other intriguing articles in this Special Issue focus on the use of diagnostic imaging for the diagnosis of genital diseases, particularly in the early stages of cervical cancer [5] and endometrial carcinoma [6].

Vidal Urbinati et al. demonstrated a significant correlation between vaginosonography and magnetic resonance imaging in the assessment of tumor dimensions. They highlighted the superior performance of the sonographic tool in detecting small tumors and predicting the absence of fornix infiltration [5].

In their retrospective study, Pace et al. identified several ultrasonographic features that, in conjunction with subjective hysteroscopic assessment by experienced clinicians, can suggest the presence of occult endometrial cancer in patients with a preoperative histologic diagnosis of atypical endometrial hyperplasia. These features include endometrial thickness, a larger diameter of the lesion, an interrupted endometrial–myometrial junction, and high vascular density on color Doppler imaging [6].

Furthermore, a significant section of this Special Issue is devoted to the pathology of the lower extra-cervical genital tract. Within this context, three original articles and one review have been published, focusing on various aspects such as vaginal pre-cancers and cancer [7], extramammary Paget's disease of the vulva [8], anal cancer [9], and bladder cancer [10].

The retrospective analysis conducted by Iacobone et al. aimed to investigate the correlation between colposcopic features and the development of high-grade vaginal intraepithelial neoplasia (VAIN) [7]. An accurate diagnosis is crucial for the effective management of vaginal pre-cancers and cancers. The study found that certain colposcopic findings, such as grade 2, papillary, and vascular patterns, can serve as predictive factors for high-grade VAIN. Moreover, HPV genotyping can contribute to risk stratification and facilitate the prompt identification of women at a higher risk of persistence, recurrence, and progression to vaginal cancer in cases of high-grade VAIN.

Another highly intriguing article authored by Iacobone et al. [8] explores cervico-vaginal involvement in extramammary Paget's disease of the vulva, a distinctive and uncommon condition. This article provides a comprehensive examination of both the diagnostic aspects and the management strategies related to this pathology, highlighting the importance of recognizing its significance in women with a long-standing history of vulvar Paget's disease. The article emphasizes the value and reliability of cytology, coupled with immunocytochemistry, as a prompt and indispensable tool for early diagnosis.

In this Special Issue, Guarendian et al. [9] employed whole-genome sequencing, an innovative method that is transforming tumor genetics management. Their findings, utilizing this advanced approach, indicate that HPV 16 sub-lineages do not exhibit association with disease versus asymptomatic carriage, nor do they demonstrate independent associations with outcomes in anal cancer patients.

Additionally, a captivating systematic review on the prevalence of HPV infection in bladder cancer is presented within this Special Issue. In this article, Muresu et al. highlight a potential role of HPV in the development of bladder cancer, providing indirect support for the implementation of primary preventive strategies as recommended by international authorities and study groups [10].

Finally, the article by Origoni et al. draws attention to the fundamental role of education in medicine, particularly in the training of colposcopists. This study emphasizes the significance of educating new generations of skilled gynecologists and standardizing a procedure that is inherently subjective. The adoption of colposcopy standards and quality recommendations by scientific societies is a fundamental step towards ensuring effective cervical cancer prevention [11].

All the papers presented in this Special Issue underscore the significance of research and progress in the diagnosis and management of lower genital tract diseases. The prevailing challenge lies in the exploration of increasingly sophisticated and precise tools that allow for early detection and robust management approaches.

The advancement of diagnostic techniques and the evolution of patient management hold promising potential to alleviate the burden and enhance the treatment of lower genital tract diseases.

Author Contributions: Writing—original draft, review and editing, F.B. and A.D.I. All authors have read and agreed to the published version of the manuscript.

Funding: This research received no external funding.

Institutional Review Board Statement: Not applicable.

Conflicts of Interest: The authors declare no conflict of interest.

References

1. Gabrieli, D.; Suissa-Cohen, Y.; Jaber, S.; Lev-Sagie, A. "Modified Schirmer Test" as an Objective Measurement for Vaginal Dryness: A Prospective Cohort Study. *Diagnostics* **2022**, *12*, 574. [CrossRef] [PubMed]
2. Martinelli, M.; Giubbi, C.; Sechi, I.; Bottari, F.; Iacobone, A.; Musumeci, R.; Perdoni, F.; Muresu, N.; Piana, A.; Fruscio, R.; et al. Evaluation of BD Onclarity™ HPV Assay on Self-Collected Vaginal and First-Void Urine Samples as Compared to Clinician-Collected Cervical Samples: A Pilot Study. *Diagnostics* **2022**, *12*, 3075. [CrossRef]
3. Nikolic, N.; Basica, B.; Mandic, A.; Surla, N.; Gusman, V.; Medic, D.; Petrovic, T.; Strbac, M.; Petrovic, V. E6/E7 mRNA Expression of the Most Prevalent High-Risk HPV Genotypes in Cervical Samples from Serbian Women. *Diagnostics* **2023**, *13*, 917. [CrossRef] [PubMed]
4. Bottari, F.; Iacobone, A.; Radice, D.; Preti, E.; Preti, M.; Franchi, D.; Boveri, S.; Sandri, M.; Passerini, R. HPV Tests Comparison in the Detection and Follow-Up after Surgical Treatment of CIN2+ Lesions. *Diagnostics* **2022**, *12*, 2359. [CrossRef] [PubMed]
5. Vidal Urbinati, A.; Pino, I.; Iacobone, A.; Radice, D.; Azzalini, G.; Guerrieri, M.; Preti, E.; Martella, S.; Franchi, D. Vaginosonography versus MRI in Pre-Treatment Evaluation of Early-Stage Cervical Cancer: An Old Tool for a New Precision Approach? *Diagnostics* **2022**, *12*, 2904. [CrossRef]
6. Pace, L.; Actis, S.; Mancarella, M.; Novara, L.; Mariani, L.; Perrini, G.; Govone, F.; Testi, A.; Campisi, P.; Ferrero, A.; et al. Clinical, Sonographic, and Hysteroscopic Features of Endometrial Carcinoma Diagnosed after Hysterectomy in Patients with a Preoperative Diagnosis of Atypical Hyperplasia: A Single-Center Retrospective Study. *Diagnostics* **2022**, *12*, 3029. [CrossRef] [PubMed]
7. Iacobone, A.; Radice, D.; Guerrieri, M.; Spolti, N.; Grossi, B.; Bottari, F.; Boveri, S.; Martella, S.; Vidal Urbinati, A.; Pino, I.; et al. Which Risk Factors and Colposcopic Patterns Are Predictive for High-Grade VAIN? A Retrospective Analysis. *Diagnostics* **2023**, *13*, 176. [CrossRef] [PubMed]
8. Iacobone, A.; Guerrieri, M.; Preti, E.; Spolti, N.; Radici, G.; Peveri, G.; Bagnardi, V.; Tosti, G.; Maggioni, A.; Bottari, F.; et al. Tips and Tricks for Early Diagnosis of Cervico-Vaginal Involvement from Extramammary Paget's Disease of the Vulva: A Referral Center Experience. *Diagnostics* **2023**, *13*, 464. [CrossRef] [PubMed]
9. Guerendiain, D.; Mühr, L.; Grigorescu, R.; Holden, M.; Cuschieri, K. Mapping HPV 16 Sub-Lineages in Anal Cancer and Implications for Disease Outcomes. *Diagnostics* **2022**, *12*, 3222. [CrossRef] [PubMed]
10. Muresu, N.; Di Lorenzo, B.; Saderi, L.; Sechi, I.; Del Rio, A.; Piana, A.; Sotgiu, G. Prevalence of Human Papilloma Virus Infection in Bladder Cancer: A Systematic Review. *Diagnostics* **2022**, *12*, 1759. [CrossRef] [PubMed]
11. Origoni, M.; Cantatore, F.; Sopracordevole, F.; Clemente, N.; Spinillo, A.; Gardella, B.; De Vincenzo, R.; Ricci, C.; Landoni, F.; Di Meo, M.; et al. Colposcopy Accuracy and Diagnostic Performance: A Quality Control and Quality Assurance Survey in Italian Tertiary-Level Teaching and Academic Institutions—The Italian Society of Colposcopy and Cervico-Vaginal Pathology (SICPCV). *Diagnostics* **2023**, *13*, 1906. [CrossRef] [PubMed]

Disclaimer/Publisher's Note: The statements, opinions and data contained in all publications are solely those of the individual author(s) and contributor(s) and not of MDPI and/or the editor(s). MDPI and/or the editor(s) disclaim responsibility for any injury to people or property resulting from any ideas, methods, instructions or products referred to in the content.

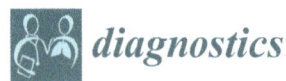

Article

"Modified Schirmer Test" as an Objective Measurement for Vaginal Dryness: A Prospective Cohort Study

Dana Gabrieli [1,*,†], Yael Suissa-Cohen [2,†], Sireen Jaber [2] and Ahinoam Lev-Sagie [1,2]

1 Faculty of Medicine, Hebrew University of Jerusalem, Jerusalem 9780214, Israel; levsagie@netvision.net.il
2 Department of Obstetrics and Gynecology, Hadassah-Hebrew University Medical Center, Mount Scopus, Jerusalem 9765422, Israel; yaelshi.suissa@mail.huji.ac.il (Y.S.-C.); sireenjaber@gmail.com (S.J.)
* Correspondence: danagabrieli@gmail.com
† These authors contributed equally to this work.

Abstract: None of the currently available parameters allow for a direct and objective measurement of vaginal moisture. We used a calibrated filter paper strip as a measurement tool for the quantification of vaginal fluid, in a similar manner as the ophthalmic "Schirmer test" (used for eye moisture measurement). The study aimed to evaluate the validity of this new, objective tool, to measure vaginal moisture. We compared vaginal moisture measurements using the "modified Schirmer test" in symptomatic women with genitourinary syndrome of menopause to those of women without vaginal dryness. The mean "modified Schirmer test" measurement in the control group was 21.7 mm compared to 3.3 mm in the study group, yielding a statistically significant difference ($p < 0.001$). Strong correlations were found between "modified Schirmer test" measurements and pH (correlation coefficient −0.714), Vaginal Health Index [VHI (0.775)], and Visual Analogue Score (VAS) of dryness during intercourse (−0.821). Our findings suggest that the "modified Schirmer test" can be used as an objective measurement for the assessment of vaginal fluid level. This test may also prove useful for evaluation of non-hormonal treatments aimed to treat vaginal dryness.

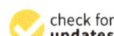

Citation: Gabrieli, D.; Suissa-Cohen, Y.; Jaber, S.; Lev-Sagie, A. "Modified Schirmer Test" as an Objective Measurement for Vaginal Dryness: A Prospective Cohort Study. *Diagnostics* 2022, 12, 574. https://doi.org/10.3390/diagnostics12030574

Academic Editors: Fabio Bottari and Anna Daniela Iacobone

Received: 28 January 2022
Accepted: 21 February 2022
Published: 23 February 2022

Publisher's Note: MDPI stays neutral with regard to jurisdictional claims in published maps and institutional affiliations.

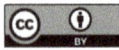

Copyright: © 2022 by the authors. Licensee MDPI, Basel, Switzerland. This article is an open access article distributed under the terms and conditions of the Creative Commons Attribution (CC BY) license (https://creativecommons.org/licenses/by/4.0/).

Keywords: genitourinary syndrome of menopause (GSM); vaginal dryness; vaginal atrophy; vaginal health index (VHI); estrogen; vaginal maturation index (VMI); fractional CO_2 laser

1. Introduction

Urogenital atrophy, also referred to as genitourinary syndrome of menopause (GSM) [1], is caused by decreased estrogen levels in women's urogenital tissues. Symptoms include vulvovaginal discomfort described as dryness, itching, burning, irritation, and soreness; sexual dysfunction due to decreased lubrication and dyspareunia; and urinary complaints such as urgency, frequency, and recurrent urinary tract infections [2,3].

Among menopausal women, prevalence of GSM is estimated at approximately 50–60%, making it one of the most frequent causes of genital complaints in this age group [4]. The diagnosis is clinical, based on a combination of symptoms and signs upon physical examination, including thin, pale, smooth, and shiny vaginal epithelium with diminished elasticity [2]. Estrogen supplementation (topically or systemically) is considered the most efficient treatment [5,6]. Following estrogen administration, epithelial maturation occurs, with subsequent changes in epithelial thickness, pH level, and tissue elasticity [6,7].

Treatment efficacy is evaluated in clinical trials using a range of measurements that represent the changes occurring in the vagina in response to the presence or absence of estrogen. The commonly used measures include pH level, vaginal health index (VHI, Table 1) and the vaginal maturation index (VMI) [8]. Other tools used to assess treatment are a variety of questionnaires or scores, relying on patient's self-report, assessing symptoms' severity or quality of life parameters. Available questionnaires include the Most Bothersome Symptoms (MBS), the Day-to-Day Impact on Vaginal Aging (DIVA) Questionnaire, the Vulvovaginal Symptoms Questionnaire (VSQ), and the Vulvar Pain Assessment Questionnaire (VPAQ) [8]. Alternatively, an array of scores rate severity of symptoms, enabling subjective comparison. Available scores include the Vaginal and Vulvar Assessment Scale, the Female Sexual Function Index (FSFI), and the Female Sexual Distress Scale-Revised (FSDS-R) [8].

As many women with GSM are reluctant to use local estrogen due to various concerns [9], alternatives for topical hormonal treatment are sought. Studies have been evaluating the effectiveness of alternative therapies that do not include estrogen, such as hydrating agents, hormonal non-estrogens including DHEA [6], and energy based treatments, such as the fractional CO_2 laser [9,10], non-ablative vaginal Er:YAG laser (VEL) [11] and radiofrequency procedures [12].

Introduction of energy-based treatments for GSM in recent years resulted in studies evaluating the efficacy of these treatments. These modalities are claimed to improve GSM in an estrogen independent mechanism, such as connective tissue remodulation and neovascularization [9,11–14]. Nevertheless, most of the published research evaluated treatment outcomes using one or more estrogen-dependent measures (i.e., pH, VMI, and VHI). Despite reporting positive effects on symptoms and a relative improvement in the VHI index, pH levels and cytological measures, unsurprisingly, often do not show a clinically significant difference [15–19].

As none of the currently available parameters allow a direct and objective measurement of the vaginal condition and moisture, there is a need for such tools. Ideally, such measures should be objective, allow assessment of GSM-associated signs, and incorporate parameters relevant to new treatment modalities, which do not depend on estrogen or its effects on the vaginal tissue.

Considering patients' reports of increased vaginal secretions following estrogen supplementation as well as following laser treatment, we opted to develop and test a vaginal dryness/moisture measurement tool. The tool we used was a calibrated filter paper strip, similar to the one used to perform the ophthalmic "Schirmer test" for eye moisture measurement.

Our goal was to evaluate the validity of this objective measurement tool for vaginal moisture by comparing measurements in symptomatic women suffering from GSM-associated vaginal dryness to measurements in healthy women without vaginal dryness.

2. Materials and Methods

This prospective cohort study consisted of women evaluated between January 2021 and June 2021 in an outpatient gynecologic clinic at Hadassah University Medical Center, Jerusalem, Israel. The study consisted of two groups: (1) menopausal women with complaints characteristic of GSM, including dryness, and (2) premenopausal women without vulvovaginal symptoms, who denied dryness.

An additional inclusion criterion included age > 18 years. Exclusion criteria included urinary incontinence, vaginal prolapse, vulvovaginal infection, vulvar skin disease, diagnosed Sjogren Syndrome, pregnancy, and vaginal bleeding.

The study was approved by the Institutional Review Board (Number 0923-20-HMO) and all participants signed informed consent.

Measurement of vaginal moisture was performed by placing a calibrated filter paper test strip, in a standard manner (see below) for 5 min. In all cases, to keep uniformity, the tip of the paper was located adjacent to the hymenal tissue (or its remnants) on the right side of the vaginal opening (at the "7 o'clock" location) (Figure 1).

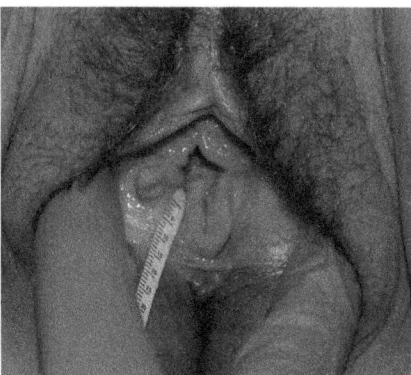

Figure 1. Modified Schirmer test—paper strip location. Measurement of vaginal moisture is performed by placing the tip of a calibrated filter paper test strip adjacent to the remnants of the hymenal tissue on the right side of the vaginal opening, at the "7 o'clock" location.

The paper was placed using a Q-tip while the patient was lying on a gynecological bed, and it was left in place for 5 min. After 5 min, the paper strip was gently removed. Fluid amount was measured by the length of the moistened area of the strip in millimeters (Figure 2).

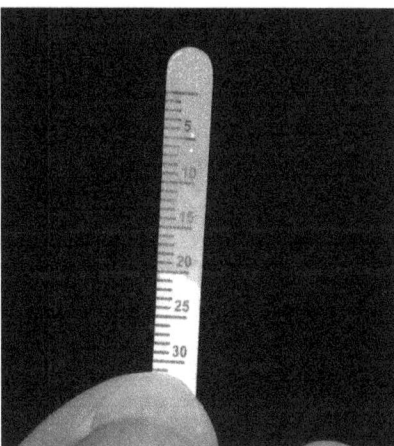

Figure 2. Modified Schirmer test paper strip measurement modality. Fluid amount is measured by the length of the moistened area of the strip in millimeters, i.e., 20 mm.

The test is based on the principle of capillary action, which allows the fluid from the vagina to be absorbed along the length of a paper test strip in an identical fashion as a horizontal capillary tube. The hypothesis is that the rate of travel along the test strip for 5 min time represents the amount of fluid in the vagina.

To evaluate the association between the "modified Schirmer test" and other measures, the following data were collected for each patient: vaginal pH was measured using a pH-indicator strip (pH range 3–8, Merck, Germany), VHI score was calculated (Table 1) and documented, and patients were requested to score the degree of daily vaginal dryness as well as dryness during intercourse, using a 0–10 visual analogue scale (VAS), with 0 representing no dryness, and 10 being the worst possible dryness.

Table 1. The vaginal health index (VHI) (adapted from Bachmann et al. [20]).

Score	1	2	3	4	5
Elasticity	None	Poor	Fair	Good	Excellent
Fluid Volume (Pooling of Secretions)	None	Scant amount, vault not entirely covered	Superficial amount, vault entirely covered	Moderate amount of dryness (small areas of dryness on cotton-tip applicator)	Normal amount (fully saturates on cotton-tip applicator)
pH	6.1 or above	5.6–6.0	5.1–5.5	4.7–5.0	4.6 or below
Epithelial Integrity	Petechiae noted before contact	Bleeds with light contact	Bleeds with scraping	Not friable, thin epithelium	Normal
Moisture (Coating)	None, surface inflamed	None, surface not inflamed	Minimal	Moderate	Normal

Estimation of sample size was based on the expected difference in "modified Schirmer test" measurements between symptomatic menopausal women and asymptomatic non-menopausal women, calculated using available preliminary data collected for another study (NCT03063684). Given standard deviation measurements of 8.8 mm in the control group compared to 0.79 mm in the GSM group, to prove any difference of 4 mm or higher between the two groups statistically significant, with a significance of 5% (unilateral) and a power of 80%, the calculated number of women needed in each group was 30.

Data were analyzed using the SSPS software (SSPS Science, Chicago, IL, USA). Comparison of "modified Schirmer test" results between the two groups was performed using a t-test. Correlation analysis was performed using Pearson's rank correlation. Statistical significance was set at $p < 0.05$.

3. Results

Sixty women were enrolled, and their characteristics are detailed in Table 2. Out of the 30 women who were enrolled in the control group, two were excluded from the final analysis because they did not meet the inclusion criteria, as despite verbally denying any vaginal complaints, their VAS during intercourse score was 4 or higher.

Table 2. Patients' characteristics.

Study Group		Control (N = 28)	GSM (N = 30)
Age	Mean (Std. Deviation)	38.2 (6.7)	48.3 (7.1)
	Median (Range)	36.5 (28–52)	47.5 (36–63)
Gravidity	Mean (Std. Deviation)	3.1 (1.9)	4.1 (2.1)
	Median (Range)	3 (0–9)	4 (2–10)
Vaginal Deliveries	Mean (Std. Deviation)	1.8 (1.4)	3 (1.3)
	Median (Range)	2 (0–4)	3 (1–8)
Hormonal Status	Menstruation (%)	19 (67.9)	0 (0)
	Amenorrhea with Hormonal IUD (%)	7 (25)	0 (0)
	Perimenopause (%)	2 (7.1)	0 (0)
	Menopause (%)	0 (0)	30 (100)
Contraception	None (%)	8 (28.6)	30 (100)
	BTL (%)	2 (7.1)	0 (0)
	Condoms (%)	4 (14.3)	0 (0)
	Copper IUD (%)	4 (14.3)	0 (0)
	Hormonal IUD (%)	7 (25)	0 (0)
	HCs (%)	3 (10.7)	0 (0)

GSM = genitourinary syndrome of menopause, IUD = intra-uterine device, BTL = bilateral tubal ligation, HCs = hormonal contraceptives.

In the GSM group, 28 women were previously diagnosed with breast cancer, and 23 of them were treated with aromatase inhibitors.

"Modified Schirmer test" measurements, pH levels, VHI, and VAS are presented in Table 3. Comparison of "modified Schirmer test" measurements between the two study groups is presented in Table 3 and Figure 3. The differences between the measurements in the study group and the control group were statistically significant.

Table 3. Measurements of parameters evaluating vaginal atrophy.

Study Group	Control (N = 28)		Atrophy (N = 30)		t-Test for Equality of Means
	Mean (Std. Deviation)	Median (Range)	Mean (Std. Deviation)	Median (Range)	
Modified Schirmer (mm)	21.7 (9.3)	20.5 (9–40)	3.3 (3.9)	2 (0–12)	$p < 0.001$
pH	4.1 (0.4)	4 (4–6)	6.9 (0.85)	7 (5–8)	$p < 0.001$
VHI	24.3 (1.0)	25 (22–25)	12.3 (2.3)	12.5 (8–18)	$p < 0.001$
VAS daily dryness	0.4 (0.8)	0 (0–3)	6.0 (3.8)	7.5 (0–10)	$p < 0.001$
VAS intercourse dryness	0.9 (1.1)	0 (0–3)	9.7 (0.5)	10 (8–10)	$p < 0.001$

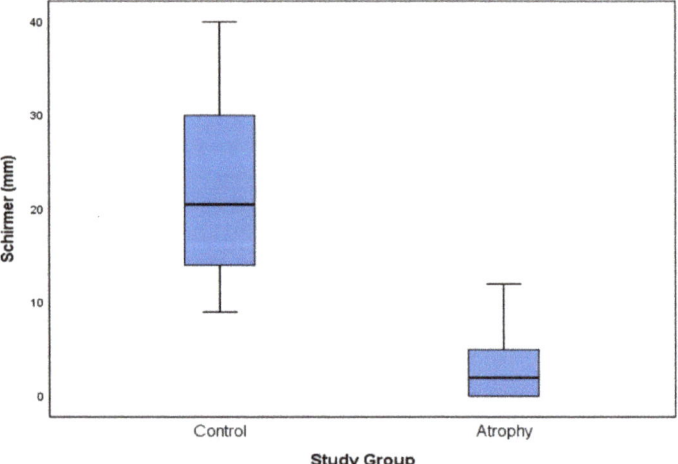

Figure 3. Modified Schirmer measurements in control and study groups. The figure graphically presents the differences between "modified Schirmer test" measurements in the control and the GSM groups. The horizontal line within the box indicates the median, boundaries of the box indicate the 1st and 3rd quartile, and whiskers indicate the minimum and maximum values.

A statistically significant difference was observed between the two groups regarding the number of vaginal deliveries. We therefore performed a covariate analysis, correcting for vaginal deliveries, to establish that the distinction in the "modified Schirmer test" measurements was not a result of the difference in vaginal deliveries alone. The analysis yielded a statistically significant difference after the correction as well.

Correlations between all measured parameters of the entire study population, expressed by Pearson's correlation coefficient, are shown in Table 4. The modified Schirmer measurements showed strong correlations to pH, VHI, and intercourse-VAS. All correlations were statistically significant ($p < 0.001$).

Table 4. Correlations between the different measures. Pearson's correlation coefficient is a measure of the linear correlation between these parameters. Correlation coefficients of 1 or −1 represent perfect correlations, whereas a correlation coefficient of 0 represents no correlation. Thus, the closer to 1 or −1 the value of the coefficient is, the stronger the correlation.

		Modified Schirmer (mm)	pH	VHI	VAS Daily Dryness
Correlation Coefficient (Significance)	pH	−0.714 (0.0)			
	VHI	0.775 (0.0)	−0.901 (0.0)		
	VAS daily dryness	−0.544 (0.0)	0.711 (0.0)	−0.709 (0.0)	
	VAS intercourse dryness	−0.821 (0.0)	0.885 (0.0)	−0.936 (0.0)	0.731 (0.0)

4. Discussion

The purpose of this study was to test a new, objective measurement modality for vaginal moisture/dryness and to evaluate its validity. To achieve this, we used a calibrated filter-paper test strip, similar to the one used for the ophthalmic Schirmer test, in a standardized manner comparing symptomatic women suffering from GSM-associated vaginal dryness to women without dryness. The comparison yielded a statistically significant difference between the groups, suggesting that this test is correlated with symptoms and is useful in distinguishing symptomatic vaginal dryness from normal vaginal moisture.

Furthermore, the "modified Schirmer test" measurements showed strong and statistically significant correlations to the currently used indices of vaginal atrophy, i.e., pH, VHI, and VAS scores. These correlations imply a non-inferiority of the test compared to currently accepted measures.

It is important to note that the two study groups were significantly diverse in most characteristics (age, hormonal status, contraception, and lubricant use), as they represent essentially different phases of women's lives in terms of hormonal status.

We found no statistically significant distinction in the "modified Schirmer test" measurements between women who reported using hormonal contraceptives and those who reported using non-hormonal contraceptives; neither did we find differences between women with diverse hormonal statuses in the control group (i.e., normal menstruation, amenorrhea associated with hormonal IUD, and perimenopause). This could be a resultant of the small sample size, as these were subgroups of the entire control group. Although larger studies are needed to confirm our findings, the finding that this test is not altered by hormonal status or contraceptive modalities may indicate yet another advantage of its use, as it provides a direct and hormonal-independent indication of the vaginal moisture level.

Clinical trials evaluate treatment efficacy for GSM mostly using measures that represent vaginal changes occurring in response to the presence or absence of estrogen. Most frequently, these include pH level, the VHI, and the VMI [13]. Vaginal pH level is mainly determined by the presence or absence of lactobacilli. These bacteria produce lactic acid as they catabolize glycogen, which in turn decreases the vaginal pH level to 3.5–4.5. As glycogen is found in mature epithelial cells yet absent in para-basal epithelial cells (which represent atrophy), a vaginal pH level >5 in the absence of other causes (such as infection or presence of semen, cervical mucous, or blood) is indicative of glycogen absence, thus, of decreased estrogen and resultant atrophy [3,8]. The VHI, first described by Bachmann in 1992 [20], is widely used even though it has not been validated (Gloria Bachmann, personal communication) and uses mostly subjective parameters. The VHI is comprised of five parameters, observed during examination per speculum, graded from 1 to 5 each. Four parameters are not well defined and are subjective to inter and intra observer differences: vaginal elasticity, fluid volume (measured by fluid pooling in the fornix), epithelial integrity, and epithelial moisture, whereas only one measurement is objective—the vaginal pH [21]. According to the VHI, atrophy is defined as a score lower than 15 [21]. The VHI does not include clear examination instructions and is, therefore, dependent on examiner's interpretation, thus lacking uniformity. Like other measures used, it is, at least partially, an estrogen-dependent index, as pH level comprises one fifth of its value.

VMI is another tool that represents vaginal estrogen influence on epithelial cytology, through calculating the relative percentage of superficial (mature) cells compared to intermediate and para-basal epithelial cells [3,8].

The main strength of our study is the introduction of a new measurement, which is easy to use and interpret. To our knowledge, previous studies that aimed to test the amount of vaginal discharge included usage of swabbing the entire vagina during an exam and weighing the swab [22], weighing tampons after inserting them for 8 h [23], by aspiration of vaginal fluid [24], or by pad weighing [25]. Nevertheless, these modalities are either effort- and time-consuming or lack precision, as the weighed fluid is not necessarily comprised of vaginal discharge alone and may also contain sweat or urine. Other drawbacks include patient discomfort and functionality. In addition, none of these measures were studied in relation to vaginal atrophy.

Furthermore, the current tool may allow an objective and direct evaluation of dryness symptoms when there is a discrepancy between symptoms and findings. For example, in patients who complain of dryness but have an apparently normal examination, this tool may allow confirmation of a normal amount of discharge, suggesting a sensory issue or vulvodynia and directing further evaluation or suitable treatment.

Our study is limited for several reasons, including the small number of participants, the lack of measures among asymptomatic menopausal women, and the lack of measurement comparison before and after treatment. The "modified Schirmer test" should be further evaluated in larger scale studies, which will generate more accurate and specific ranges of measurements, representing and distinguishing between menopause-associated-vaginal-atrophy, menopause without atrophy, and an estrogenized state. Furthermore, larger sample sizes may allow the division of measurement ranges into subranges, such as pre-menopausal women using hormonal contraceptives with and without vaginal dryness, compared to age-matched women who are not using hormonal contraceptives.

The main advantage of the "modified Schirmer test" is its potential to serve as an objective test in assessing vaginal dryness/moisture level in relation to non-estrogenic treatments for vaginal dryness. Therefore, the validity of this test should be further studied by comparison of measurements before and after treatments aimed to relieve vaginal atrophy.

5. Conclusions

Our findings suggest that the "modified Schirmer test" can be used as an objective indicator of vaginal moisture level, distinguishing women who suffer from vaginal dryness from those who do not. This test may also prove useful for evaluation of non-hormonal treatment results in longitudinal research, where direct and objective measures of vaginal moisture are sought to complement the subjective VAS score.

Author Contributions: Conceptualization, A.L.-S.; methodology, D.G. and A.L.-S.; data curation, Y.S.-C., S.J. and A.L.-S.; formal analysis, D.G.; writing—original draft, review, and editing, D.G. and A.L.-S. All authors have read and agreed to the published version of the manuscript.

Funding: This research received no external funding.

Institutional Review Board Statement: The study was conducted in accordance with the Declaration of Helsinki and approved by the Institutional Review Board of Hadassah Medical Center, Jerusalem, Israel (Number 0923-20-HMO, approved 31 December 2020).

Informed Consent Statement: Written informed consent was obtained from all subjects involved in the study.

Data Availability Statement: The data presented in this study are available on request from the corresponding author.

Conflicts of Interest: The authors declare no conflict of interest.

References

1. Portman, D.J.; Gass, M.L.S. Genitourinary syndrome of menopause: New terminology for vulvovaginal atrophy from the International Society for the Study of Women's Sexual Health and The North American Menopause Society. *Menopause* **2014**, *21*, 1063–1068. [CrossRef]
2. Bachmann, G.A.; Nevadunsky, N.S. Diagnosis and treatment of atrophic vaginitis. *Am. Fam. Physician* **2000**, *61*, 3090–3096. [PubMed]
3. Sturdee, D.W.; Panay, N. Recommendations for the management of postmenopausal vaginal atrophy. *Climacteric* **2010**, *13*, 509–522. [CrossRef]
4. Parish, S.J.; Nappi, R.E.; Krychman, M.L.; Kellogg-Spadt, S.; Simon, J.A.; Goldstein, J.A.; Kingsberg, S.A. Impact of vulvovaginal health on postmenopausal women: A review of surveys on symptoms of vulvovaginal atrophy. *Int. J. Womens Health* **2013**, *5*, 437–447. [CrossRef] [PubMed]
5. Tan, O.; Bradshaw, K.; Carr, B.R. Management of vulvovaginal atrophy-related sexual dysfunction in postmenopausal women: An up-to-date review. *Menopause* **2012**, *19*, 109–117. [CrossRef] [PubMed]
6. Management of symptomatic vulvovaginal atrophy: 2013 position statement of The North American Menopause Society. *Menopause* **2013**, *20*, 888–902. [CrossRef]
7. Bachmann, G.; Bouchard, C.; Hoppe, D.; Ranganath, R.; Altomare, C.; Vieweg, A.; Graepel, J.; Helzner, E. Efficacy and safety of low-dose regimens of conjugated estrogens cream administered vaginally. *Menopause* **2009**, *16*, 719–727. [CrossRef]
8. Pérez-López, F.R.; Vieira-Baptista, P.; Phillips, N.; Cohen-Sacher, B.; Fialho, S.C.A.V.; Stockdale, C.K. Clinical manifestations and evaluation of postmenopausal vulvovaginal atrophy. *Gynecol. Endocrinol.* **2021**, *37*, 740–745. [CrossRef]
9. Perino, A.; Calligaro, A.; Forlani, F.; Tiberio, C.; Cucinella, G.; Svelato, A.; Saitta, S.; Calagna, G. Vulvo-vaginal atrophy: A new treatment modality using thermo-ablative fractional CO_2 laser. *Maturitas* **2015**, *80*, 296–301. [CrossRef]
10. Gaspar, A.; Addamo, G.; Brandi, H. Vaginal Fractional CO_2 Laser: A Minimally Invasive Option for Vaginal Rejuvenation. *Am. J. Cosmet. Surg.* **2011**, *28*, 156–162. [CrossRef]
11. Gambacciani, M.; Palacios, S. Laser therapy for the restoration of vaginal function. *Maturitas* **2017**, *99*, 10–15. [CrossRef]
12. Stachowicz, A.M.; Hoover, M.L.; Karram, M.M. Clinical utility of radiofrequency energy for female genitourinary dysfunction: Past, present, and future. *Int. Urogynecol. J.* **2021**, *32*, 1345–1350. [CrossRef]
13. Singh, P.; Chong, C.Y.L.; Han, H.C. Effects of Vulvovaginal Laser Therapy on Postmenopausal Vaginal Atrophy: A Prospective Study. *J. Gynecol. Surg.* **2019**, *35*, 99–104. [CrossRef]
14. Salvatore, S.; Maggiore, U.L.; Athanasiou, S.; Origoni, M.; Candiani, M.; Calligaro, A.; Zerbinati, N. Histological study on the effects of microablative fractional CO_2 laser on atrophic vaginal tissue: An ex vivo study. *Menopause* **2015**, *22*, 845–849. [CrossRef] [PubMed]
15. Cruz, V.L.; Steiner, M.L.; Pompei, L.M.; Strufaldi, R.; Fonseca, F.L.; Santiago, L.H.; Wajsfeld, T.; Fernandes, C.E. Randomized, double-blind, placebo-controlled clinical trial for evaluating the efficacy of fractional CO_2 laser compared with topical estriol in the treatment of vaginal atrophy in postmenopausal women. *Menopause* **2017**, *25*, 21–28. [CrossRef] [PubMed]
16. Athanasiou, S.; Pitsouni, E.; Falagas, M.E.; Salvatore, S.; Grigoriadis, T. CO_2-laser for the genitourinary syndrome of menopause. How many laser sessions? *Maturitas* **2017**, *104*, 24–28. [CrossRef] [PubMed]
17. Pitsouni, E.; Grigoriadis, T.; Tsiveleka, A.; Zacharakis, D.; Salvatore, S.; Athanasiou, S. Microablative fractional CO_2-laser therapy and the genitourinary syndrome of menopause: An observational study. *Maturitas* **2016**, *94*, 131–136. [CrossRef]
18. Takacs, P.; Sipos, A.G.; Kozma, B.; Cunningham, T.D.; Larson, K.; Lampé, R.; Poka, R. The Effect of Vaginal Microablative Fractional CO_2 Laser Treatment on Vaginal Cytology. *Lasers Surg. Med.* **2020**, *52*, 708–712. [CrossRef]
19. Filippini, M.; Luvero, D.; Salvatore, S.; Pieralli, A.; Montera, R.; Plotti, F.; Candiani, M.; Angioli, R. Efficacy of fractional CO_2 laser treatment in postmenopausal women with genitourinary syndrome: A multicenter study. *Menopause* **2020**, *27*, 43–49. [CrossRef]
20. Bachmann, G.A.; Notelovitz, M.; Kelly, S.J.; Owens, A.; Thompson, C. Long-term nonhormonal treatment of vaginal dryness. *Clin. Pract. Sex* **1992**, *8*, 3–8.
21. Pieralli, A.; Fallani, M.G.; Becorpi, A.; Bianchi, C.; Corioni, S.; Longinotti, M.; Tredici, Z.; Guaschino, S. Fractional CO_2 laser for vulvovaginal atrophy (VVA) dyspareunia relief in breast cancer survivors. *Arch. Gynecol. Obstet.* **2016**, *294*, 841–846. [CrossRef]
22. Stone, A.; Gamble, C.J. The quantity of vaginal fluid. *Am. J. Obstet. Gynecol.* **1959**, *78*, 279–281. [CrossRef]
23. Godley, M.J. Quantitation of vaginal discharge in healthy volunteers. *BJOG Int. J. Obstet. Gynaecol.* **1985**, *92*, 739–742. [CrossRef] [PubMed]
24. Eschenbach, D.A.; Thwin, S.S.; Patton, D.L.; Hooton, T.M.; Stapleton, A.E.; Agnew, K.; Winter, C.; Meier, A.; Stamm, W.E. Influence of the normal menstrual cycle on vaginal tissue, discharge, and microflora. *Clin. Infect. Dis.* **2000**, *30*, 901–907. [CrossRef]
25. Wall, L.L.; Couchman, G.M.; McCoy, M.C. Vaginal discharge as a confounding factor in the diagnosis of urinary incontinence by perineal pad testing. *Int. Urogynecology J.* **1991**, *2*, 219–221. [CrossRef]

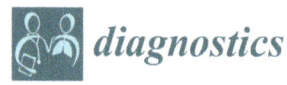

Article

Evaluation of BD Onclarity™ HPV Assay on Self-Collected Vaginal and First-Void Urine Samples as Compared to Clinician-Collected Cervical Samples: A Pilot Study

Marianna Martinelli [1], Chiara Giubbi [1], Illari Sechi [2], Fabio Bottari [3,4], Anna Daniela Iacobone [4,5], Rosario Musumeci [1], Federica Perdoni [1], Narcisa Muresu [6], Andrea Piana [2], Robert Fruscio [7], Fabio Landoni [7] and Clementina Elvezia Cocuzza [1,*]

1 Department of Medicine and Surgery, University of Milano-Bicocca, 20900 Monza, Italy
2 Department of Medical, Surgical and Experimental Sciences, University of Sassari, 07100 Sassari, Italy
3 Division of Laboratory Medicine, European Institute of Oncology IRCCS, 20141 Milan, Italy
4 Department of Biomedical Sciences, University of Sassari, 07100 Sassari, Italy
5 Preventive Gynecology Unit, European Institute of Oncology IRCCS, 20141 Milan, Italy
6 Department of Humanities and Social Sciences, University of Sassari, 07100 Sassari, Italy
7 Clinic of Obstetrics and Gynecology, Department of Medicine and Surgery, San Gerardo Hospital, University of Milan Bicocca, 20900 Monza, Italy
* Correspondence: clementina.cocuzza@unimib.it; Tel.: +39-02-64488358

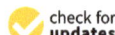

Citation: Martinelli, M.; Giubbi, C.; Sechi, I.; Bottari, F.; Iacobone, A.D.; Musumeci, R.; Perdoni, F.; Muresu, N.; Piana, A.; Fruscio, R.; et al. Evaluation of BD Onclarity™ HPV Assay on Self-Collected Vaginal and First-Void Urine Samples as Compared to Clinician-Collected Cervical Samples: A Pilot Study. *Diagnostics* **2022**, *12*, 3075. https://doi.org/10.3390/diagnostics12123075

Academic Editor: Laurent Bélec

Received: 9 November 2022
Accepted: 30 November 2022
Published: 7 December 2022

Publisher's Note: MDPI stays neutral with regard to jurisdictional claims in published maps and institutional affiliations.

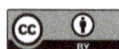

Copyright: © 2022 by the authors. Licensee MDPI, Basel, Switzerland. This article is an open access article distributed under the terms and conditions of the Creative Commons Attribution (CC BY) license (https://creativecommons.org/licenses/by/4.0/).

Abstract: The accuracy of available HPV molecular assays on self-samples needs to be evaluated as compared to clinician-collected samples. This pilot study aimed to investigate the BD Onclarity™ HPV assay on vaginal and first-void urine samples. Sixty-four women referred to colposcopy for cervical dysplasia performed a vaginal self-collection and provided a first-void urine sample, after informed consent. A cervical specimen was collected during the clinician examination. All samples were tested using BD Onclarity™ HPV assay on the BD Viper™ LT System. Overall positive agreement (OPA) between cervical and self-sample results was evaluated using Cohen's kappa value (κ). Using a clinical cut-off of 38.3 Ct for HPV 16 and 34.2 Ct for other HR genotypes, compared to cervical sample, the self-collected vaginal sample OPA was 85.9%, and κ = 0.699. Without a clinical cut-off, the OPA was 95.3%, and the κ = 0.890. Data obtained comparing cervical and urine samples showed an OPA of 87.5% with a κ = 0.79 using a clinical cut-off, and an OPA of 90.6% with a κ = 0.776 without a clinical cut-off. Data showed a substantial agreement between both self-collected and clinician-collected samples. A specific clinical cut-off analysis should be considered based on type of sample analysed.

Keywords: human papillomavirus; self-collection; vaginal self-sample; first-void urine; cervical cancer screening; diagnostic accuracy

1. Introduction

Cervical cancer is one of the most important malignancies affecting women and caused about 342,000 deaths in 2020. It is well-known that this type of tumour is caused by persisting infection of high-risk human papillomavirus (hrHPV). Recently, the World Health Organization (WHO) developed a global strategy for cervical cancer elimination to be reached by 2030, and one of the points of this strategy is to reach the 70% of women screened using a high-performance test by the age of 35, and again by the age of 45 [1].

Eighty-five percent of cervical cancer deaths occur in developing countries, where it still represents the first leading cancer death cause. Self-sampling could be an additional strategy to reach unscreened and under-screened women, especially in middle- and low-income countries.

As of now, the global use of HPV self-sampling is still limited. Only 17 countries with identified screening programs recommend the use of self-sampling in primary screening or to reach non-responder women. However, the COVID-19 pandemic has accelerated worldwide self-sampling introduction, which is now considered an important strategy to increase screening coverage in the coming years [2].

The importance of self-sampling in improving adherence to cervical cancer screening has been well documented in the last few years, especially for women not participating in prevention programs due to different socio-cultural reasons [3,4]. The main barrier is related to the need for a physician or healthcare worker for cervical specimen collection [5]. The use of alternative and less invasive samples, such as self-collected vaginal and first-void urine samples, represents the best choice to overcome this issue.

Different devices are commercially available and seem to be suitable for this purpose. However, the accuracy of clinically validated PCR-based human papillomavirus detection kits on self-samples needs to be evaluated as compared to clinician-collected samples, as already reported in a recent meta-analysis by Arbyn et al. [6]. Previous studies have already shown that HPV testing conducted on vaginal self-samples has a similar sensitivity compared to testing on physician-collected cervical samples for the detection of cervical intraepithelial neoplasia grade 2 or higher (CIN2+) [6–8]. Nevertheless, the sample preparation and preanalytical processes used are highly different [9]. Different assays suggest in their manufacturer instructions to start from different specimen volumes for hrHPV detection, and this could influence the result obtained, especially for self-collected samples. Moreover, the results obtained from samples collected using dry vaginal swabs could be conditioned from the solution volume used for swab resuspension.

Urine seems to be a good, non-invasive, and more acceptable material for the detection of HPV and sexually transmitted infections [10–12]. Moreover, because first-void urine contains exfoliated cells from the cervix [13], it could be considered a specimen alternative to a clinician-collected cervical sample for the molecular detection of HPV. Furthermore, several studies have recently been published reporting consistent results from the use of urine samples for HPV detection [14–18]. Also for this kind of sample, the performance of urine-based HPV testing for CIN2+ detection is affected by the various HPV assays and non-standardized urine collection methods [14].

The objective of this pilot study was to evaluate accuracy of the BD Onclarity™ HPV assay on self-collected vaginal and first-void urine samples as compared to clinician-collected cervical samples.

The BD Onclarity™ assay has been internationally validated for liquid-phase cytology samples for use in primary HPV screening according to both the Mejer guidelines and the VALGENT genotyping protocol [19,20]; in this study we evaluated the performance of this test, already extensively studied in a screening setting, on self-collected samples in order to assess its usefulness to increase adherence to screening programs.

In particular, in this pilot study, we decided to use the same BD Onclarity™ protocol that is used for cervical specimens, without making changes, in order to discover whether the same protocol could also work for different samples compared to a liquid-phase cytology sample.

2. Materials and Methods

2.1. Study Design and Sample Collection

For this pilot study of diagnostic accuracy, a group of 64 women (mean age: 38.4 years) with a recent diagnosis of cervical dysplasia attending the Colposcopy Clinic of San Gerardo Hospital (Monza, Italy) were enrolled. The study protocol was approved by the Ethics Committee of the University of Milano-Bicocca, Monza, Italy (Protocol n. 0037320/2017 and 0086409/2018). All subjects provided written and informed consent to participate in the study. Patients were excluded in case of immunodeficiency, HIV infection, presumed or confirmed pregnancy, diagnosis of any malignancies, and/or chemotherapy in the previous 6 months.

All women were adequately informed about the study by Colposcopy Clinic staff and were asked to autonomously collect a vaginal self-sample using a FLOQSwab® (5E046S,

Copan, Brescia, Italy) and a first-void urine (FVU) sample using a Colli-pee® 20 mL (Novosanis, Wijnegem, Belgium) before colposcopy examination. The information brochure of the study and the instructions on how to use the devices were given to all participants.

During the colposcopy examination, the gynaecologist collected one cervical sample using an L-shaped FLOQSwab® (Copan). All physician-collected cervical and self-collected vaginal and urine samples were sent to the Clinical Microbiology Laboratory of the Department of Medicine and Surgery, University of Milano-Bicocca, Italy, for preanalytical processing within 24 h of collection.

2.2. Preanalytical Sample Processing

Cervical samples were collected using an L-shaped FLOQSwab® (Copan, Brescia, Italy) and transported in a tube with 20 mL of PreservCyt® Solution (HOLOGIC, Marlborough, MA, USA). All samples were well shaken using vortex for 30 seconds, and 1.5 mL aliquots were made.

Vaginal self-samples were obtained using a FLOQSwab® (Copan, Brescia, Italy) and transported dry to the laboratory. Each specimen was suspended in 5.5 mL of PreservCyt® Solution (HOLOGIC, Marlborough, MA, USA), and 5 aliquots were made.

The Colli-Pee® 20 mL device allowed for capturing a first-void urine volume of 13 mL (+/−2 mL), in a collection device containing 7 mL of preservative urine conservation medium (UCM), leading to a final volume of 20 mL (+/−2 mL) [15]. Urine samples were aliquoted after arrival at the laboratory. One aliquot of each type of sample was sent to the Division of Laboratory Medicine of the European Institute of Oncology, Milan, Italy, for HPV testing.

2.3. BD Onclarity™ HPV Assay

The BD Onclarity™ HPV assay (BD, USA), which detects 14 high-risk (HR) genotypes, provides the capability of extended genotyping through individual detection of HPV 31, 51, and 52 (in addition to 16, 18, and 45) and pooled detection of 33/58, 35/39/68, and 56/59/66. An endogenous human beta-globin sequence is detected as a sample validity control, sample extraction, and amplification efficiency [20–22].

All samples were tested following manufacturer instructions: BD Onclarity™ uses 0.5 mL of sample (cervical, vaginal, or urine sample) which is added to a suitable solution produced by BD (the LBC tube) to reach a final volume of 2.2 mL, of which 0.8 mL of sample is automatically taken by the instrument to perform nucleic acid extraction using the extraction chemistry developed by BD (BD FOX ™). The extracted DNA is then eluted to a final volume of 400 microliters, and 50 microliters is automatically pipetted into each of the three wells containing the dried master mix in order to perform real-time PCR.

The clinical cut-off is set to be related to CIN2+ disease, and an algorithm verifies the adequacy of the sample using the amplification of the human beta-globin gene. In particular, the software interprets the amplification curves on the basis of the following threshold cycles (Ct): 38.3 Ct for HPV16, 34.2 Ct for other HR-HPVs, and 34.2 Ct for beta-globin. Samples which were judged invalid were re-tested a second time (9 cervical samples, 2 vaginal swabs, and 4 urines).

2.4. Statistical Analysis

The overall percentage agreement (OPA) between cervical and self-sample results was evaluated using Cohen's kappa value (κ) using the GraphPad QuickCalcs software (updated in 2014, available at http://graphpad.com/quickcalcs accessed on 30 October 2022). Agreement was interpreted as slight (κ < 0.200), fair (0.200 < κ < 0.401), moderate (0.400 < κ < 0.601), good (0.600 < κ < 0.801), very good (0.800 < κ < 1.000), or perfect (κ = 1.000). Sample results were evaluated using two different cut-offs: (i) clinical cut-off of 38.3 Ct (cycle threshold) for HPV 16 and 34.2 Ct for other HR genotypes, as indicated in the package insert and (ii) without the clinical cut-off (accepting positivity up to 40 Ct).

3. Results

3.1. Study Population

The 64 women enrolled in this study were referred to colposcopy because of a recent diagnosis of cervical dysplasia confirmed by Pap smear examination. Clinical data regarding Pap test, colposcopy, and biopsy results are reported in Table 1. Twenty-three out of the sixty-four women showed abnormal colposcopy findings, and cervical guided biopsies were taken to histologically define the grade of the lesion; 18/23 (78.3%) biopsies showed the presence of a CIN2+ lesion.

Table 1. Clinical data of patients enrolled. Low-grade intraepithelial lesion (LSIL); atypical squamous cells of undetermined significance (ASCUS); high-grade intraepithelial lesion (HSIL); atypical glandular cells of undetermined significance (AGCUS); cervical intraepithelial neoplasia (CIN).

Pap Test Result	n (64)	%
ASCUS	15	23.4%
LSIL	24	37.5%
AGCUS	5	7.8%
ASCH	6	9.4%
HSIL	14	21.9%
Colposcopy Result	n (64)	%
ABNORMAL	23	35.9%
NORMAL	41	64.1%
Biopsy Result	n (23)	%
NEG	2	8.7%
CIN 1	3	13.0%
CIN 2	3	13.0%
CIN 3	14	60.9%
Cervical Cancer	1	4.3%

3.2. HPV Positivity and Genotype Distribution among Samples Collected

HPV positivity results considering and not considering the clinical cut-off are reported in Figure 1. A very high rate of HPV positivity in cervical samples was found among the women enrolled: 67.2% (43/64) and 73.4% (47/64) considering and not considering the clinical cut-off, respectively. Considering just results obtained regarding HPV genotypes individually detected, HPV 16 was the most prevalent genotype identified among samples analysed, followed by HPV 31. Using the clinical cut-off, multiple genotype infections were observed in 14% (9/64), 18.7% (12/64), and 21.8% (14/64) of cervical, vaginal, and urine samples, respectively. Not considering the clinical cut-off, the percentages obtained were 31.2% (20/64), 28.1% (18/64), and 35.9% (23/64) for cervical, vaginal, and urine samples, respectively (Figure 2).

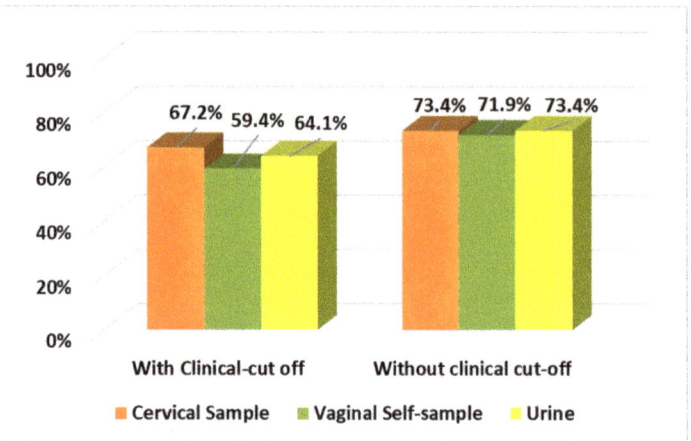

Figure 1. HPV positivity analysed considering and not considering clinical cut-off.

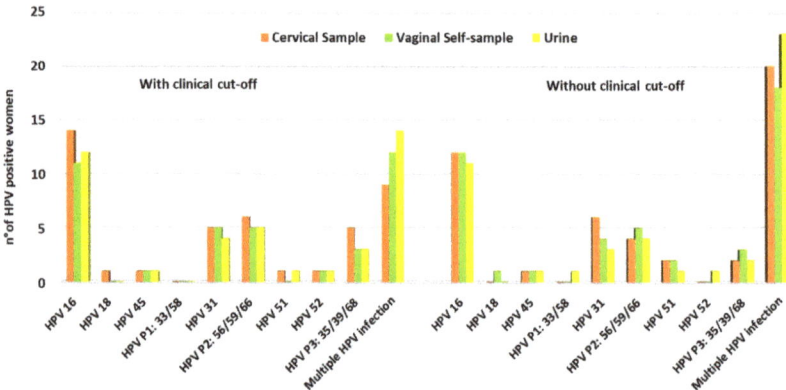

Figure 2. HPV genotype distribution analysed considering and not considering clinical cut-off.

3.3. HPV Overall Positive Agreement between Cervical and Vaginal Self-Samples

Using clinical cut-offs of 38.3 Ct for HPV 16 and 34.2 Ct for other HR genotypes, compared to the cervical samples, the self-collected vaginal sample PPA (positive percentage agreement) was 36/43 = 83.7%; the NPA (negative percentage agreement) was 19/21 = 90.5%. The OPA was 85.9% (55/64), and the Cohen's kappa was 0.699 (good agreement).

However, differences in collection procedures, preanalytical procedures, and the nature of the investigated samples may influence HPV detection rates on self-collected samples as compared to cervical specimens. Therefore, data analysis was performed without the clinical cut-off (accepting positivity up to Ct 40). Without the clinical cut-off, the PPA between self-collected vaginal samples and cervical samples was 45/47 = 95.7%; the NPA was 16/17 = 94.1%. The OPA was 95.3% (61/64), and the Cohen's kappa was 0.882 (almost perfect agreement).

Using the package insert cut-offs of 38.3 Ct for HPV 16 and 34.2 Ct for other HR genotypes for the cervical samples and a cut-off of 40 Ct for the vaginal samples, to account for the excessive dilution, the self-collected sample PPA was 43/43 = 100%; the NPA was 18/21 = 85.7%. The OPA was 95.3%, and the Cohen's kappa was 0.890 (almost perfect agreement). All results are reported in Table 2.

Table 2. Agreement in HPV detection of cervical and self-collected samples using different cut-off values.

Ct Cut-Off Value	Vaginal Self-Sample				Urine			
	PPA% (n)	PNA% (n)	OPA% (n)	κ	PPA% (n)	PNA% (n)	OPA% (n)	κ
<38.3 Ct for HPV 16 (for all sample types) <34.2 Ct for the other HPVs (for all sample types)	83.7% (36/43)	90.5% (19/21)	85.9% (55/64)	0.699	90.7% (39/43)	90.5% (19/21)	90.6% (58/64)	0.792
<40 Ct for HPV 16 and other HPVs (for all sample types)	95.7% (45/47)	94.1% (16/17)	95.3% (61/64)	0.882	91.5% (43/47)	76.5% (13/17)	87.5% (56/64)	0.680
<38.3 Ct for HPV 16 (for cervical samples) <34.2 Ct for the other HPVs (for cervical samples) <40 Ct for HPV 16 and other HPVs (for self-samples)	100% (43/43)	85.7% (18/21)	95.3% (61/64)	0.890	97.7% (42/43)	76.2% (16/21)	90.6 (58/64)	0.776

3.4. HPV Overall Positive Agreement between Cervical and First-Void Urine Samples

Using the clinical cut-offs, the PPA between first-void urine sample and cervical samples was 39/43 = 90.7% and the NPA 19/21 = 90.5%. The OPA was 87.5%, and the Cohen's kappa was 0.79 (good agreement).

Without any clinical cut-off, the PPA was 43/47 = 91.5%; the NPA was 13/17 = 76.5%. The OPA was 95.3%, and the Cohen's kappa was 0.680 (good agreement).

Using the package insert cut-offs of 38.3 Ct for HPV 16 and 34.2 Ct for other HR genotypes for the cervical samples and a clinical cut-off of 40 Ct for the urine samples, the PPA of self-collected urine samples was 42/43 = 97.7%; the NPA was 16/21 = 76.2%. The OPA was 90.6% (58/64), and the Cohen's kappa was 0.776 (good agreement). The results are reported in Table 2.

3.5. Correlation between HPV Positivity and Clinical Outcome

Comparing the results obtained from hrHPV testing with the clinical data, we evaluated the overall HPV positivity considering women with abnormal colposcopy findings and women with CIN2+ biopsy. Results for the cervical, vaginal, and urine samples with and without a clinical cut-off are presented in Tables 3 and 4. In Figures 3 and 4 are reported the HPV genotypes' distribution among women with abnormal colposcopy (Figure 3) and among women with CIN2+ lesions (Figure 4).

Table 3. HPV-positive women related to colposcopy results.

		With Clinical Cut-Off		Without Clinical Cut-Off	
	Colposcopy Results (Tot. 64)	Total HPV-Positive Women (n)	Total HPV-Positive Women (%)	Total HPV-Positive Women (n)	Total HPV-Positive Women (%)
Cervical Sample	ABNORMAL	20	31.3%	20	31.3%
	NORMAL	23	35.9%	25	39.1%
Vaginal self-sample	ABNORMAL	18	28.1%	21	32.8%
	NORMAL	20	31.3%	25	39.1%
Urine	ABNORMAL	18	28.1%	20	31.3%
	NORMAL	23	35.9%	27	42.2%

Table 4. HPV-positive women related to biopsy results.

		With Clinical Cut-Off		Without Clinical Cut-Off	
	Biopsy Results (Tot. 23)	Total HPV-Positive Women (*n*)	Total HPV-Positive Women (%)	Total HPV-Positive Women (*n*)	Total HPV-Positive Women (%)
Cervical Sample	CIN2+	17	73.9%	18	78.3%
	CIN2−	3	13.0%	4	17.4%
Vaginal self-sample	CIN2+	15	65.2%	18	78.3%
	CIN2−	3	13.0%	3	13.0%
Urine	CIN2+	16	69.6%	17	73.9%
	CIN2−	2	8.7%	3	13.0%

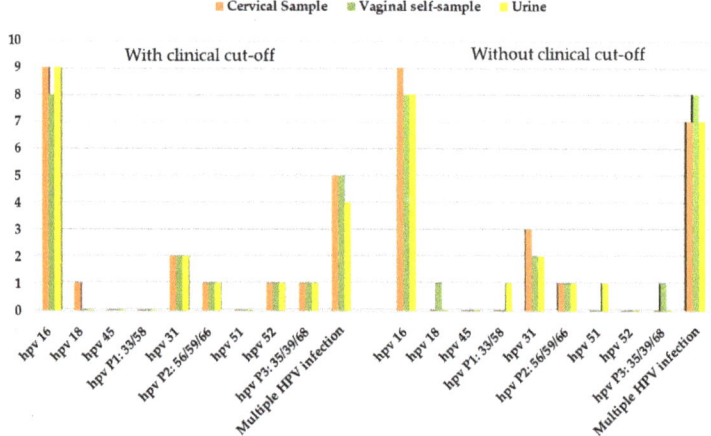

Figure 3. HPV genotypes' distribution among women with abnormal colposcopy findings.

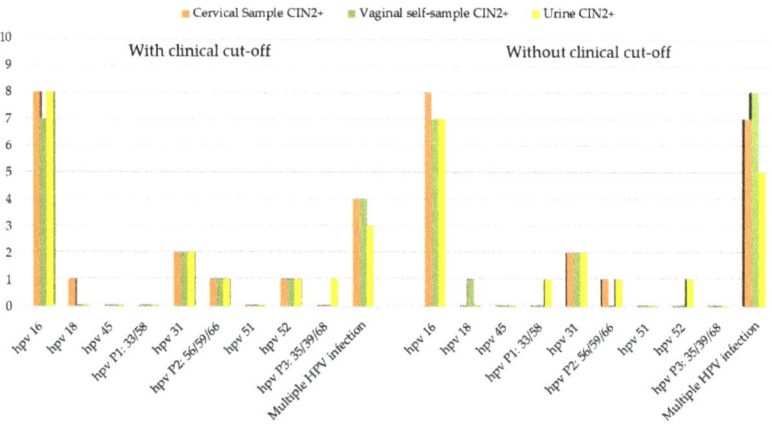

Figure 4. HPV genotypes' distribution among women with CIN2+ lesions.

4. Discussion

There is presently great interest in the use of self-collected samples as an alternative strategy in cervical cancer screening. The introduction of self-sampling in screening has been demonstrated to be more acceptable to women, resulting in improved participation in prevention programs [4,23].

Nowadays, several devices for self-sampling are commercially available, with different performances in sample collection [24–26]. The majority of HPV molecular assays are validated on cervical samples, the gold standard in cervical cancer screening [27]. However HPV assays may give different results when tested on self-taken vaginal and urine samples. Consequently, in order to obtain reproducible results, a specific HPV assay-sample-type validation is necessary [28].

The aim of this study was to evaluate accuracy of the BD Onclarity™ HPV assay on self-collected vaginal samples using a FLOQSwab® and first-void urine using the Colli-Pee® 20 mL device.

The results of the study showed a good overall positive agreement between self-collected specimens and clinician-collected samples, confirming data already reported in the expanded meta-analysis by Arbyn et al. [6,7]. Recently, a new meta-analysis of test agreement between HPV tests using self-taken vs. clinician-collected samples based on 26 studies (10,071 participants) was published, updating a previous meta-analysis on test accuracy for cervical precancers [29].

The validity of urine samples has been widely debated. On the one hand, this type of sample is easy to collect, overcomes some cultural barriers, and could be useful for surveillance in young populations [30]; on the other hand, the DNA in first-void urine is not always appropriately preserved, thus not allowing the obtaining of an adequate quantity of nucleic acids for HPV analysis [31]. Moreover, urine may collect cells from other nearby anatomical sites, accounting for the higher HPV detection rates and/or multiple infections when compared to cervical samples.

In this study, results from urine samples collected using the Colli-Pee® 20 mL are comparable to results for cervical and vaginal samples, confirming—as previously reported in the literature—the validity of this device for the collection and storage of first-void urine using a preservative medium [15–18,32].

A limitation of the study is that the results come from samples collected from a population of women referred to colposcopy and not from a primary screening setting. However, the purpose of the study was to understand whether the BD Onclarity™ HPV assay could be used in combination with self-samples; hence, it was necessary to have a sufficient number of HPV-positive women to answer this question. For the same reason, previous studies aiming to evaluate HPV testing on clinician-collected vs. self-collected samples have been conducted in a colposcopy setting [18,33,34]. The other main limitation of this study is the small sample size, with participating women being enrolled at only one colposcopy centre. This analysis should therefore be considered a pilot study, and the data obtained could represent the starting point for further larger validation studies on new self-collection devices paired with the BD Onclarity™ HPV assay. Previous published reports also showed similar limitations regarding sample size as well as a lack of standardized preanalytical methods [14,20,32].

In the present study, vaginal swabs resuspended in 5.5 mL of PreservCyt and 20 mL of first-void urine samples were processed using the same preanalytical protocol as cervical samples by placing 0.5 mL of each sample's starting volume in tubes containing 1.7 mL of BD preserve fluid. Differences in collection procedures, preanalytical procedures, and the nature of the investigated samples may influence HPV detection rates on self-collected samples as compared to cervical specimens, on which the BD Onclarity™ HPV assay protocol and clinical cut-offs had been previously validated. For this reason, we have analysed the data obtained both with the cut-offs set by the manufacturer for cervical samples and without the pre-set cut-offs, still obtaining comparable results in terms of concordance and agreement. However, the different results obtained underline the importance of considering using different testing protocols and analytical cut-offs based on the sample type.

No invalid samples were observed in this pilot study after retesting, irrespective of the sample type. The good sample adequacy observed for vaginal and first-void urine samples may have resulted from collection at the point of care and to reduced time from collection to laboratory testing.

HPV genotyping in self-collected samples represents another strength of the BD Onclarity™ HPV assay, as genotyping could be a good strategy for the triage of HR-HPV-positive women in order to identify those at greater risk of cervical cancer progression, such as HPV 16 and/or 18 positive women. The use of HPV genotyping assays could be very important, particularly for screening programs based on self-sampling due to the impossibility to performing cytology triage on the same sample. Moreover, HPV genotyping on self-taken samples could be helpful to look for persistence of the same HPV genotype at follow-up and as test-of-cure, without the need for a clinician-collected sample at each visit. The possibility of performing a reliable test to verify the success of surgical treatment or the risk of relapse on a self-taken sample can represent another great advantage for women to consider.

Due to the low number of positive samples, we did not perform a statistical analysis of specimens' agreement considering specific HPV genotypes. However, these preliminary results showed a good concordance, especially for HPV 16, even if a further study enrolling a larger number of patients is necessary to obtain statistically significant results.

Up to now, the importance of self-sampling has been stressed to increase adherence to cervical cancer screening programs for women not participating due to socio-cultural or physical barriers. The SARS-CoV-2 pandemic has added another valuable reason to enhance the use of self-sample tests collected at home by women, thus avoiding the need to go to hospital and the risk of COVID exposure and infection [35].

5. Conclusions

Overall, data analysis without adjustment resulted in substantial agreement between the self-collected and clinic-collected samples, with PPA values of 83.7% and 90.7% for vaginal and urine samples, respectively. With correction for excess dilution in the sample preparation, there was almost perfect agreement, with PPA values of 100% and 97.7% for vaginal and urine samples, respectively. In conclusion, data from this pilot study are promising for the employment of the BD Onclarity™ HPV assay on vaginal samples and first-void urine samples, with an accuracy almost equivalent to clinician-collected cervical samples.

Author Contributions: Conceptualization, C.E.C.; methodology, M.M., I.S., F.P., N.M. and F.B.; formal analysis, M.M., F.B. and C.G.; data curation, M.M., C.G., R.M., N.M. and C.E.C.; writing—original draft preparation, M.M., C.G., A.D.I., F.B. and C.E.C.; writing—review and editing, M.M., C.G., A.D.I., F.B., R.M., R.F., F.L., N.M., A.P., I.S. and C.E.C.; supervision, C.E.C. All authors have read and agreed to the published version of the manuscript.

Funding: This research received no external funding. BD Onclarity™ HPV assays were donated by BD; FLOQSwab® L-shape and vaginal self-samples were donated by Copan; Colli-pee® devices were donated by Novosanis.

Institutional Review Board Statement: The study was conducted in accordance with the Declaration of Helsinki and approved by the Ethics Committee of the University of Milano-Bicocca (Protocol n. 0037320/2017 and 0086409/2018).

Informed Consent Statement: Informed consent was obtained from all subjects involved in the study.

Conflicts of Interest: The authors declare no conflict of interest.

References

1. Global Strategy to Accelerate the Elimination of Cervical Cancer as a Public Health Problem. Available online: https://www.who.int/publications-detail-redirect/9789240014107 (accessed on 28 September 2021).
2. Serrano, B.; Ibáñez, R.; Robles, C.; Peremiquel-Trillas, P.; de Sanjosé, S.; Bruni, L. Worldwide Use of HPV Self-Sampling for Cervical Cancer Screening. *Prev. Med.* **2022**, *154*, 106900. [CrossRef]
3. Lam, J.U.H.; Elfström, K.M.; Ejegod, D.M.; Pedersen, H.; Rygaard, C.; Rebolj, M.; Lynge, E.; Juul, K.E.; Kjær, S.K.; Dillner, J.; et al. High-Grade Cervical Intraepithelial Neoplasia in Human Papillomavirus Self-Sampling of Screening Non-Attenders. *Br. J. Cancer* **2018**, *118*, 138–144. [CrossRef]

4. Verdoodt, F.; Jentschke, M.; Hillemanns, P.; Racey, C.S.; Snijders, P.J.F.; Arbyn, M. Reaching Women Who Do Not Participate in the Regular Cervical Cancer Screening Programme by Offering Self-Sampling Kits: A Systematic Review and Meta-Analysis of Randomised Trials. *Eur. J. Cancer* **2015**, *51*, 2375–2385. [CrossRef]
5. Chorley, A.J.; Marlow, L.A.V.; Forster, A.S.; Haddrell, J.B.; Waller, J. Experiences of Cervical Screening and Barriers to Participation in the Context of an Organised Programme: A Systematic Review and Thematic Synthesis: Experiences of Cervical Screening and Barriers to Participation. *Psycho-Oncology* **2017**, *26*, 161–172. [CrossRef]
6. Arbyn, M.; Verdoodt, F.; Snijders, P.J.F.; Verhoef, V.M.J.; Suonio, E.; Dillner, L.; Minozzi, S.; Bellisario, C.; Banzi, R.; Zhao, F.-H.; et al. Accuracy of Human Papillomavirus Testing on Self-Collected versus Clinician-Collected Samples: A Meta-Analysis. *Lancet Oncol.* **2014**, *15*, 172–183. [CrossRef]
7. Arbyn, M.; Smith, S.B.; Temin, S.; Sultana, F.; Castle, P. Detecting Cervical Precancer and Reaching Underscreened Women by Using HPV Testing on Self Samples: Updated Meta-Analyses. *BMJ* **2018**, *363*, k4823. [CrossRef]
8. Snijders, P.J.F.; Verhoef, V.M.J.; Arbyn, M.; Ogilvie, G.; Minozzi, S.; Banzi, R.; van Kemenade, F.J.; Heideman, D.A.M.; Meijer, C.J.L.M. High-Risk HPV Testing on Self-Sampled *versus* Clinician-Collected Specimens: A Review on the Clinical Accuracy and Impact on Population Attendance in Cervical Cancer Screening. *Int. J. Cancer* **2013**, *132*, 2223–2236. [CrossRef]
9. Hawkes, D.; Keung, M.H.T.; Huang, Y.; McDermott, T.L.; Romano, J.; Saville, M.; Brotherton, J.M.L. Self-Collection for Cervical Screening Programs: From Research to Reality. *Cancers* **2020**, *12*, 1053. [CrossRef]
10. Frati, E.; Fasoli, E.; Martinelli, M.; Colzani, D.; Bianchi, S.; Carnelli, L.; Amendola, A.; Olivani, P.; Tanzi, E. Sexually Transmitted Infections: A Novel Screening Strategy for Improving Women's Health in Vulnerable Populations. *Int. J. Mol. Sci.* **2017**, *18*, 1311. [CrossRef]
11. De Baetselier, I.; Smet, H.; Abdellati, S.; De Deken, B.; Cuylaerts, V.; Reyniers, T.; Vuylsteke, B.; Crucitti, T. Evaluation of the "Colli-Pee", a First-Void Urine Collection Device for Self-Sampling at Home for the Detection of Sexually Transmitted Infections, versus a Routine Clinic-Based Urine Collection in a One-to-One Comparison Study Design: Efficacy and Acceptability among MSM in Belgium. *BMJ Open* **2019**, *9*, e028145. [CrossRef]
12. Gaydos, C.A.; Quinn, T.C. Urine Nucleic Acid Amplification Tests for the Diagnosis of Sexually Transmitted Infections in Clinical Practice. *Curr. Opin. Infect. Dis.* **2005**, *18*, 55–66. [CrossRef]
13. Vorsters, A.; Van Damme, P.; Clifford, G. Urine Testing for HPV: Rationale for Using First Void. *BMJ* **2014**, *349*, g6252. [CrossRef]
14. Rohner, E.; Rahangdale, L.; Sanusi, B.; Knittel, A.K.; Vaughan, L.; Chesko, K.; Faherty, B.; Tulenko, S.E.; Schmitt, J.W.; Romocki, L.S.; et al. Test Accuracy of Human Papillomavirus in Urine for Detection of Cervical Intraepithelial Neoplasia. *J. Clin. Microbiol.* **2020**, *58*, e01443-19. [CrossRef]
15. Pattyn, J.; Van Keer, S.; Biesmans, S.; Ieven, M.; Vanderborght, C.; Beyers, K.; Vankerckhoven, V.; Bruyndonckx, R.; Van Damme, P.; Vorsters, A. Human Papillomavirus Detection in Urine: Effect of a First-Void Urine Collection Device and Timing of Collection. *J. Virol. Methods* **2019**, *264*, 23–30. [CrossRef]
16. Van Keer, S.; Tjalma, W.A.A.; Pattyn, J.; Biesmans, S.; Pieters, Z.; Van Ostade, X.; Ieven, M.; Van Damme, P.; Vorsters, A. Human Papillomavirus Genotype and Viral Load Agreement between Paired First-Void Urine and Clinician-Collected Cervical Samples. *Eur. J. Clin. Microbiol. Infect. Dis.* **2018**, *37*, 859–869. [CrossRef]
17. Van Keer, S.; Peeters, E.; Vanden Broeck, D.; De Sutter, P.; Donders, G.; Doyen, J.; Tjalma, W.A.A.; Weyers, S.; Vorsters, A.; Arbyn, M. Clinical and Analytical Evaluation of the RealTime High Risk HPV Assay in Colli-Pee Collected First-Void Urine Using the VALHUDES Protocol. *Gynecol. Oncol.* **2021**, *162*, 575–583. [CrossRef]
18. Leeman, A.; del Pino, M.; Molijn, A.; Rodriguez, A.; Torné, A.; de Koning, M.; Ordi, J.; van Kemenade, F.; Jenkins, D.; Quint, W. HPV Testing in First-Void Urine Provides Sensitivity for CIN2+ Detection Comparable with a Smear Taken by a Clinician or a Brush-Based Self-Sample: Cross-Sectional Data from a Triage Population. *BJOG Int. J. Obstet. Gynaecol.* **2017**, *124*, 1356–1363. [CrossRef]
19. Cuschieri, K.; Geraets, D.T.; Moore, C.; Quint, W.; Duvall, E.; Arbyn, M. Clinical and Analytical Performance of the Onclarity HPV Assay Using the VALGENT Framework. *J. Clin. Microbiol.* **2015**, *53*, 3272–3279. [CrossRef]
20. Ejegod, D.M.; Junge, J.; Franzmann, M.; Kirschner, B.; Bottari, F.; Sideri, M.; Sandri, M.-T.; Bonde, J. Clinical and Analytical Performance of the BD Onclarity™ HPV Assay for Detection of CIN2+ Lesions on SurePath Samples. *Papillomavirus Res.* **2016**, *2*, 31–37. [CrossRef]
21. Bottari, F.; Iacobone, A.D. Profile of the BD HPV Onclarity™ Assay. *Expert Rev. Mol. Diagn.* **2019**, *19*, 565–570. [CrossRef]
22. Arbyn, M.; Snijders, P.J.F.; Meijer, C.J.L.M.; Berkhof, J.; Cuschieri, K.; Kocjan, B.J.; Poljak, M. Which High-Risk HPV Assays Fulfil Criteria for Use in Primary Cervical Cancer Screening? *Clin. Microbiol. Infect.* **2015**, *21*, 817–826. [CrossRef] [PubMed]
23. Racey, C.S.; Withrow, D.R.; Gesink, D. Self-Collected HPV Testing Improves Participation in Cervical Cancer Screening: A Systematic Review and Meta-Analysis. *Can. J. Public Health* **2013**, *104*, e159–e166. [CrossRef] [PubMed]
24. Sechi, I.; Cocuzza, C.; Martinelli, M.; Muresu, N.; Castriciano, S.; Sotgiu, G.; Piana, A. Comparison of Different Self-Sampling Devices for Molecular Detection of Human Papillomavirus (HPV) and Other Sexually Transmitted Infections (STIs): A Pilot Study. *Healthcare* **2022**, *10*, 459. [CrossRef] [PubMed]
25. Ertik, F.C.; Kampers, J.; Hülse, F.; Stolte, C.; Böhmer, G.; Hillemanns, P.; Jentschke, M. CoCoss-Trial: Concurrent Comparison of Self-Sampling Devices for HPV-Detection. *Int. J. Environ. Res. Public Health* **2021**, *18*, 10388. [CrossRef] [PubMed]

26. Bokan, T.; Ivanus, U.; Jerman, T.; Takac, I.; Arko, D. Long Term Results of Follow-up after HPV Self-Sampling with Devices Qvintip and HerSwab in Women Non-Attending Cervical Screening Programme. *Radiol. Oncol.* **2021**, *55*, 187–195. [CrossRef] [PubMed]
27. Arbyn, M.; Simon, M.; Peeters, E.; Xu, L.; Meijer, C.J.L.M.; Berkhof, J.; Cuschieri, K.; Bonde, J.; Ostrbenk Vanlencak, A.; Zhao, F.-H.; et al. 2020 List of Human Papillomavirus Assays Suitable for Primary Cervical Cancer Screening. *Clin. Microbiol. Infect.* **2021**, *27*, 1083–1095. [CrossRef] [PubMed]
28. Arbyn, M.; Peeters, E.; Benoy, I.; Vanden Broeck, D.; Bogers, J.; De Sutter, P.; Donders, G.; Tjalma, W.; Weyers, S.; Cuschieri, K.; et al. VALHUDES: A Protocol for Validation of Human Papillomavirus Assays and Collection Devices for HPV Testing on Self-Samples and Urine Samples. *J. Clin. Virol.* **2018**, *107*, 52–56. [CrossRef] [PubMed]
29. Arbyn, M.; Castle, P.E.; Schiffman, M.; Wentzensen, N.; Heckman-Stoddard, B.; Sahasrabuddhe, V.V. Meta-analysis of Agreement/Concordance Statistics in Studies Comparing Self- vs Clinician-collected Samples for HPV Testing in Cervical Cancer Screening. *Int. J. Cancer* **2022**, *151*, 308–312. [CrossRef]
30. Bianchi, S.; Frati, E.R.; Panatto, D.; Martinelli, M.; Amicizia, D.; Zotti, C.M.; Martinese, M.; Bonanni, P.; Boccalini, S.; Coppola, R.C.; et al. Detection and Genotyping of Human Papillomavirus in Urine Samples from Unvaccinated Male and Female Adolescents in Italy. *PLoS ONE* **2013**, *8*, e79719. [CrossRef]
31. Daponte, A.; Michail, G.; Daponte, A.-I.; Daponte, N.; Valasoulis, G. Urine HPV in the Context of Genital and Cervical Cancer Screening—An Update of Current Literature. *Cancers* **2021**, *13*, 1640. [CrossRef]
32. Cadman, L.; Reuter, C.; Jitlal, M.; Kleeman, M.; Austin, J.; Hollingworth, T.; Parberry, A.L.; Ashdown-Barr, L.; Patel, D.; Nedjai, B.; et al. A Randomized Comparison of Different Vaginal Self-Sampling Devices and Urine for Human Papillomavirus Testing—Predictors 5.1. *Cancer Epidemiol. Biomark. Prev.* **2021**, *30*, 661–668. [CrossRef]
33. Cho, H.-W.; Hong, J.H.; Min, K.J.; Ouh, Y.-T.; Seong, S.J.; Moon, J.H.; Cho, S.H.; Lee, J.K. Performance and Diagnostic Accuracy of Human Papillomavirus Testing on Self-Collected Urine and Vaginal Samples in a Referral Population. *Cancer Res. Treat.* **2021**, *53*, 829–836. [CrossRef]
34. Ørnskov, D.; Jochumsen, K.; Steiner, P.H.; Grunnet, I.M.; Lykkebo, A.W.; Waldstrøm, M. Clinical Performance and Acceptability of Self-Collected Vaginal and Urine Samples Compared with Clinician-Taken Cervical Samples for HPV Testing among Women Referred for Colposcopy. A Cross-Sectional Study. *BMJ Open* **2021**, *11*, e041512. [CrossRef]
35. Lozar, T.; Nagvekar, R.; Rohrer, C.; Dube Mandishora, R.S.; Ivanus, U.; Fitzpatrick, M.B. Cervical Cancer Screening Postpandemic: Self-Sampling Opportunities to Accelerate the Elimination of Cervical Cancer. *Int. J. Women Health* **2021**, *13*, 841–859. [CrossRef]

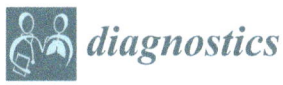

Article

E6/E7 mRNA Expression of the Most Prevalent High-Risk HPV Genotypes in Cervical Samples from Serbian Women

Natasa Nikolic [1,*], Branka Basica [1], Aljosa Mandic [2,3], Nela Surla [1], Vera Gusman [1,4], Deana Medic [1,4], Tamas Petrovic [5], Mirjana Strbac [1] and Vladimir Petrovic [1,6]

1. Institute of Public Health of Vojvodina, 21000 Novi Sad, Serbia
2. Clinic for Oncological Surgery, Oncology Institute of Vojvodina, 21208 Sremska Kamenica, Serbia
3. Department of Gynaecology and Obstetrics, Faculty of Medicine, University of Novi Sad, 21000 Novi Sad, Serbia
4. Department of Microbiology with Parasitology and Immunology, Faculty of Medicine, University of Novi Sad, 21000 Novi Sad, Serbia
5. Scientific Veterinary Institute Novi Sad, 21000 Novi Sad, Serbia
6. Department of Epidemiology, Faculty of Medicine, University of Novi Sad, 21000 Novi Sad, Serbia
* Correspondence: natasa.nikolic@izjzv.org.rs

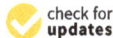

Citation: Nikolic, N.; Basica, B.; Mandic, A.; Surla, N.; Gusman, V.; Medic, D.; Petrovic, T.; Strbac, M.; Petrovic, V. E6/E7 mRNA Expression of the Most Prevalent High-Risk HPV Genotypes in Cervical Samples from Serbian Women. Diagnostics 2023, 13, 917. https://doi.org/10.3390/diagnostics13050917

Academic Editors: Fabio Bottari and Anna Daniela Iacobone

Received: 16 December 2022
Revised: 21 February 2023
Accepted: 22 February 2023
Published: 28 February 2023

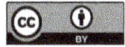

Copyright: © 2023 by the authors. Licensee MDPI, Basel, Switzerland. This article is an open access article distributed under the terms and conditions of the Creative Commons Attribution (CC BY) license (https://creativecommons.org/licenses/by/4.0/).

Abstract: Cervical cancer caused by persistent infection with HR HPV genotypes is the second leading cause of death in women aged 15 to 44 in Serbia. The expression of the E6 and E7 HPV oncogenes is considered as a promising biomarker in diagnosing high-grade squamous intraepithelial lesions (HSIL). This study aimed to evaluate HPV mRNA and DNA tests, compare the results according to the severity of the lesions, and assess the predictive potential for the diagnosis of HSIL. Cervical specimens were obtained at the Department of Gynecology, Community Health Centre Novi Sad, Serbia, and the Oncology Institute of Vojvodina, Serbia, during 2017–2021. The 365 samples were collected using the ThinPrep Pap test. The cytology slides were evaluated according to the Bethesda 2014 System. Using a real-time PCR test, HPV DNA was detected and genotyped, while the RT-PCR proved the presence of E6 and E7 mRNA. The most common genotypes in Serbian women are HPV 16, 31, 33, and 51. Oncogenic activity was demonstrated in 67% of HPV-positive women. A comparison of the HPV DNA and mRNA tests to assess the progression of cervical intraepithelial lesions indicated that higher specificity (89.1%) and positive predictive value (69.8–78.7%) were expressed by the E6/E7 mRNA test, while higher sensitivity was recorded when using the HPV DNA test (67.6–88%). The results determine the higher probability of detecting HPV infection by 7% provided by the mRNA test. The detected E6/E7 mRNA HR HPVs have a predictive potential in assessing the diagnosis of HSIL. The oncogenic activity of HPV 16 and age were the risk factors with the strongest predictive values for the development of HSIL.

Keywords: E6; E7; HPV; cervical intraepithelial lesion; biomarker; Serbia

1. Introduction

It is estimated that approximately every fourth malignancy can be linked to an infectious agent, that is, its contribution to various stages of cancer development (reviewed in [1]). About a third of this contribution is related to the human papillomavirus (HPV) (reviewed in [2]). Today, significant evidence confirms the association of high-risk (HR) HPV as a carcinogen or promoter in developing malignant diseases in different locations: the cervix, vulva, vagina, penis, anus, and certain head and neck regions. In first place are neoplasias of the lower genital tract, such as cervical cancer [3]. According to estimates by the World Health Organization (WHO), that is, by the International Agency for Research on Cancer (IARC), 604,000 new cases and 342,000 deaths were registered around the world in 2020, which makes cervical cancer the fourth most frequently diagnosed cancer in women [4]. In Serbia, organized cervical cancer screening has been conducted since

2012, using the PAP test, based on the cytomorphological examination of cervical samples. Screening is mandatory for women aged 25 to 69. However, despite organized screening, cervical cancer remains one of the most common cancers among women in Serbia [5]. The incidence of cervical cancer in Serbia is still among the highest and is approximately twice the average in Europe (10.7 to 100,000) [6,7]. It is necessary to emphasize that data on the HPV prevalence and genotype distribution among women with normal cervical cytology, precancerous cervical lesions, and cervical cancer are missing in the updated IARC Human Papillomavirus and Related Diseases Report for Serbia [6].

HPV vaccination is a crucial prevention tool against HPV infection and HPV-related precancers and cancers [8]. If vaccination against HPV is carried out before initial sexual activities, it is one of the most effective ways to prevent cervical cancer [9]. Still, in Serbia, vaccination against HPV infection is not part of the mandatory national immunization program, but it is recommended for children aged 9 to 19 years [5].

Strong evidence for HPV as a causative aetiology of cancers of various locations was provided by the IARC, which classified HPV according to its potential to cause malignant cell alteration as follows [10]:

Group 1 (carcinogenic to humans, HR) includes HPV genotypes: 16, 18, 31, 33, 35, 39, 45, 51, 52, 56, 58, and 59;

Group 2A (probably carcinogenic) includes HPV genotype 68;

Group 2B (potentially carcinogenic) includes HPV genotypes: 26, 53, 66, 67, 70, 73, 82, 30, 34, 69, 85 and 97;

Group 3 (low risk, LR) includes HPV genotypes 6 and 11.

Persistent HPV infection is the most critical risk factor for the development of cervical cancer, which is confirmed by the presence of HR HPV in over 99% of cervical cancer samples. Concerning the oncogenic potential, infection with a particular HR HPV genotype carries a specific risk for cellular transformation and malignancy (reviewed in [3]). Namely, one of the most critical determinants of the degree of pathogenicity of different HPV genotypes is the functional differences between their oncoproteins, E6 and E7 [11].

During viral genome integration into the host cell genome, E1 or E2 are usually disrupted [12]. This gene disruption leads to uncontrolled transcription of E6 and E7 genes as the E2 repression on these oncogenes disappears [13,14]. Their protein products lead to unregulated cell proliferation, differentiation, and loss of the reparative abilities of the host cell, wherefore they are considered the main actors of virus-induced oncogenesis of cervical cancer [15,16]. Thanks to the use of cervical cancer screening tests, this cancer is classified as one of the most preventable malignancies. The most common test for this purpose is the cytological abnormality test, the Papanicolaou (PAP) test. However, considering the etiological role of HR HPV in developing cervical cancer, DNA tests have been incorporated into the primary screening of developed countries. Still, this test is characterized by high sensitivity and low specificity, which indicates the necessity of improving the test's characteristics concerning specificity [17]. In this context, the results of numerous studies state that using the HR HPV mRNA test as a basic or additional test in primary screening would improve these characteristics [18].

Given the above, this research aimed to determine the oncogenic activity of the most commonly diagnosed HR HPVs in cervical smear samples using the mRNA test and compare the results according to the severity of the cervical intraepithelial lesion. Furthermore, it aimed to examine the clinical characteristics and predictive potential in assessing the diagnosis of high-grade cervical intraepithelial lesions of HPV DNA and mRNA tests.

2. Materials and Methods

2.1. Study Population and Specimen Collection

From 2017 to 2021, cervical smears were obtained from a sample of 365 female patients (age 20–74 years) with normal and abnormal results of cervical cytology who were undergoing gynecological exams at the Department of Gynecology, Community Health Centre

Novi Sad, Serbia, and the Oncology Institute of Vojvodina, Serbia. All of the women in the study did not receive any prior treatment for cervical dysplasia or cancer, and all were unvaccinated against HPV infection. The samples were collected using the ThinPrep Pap test (Hologic Inc., Marlborough, MA, USA) according to the manufacturer's instructions and sent for further analyses to the Center of Virology, Institute of Public Health of Vojvodina, Novi Sad, Republic of Serbia.

The classification of cytological findings was performed according to the criteria of the Bethesda System 2014. It was categorized into negative for intraepithelial lesion or malignancy (NILM), atypical squamous cells of unknown significance (ASCUS), low-grade squamous intraepithelial lesions (LSIL), and high-grade squamous intraepithelial lesions (HSIL). All of the women enrolled in the study were informed about the research objective and signed an informed written consent form. The study protocol was reviewed and approved by the Medical Ethical Committee of the Institute of Public Health of Vojvodina, Novi Sad, Serbia (approval number: 01-252/3).

2.2. HR HPV Detection and Genotyping

The ThinPrep cervical smear samples were stored at 4–8 °C for up to 3 days from the sampling day. The 2 mL of collected samples were transferred to nuclease-free tubes and centrifugated at $8000 \times g$ for 5 min. The formed pellet was dissolved in 200 µL of nuclease-free water and used for nucleic acid extraction. According to the manufacturer's instructions, DNA extraction was carried out using the SaMag STD DNA Extraction Kit (Sacace Biotechnologies, Como, Italy). The extracted DNA was eluted in 100 µL elution buffer. The detection and genotyping of 12 HR HPV genotypes (16, 18, 31, 33, 35, 39, 45, 51, 52, 56, 58, and 59), marked as the HPV DNA test, were performed using the High Risk Typing Real-TM Kit (Sacace Biotechnologies, Como, Italy) following manufacturer's instructions. The E7 gene of specific HPV genotypes was amplified using primers and TaqMan probes in the multiplex reaction performed in a total of 13 µL. The β globin gene is used as an internal control. Real-time PCR was performed on the SaCycler-96 (Sacace Biotechnologies, Como, Italy). After the initial activation of the DNA polymerase at 95 °C for 15 min, five cycles of amplification were performed under the following conditions: 95 °C/5 s, 60 °C/20 s, and 72 °C/15 s, and 40 amplifications were performed under the following conditions: 95 °C/5 s, 60 °C/30 s (fluorescence detection), and 72 °C/15 s. The kinetics of the detected fluorescence signals were monitored using the SaCycler-96 software package (Sacace Biotechnologies, Como, Italy).

2.3. E6/E7 mRNA HPV Detection

E6/E7 mRNA of the most prevalent HPVs was tested in the cervical samples positive for the most prevalent HR HPVs DNA and HR HPV DNA negative samples. The HR-HPV-negative samples were included in E6/E7 mRNA testing because the study aimed to determine the mRNA test's clinical characteristics by evaluating and comparing it with the HPV DNA test. Total RNA was extracted from the prepared sample using the miRNeasy Mini Kit and QIAcube robotic workstation (Qiagen, Hilden, Germany) following the manufacturer's instructions. The total RNA was eluted in 50 µL ultrapure water free from nucleases. Following the manufacturer's recommendations, potentially present contaminants were removed using the TURBO DNA-free Kit (Invitrogen/ThermoFisher Scientific, Waltham, MA, USA). The routine procedure for removing contaminants using the kit above included the addition of 5 µL of $10 \times$ TURBO DNase Buffer and 1 µL of TURBO DNase enzyme into each sample of extracted total RNA, with incubation for 30 min at a temperature of 37 °C. After the action of the enzyme, 5 µL of inactivation reagent (Dnase Inactivation Reagent) was added, with incubation for 5 min, at room temperature and occasional vortexing. After that, centrifugation was performed (90 s, $10,000 \times g$). The supernatant was carefully transferred to a nuclease-free tube. The real-time reverse transcription PCR (RT-PCR) analysis, marked as the HPV mRNA test, was performed using specific primers and TaqMan probes to detect the E6/E7 mRNA of individual HPV genotypes. The sequences for the primers and probes (Table 1) were adopted from Lindh et al. (2007) [19] and purchased from Life Technologies (Carlsbad, CA, USA). The AgPath-ID One-Step RT-PCR Kit (Applied Biosystems, Waltham, MA, USA) was used for the real-time RT-PCR. A separate reaction mixture was prepared for each set of primers and TaqMan probes. The reaction was prepared to a final volume of 25 µL containing: 12.5 µL 2× RT-PCR Buffer, 1 µL of 25× RT-PCR Enzyme Mix, primers to a final concentration of 300 nM, the probe to a final concentration of 200 nM, 1 µL of RNase Inhibitor reagent (Applied Biosystems, Waltham, MA, USA), 5 µL of isolated total RNA, and DEPC-treated nuclease-free water (Invitrogen, Waltham, MA, USA). Real-time PCR was performed on the Applied Biosystems 7500 Real-Time PCR Systems (ThermoFisher Scientific, Waltham, MA, USA). After the reverse transcription reaction at 48 °C for 30 min, the inactivation of reverse transcriptase and the activation of Taq polymerase were performed at 95 °C for 10 min. After that, 45 cycles of PCR amplification were carried out with denaturation at 95 °C for 15 s and annealing and elongation at 58 °C for 1 min. The data were analyzed with the Applied Biosystems Software v2.0.6 (ThermoFisher Scientific, Waltham, MA, USA) and the GraphPad Prism 8 (GraphPad Software, San Diego, CA, USA).

Table 1. Primer and probe sequences used for the RT-PCR analysis.

Gene	Primer and Probe Sequences (5′–3′)
E6/E7 HPV 16	F: TTGCAGATCATCAAGAACACGTAGA R: CAGTAGAGATCAGTTGTCTCTGGTTGC P: FAM-AATCATGCATGGAGATACACCTACATTGCATGA-TAMRA
E6/E7 HPV 31	F: ATTCCACAACATAGGAGGAAGGTG R: CACTTGGGTTTCAGTACGAGGTCT P: FAM-ACAGGACGTTGCATAGCATGTTGGA-TAMRA
E6/E7 HPV 33	F: ATATTTCGGGTCGTTGGGCA R: ACGTCACAGTGCAGTTTCTCTACGT P: FAM-GGACCTCCAACACGCCGCACA-TAMRA *
E6/E7 HPV 51	F: AAAGCAAAAATTGGTGGACGA R: TGCCAGCAATTAGCGCATT P: FAM-CATGAAATAGCGGGACGTTGGACG-TAMRA

F—forward; R—reverse; P—TaqMan probe; *—antisense; FAM—6-carboxyfluorescein; TAMRA—6-carboxytetramethylrhodamine.

2.4. Statistical Analysis

All of the statistical analyses were performed using SPSS statistics software Version 21.0 (Chicago, IL, USA). Testing the difference in frequencies of attributive features was performed using the Chi-square (χ^2) test of independence and quality of the match. The Student's t-test was used to compare values between the two age groups, a numerical characteristic. A one-way analysis of variance (ANOVA) and the Bonferroni post-hoc test were applied to compare values between three or more data groups. Frequencies were used to present the analysis of the oncogenic activity of multiple HR HPV infections. Sensitivity, specificity, positive predictive value (PPV), negative predictive value (NPV), and their 95% confidence intervals (CIs) of HR HPVs DNA and E6/E7 mRNA HPVs detection and cytology test were calculated. To quantify the diagnostic capabilities of the selected test and evaluate its significance, the receiver operating characteristics (ROC) curve was used, which enables testing the significance of differences in the discriminating potential of different variables for the same binary outcome. It is based on a graphical presentation of pairs of sensitivity and specificity that can be obtained by estimating the threshold value for all values of discontinuous variables of the sample. Univariate and multivariate logistic regression were used to analyze the connection between two or more features, generating adequate statistical models. Multivariate logistic regression analysis was applied to all of the analyzed factors to construct a predictive model and named the most relevant predictors for the development of HSIL. A p-value of less than 0.05 defined as statistically significance.

3. Results

3.1. Cervical Cytology

A total of 365 specimens obtained from women in the north part of the Republic of Serbia (Vojvodina) were classified based on the Bethesda System 2014 into four categories by cytological criteria.

3.2. HR HPV DNA in Cervical Samples

The cervical samples were analyzed for 12 HR HPVs, where 246 out of 365 (67.4%) had HPV-DNA-positive results, which indicates that the overall prevalence of HPV in the study population was 67.4%. All of the HPV genotypes covered by the HPV DNA test were identified (n = 274) in the study population (246 HR-HPV-positive cervical samples). The most prevalent HPV genotype is HPV 16 which makes up 38.3% (105/274) of the total HPV-detected genotypes in 42.7% (105/246) of HP- DNA-positive samples. HPV 31 takes second place with 17.2% (47/274) of total HPV-detected genotypes in 19.1% (47/246) of HPV-DNA-positive samples. Equally represented are HPV 33 and HPV 51, each with 8.8% (24/274) of total HPV-detected genotypes in 9.8% (24/246) of HPV-DNA-positive samples (Figure 1). The results show that those HR HPVs make up 73% (200/274) of the detected genotypes, including multiple infections, which determined those cervical samples (n = 172) for further examination of oncogenic activity, according to the study's aim. Multiple HPV infections were found in 15.7%. The most common co-infections were those with HPV 16 and 31, found in 7.6% (13/172) of cases with multiple infections (Table 2).

Molecular data were compared with the cytological results and age categories of patients. The distribution of cytological groups was analyzed within the most prevalent HR-HPV-DNA-positive samples (172 cervical samples), including multiple infections. A minority of women, 16.9% (n = 29), had normal results, whereas 83.1% (n = 143) showed different abnormalities. A total of 26.7% (n = 46) of the examined women had ASCUS; in 25.6% (n = 44), LSILs were found, whereas HSILs were detected in 30.8% (n = 53). The mean age of the patients was 36.7 years. Among the specimens, the number of Serbian women who were ≤30 years, 31–44 years, and ≥45 years old accounted for 36.5% (n = 68), 36.0% (n = 62), and 24.4% (n = 42) of the samples, respectively (Table 3).

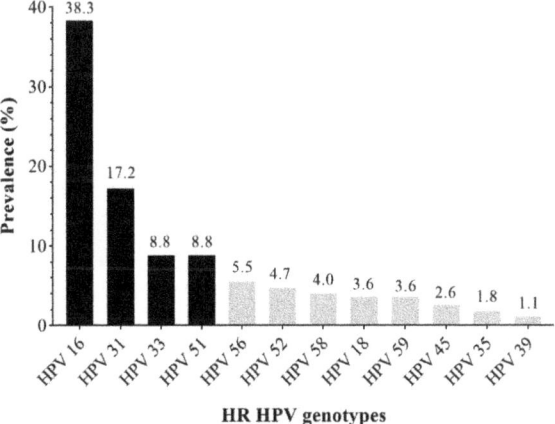

Figure 1. Genotype-specific distribution of HR HPVs.

The distribution of the most frequently detected HPVs concerning cytology is shown in Table 4. The prevalence rates of HR HPV 16 ranged from 44.8% in the group of NILM cytology to 75.5% in the HSIL group. Contrarily, the prevalence of HR HPV 31 is similar in the groups of NILM (37.9%), ASCUS (34.8%), and LSIL (31.8%), while it is lower in the group of HSIL (11.3%). HPV genotypes 33 and 51 are present in all of the cytological groups in less than 21%. The statistically significant difference in the prevalence between the number of positive findings of HPV 16 (χ^2 test; $p = 0.035$) and HPV 31 (χ^2 test; $p = 0.017$) was determined, depending on the degree of severity of the cytological findings, which was not determined for HPV 33 and 51 (χ^2 test; $p = 0.706$, $p = 0.790$, respectively) (Table 4).

Table 2. Distribution of the most prevalent HR HPVs (HR HPV 16, 31, 33, and 51) in single and multiple infections.

HPV Infection	HR HPV DNA	n (%)	n (%)
Single	16	83 (48.3)	145 (84.3)
	31	28 (16.3)	
	33	18 (10.5)	
	51	16 (9.3)	
Multiple	16, 31	13 (7.6)	27 (15.7)
	16, 51	6 (3.5)	
	31, 33	3 (1.7)	
	16, 33	2 (1.2)	
	31, 51	2 (1.2)	
	16, 31, 33	1 (0.6)	
Total:		172 (100)	172 (100)

Table 3. Cervical cytology and age of female patients diagnosed with the most prevalent HR HPVs.

Most Prevalent HR-HPV-DNA-Positive Women	n (%)
Cytology	
NILM	29 (16.9)
ASCUS	46 (26.7)
LSIL	44 (25.6)
HSIL	53 (30.8)
Total:	172 (100)
Age	
≤30	68 (36.5)
31–44	62 (36.0)
≥45	42 (24.4)
Mean age (years, SD))	36.7 (12.6)

SD—standard deviation; NILM—negative for an intraepithelial lesion or malignancy; ASCUS—atypical squamous cells of unknown significance; LSIL—low-grade squamous intraepithelial lesions; HSIL—high-grade squamous intraepithelial lesions.

A statistically significant difference was found in the number of female patients concerning the cytological findings and the age of the patients (χ^2 test; $\chi^2 = 29.500$; $p = 0.000$) (Table 5). The statistically significant difference was determined regarding the cytological findings and the age of the patients, where the female patients diagnosed with HSIL were significantly older compared to the other groups (ANOVA; $F = 9.321$; $p < 0.001$). The Bonferroni post-hoc test determined that the female patients with HSIL are statistically significantly older than those with ASCUS ($p < 0.001$), NILM ($p < 0.001$), and LSIL ($p = 0.012$) (Figure 2, Table 5). Female patients with confirmed HPV 31 are statistically significantly younger (33 years) than the other HR-HPV-DNA-positive patients (t = 2.317; $p = 0.022$). The average age of the female patients with confirmed HPV DNA 16 was 36.9 years; with HPV DNA 33, it was 34.1 years, while the average age of patients with HPV DNA 51 was 40.5 years. The statistical analyses show that the proportion of HPV 16 positivity maintained at the same level as age. Conversely, the proportion of HPV 31 positivity decreases with age. The detection of HR HPV 33 genotypes decreases with age, while HR HPV 51 increases (Table 5).

Table 4. Distribution of the most frequently detected HR HPVs according to cytology.

HR HPV DNA		Cytology				χ^2	p
		NILM	ASCUS	LSIL	HSIL		
		n (%)	n (%)	n (%)	n (%)		
HPV 16	+	13 (44.8)	28 (60.9)	24 (54.5)	40 (75.5)	8.628	0.035 *
	−	16 (55.2)	18 (39.1)	20 (45.5)	13 (24.5)		
HPV 31	+	11 (37.9)	16 (34.8)	14 (31.8)	6 (11.3)	10.214	0.017 *
	−	18 (62.1)	30 (65.2)	30 (68.2)	47 (88.7)		
HPV 33	+	6 (20.7)	6 (13.0)	5 (11.4)	7 (13.2)	1.398	0.706
	−	23 (79.3)	40 (87.0)	39 (88.6)	46 (86.8)		
HPV 51	+	4 (13.8)	5 (10,9)	8 (18.2)	7 (13.2)	1.045	0.790
	−	25 (86.2)	41 (89.1)	36 (81.8)	46 (86.8)		
Total:		29 (100)	46 (100)	44 (100)	53 (100)		

* $p < 0.05$. NILM—negative for an intraepithelial lesion or malignancy; ASCUS—atypical squamous cells of unknown significance; LSIL—low-grade squamous intraepithelial lesions; HSIL—high-grade squamous intraepithelial lesions.

Table 5. Age-specific distribution of female patients with different cytological groups and genotypes.

HR HPV-Positive Women	Age Group (Years)			Total n (%)	χ^2	p	Mean Age (years, (SD))	#	p
	≤30 n (%)	31–44 n (%)	≥45 n (%)						
Cytology									
NILM	19 (27.9)	5 (8.1)	5 (11.9)	29 (16.9)			30.9 (12.2)		0.000 ***
ASCUS	21 (30.9)	21 (33.9)	4 (9.5)	46 (26.7)	29.500	0.000 ***	33.4 (9.2)	9.321	0.000 ***
LSIL	17 (25.0)	18 (29.0)	9 (21.5)	44 (25.6)			35.9 (11.5)		0.012 *
HSIL	11 (16.2)	18 (29.0)	24 (51.1)	53 (30.8)			43.4 (6.8)		-
Total:	68 (39.5)	62 (36.1)	42 (24.4)	172 (100)					
Genotype								§	
HR HPV 16	41 (50.6)	39 (52.0)	25 (56.8)	105 (52.5)	0.147	0.929	36.9 (12.9)	0.289	0.773
HR HPV 31	24 (29.6)	15 (20.0)	8 (18.2)	47 (23.5)	3.930	0.140	33.1 (10.8)	2.317	0.022 *
HR HPV 33	10 (12.3)	10 (13.3)	4 (9.1)	24 (12.0)	0.963	0.618	34.1 (11.2)	1.077	0.283
HR HPV 51	6 (7.4)	11 (14.7)	7 15.9	24 (12.0)	2.489	0.298	40.5 (12.7)	1.610	0.109
Total:	81 (40.5)	75 (37.5)	44 (22.0)	200 (100)					

SD—Standard Deviation; #—ANOVA; §—t test; * $p < 0.05$; *** $p < 0.001$.

3.3. E6/E7 mRNA in Cervical Samples

Figure 3 shows the study design with sample processing to analyze the expression of the E6/E7 mRNA of the most prevalent HR HPV in cervical samples from Serbian women. A total of 291 cervical samples, which include HPV 16-, 31-, 33- and 51-positive (n = 172) and HR-HPV-negative samples (n = 119), were tested by the HPV mRNA test. The E6/E7 mRNA HPV was detected exclusively in HR-HPV-DNA-positive samples (Table 6). E6 and E7 transcripts of the four most frequent HR HPVs were detected in 57.5% (115/200) of the HR HPV DNA confirmed genotypes. Accordingly, the distribution of E6/E7 mRNA HR HPV 16, 31, 33, and 51 are shown in Table 6. The E6/E7 mRNA HR HPV 16 was the most abundant, which accounted for 25.5% (51/200) of HR HPV genotypes. Next in frequency was the E6/E7 mRNA HR HPV 31 in 16.5% (33/200), while the E6/E7 mRNAs HR HPV 33 and 51 were equally represented in 8% (16/200) and 7.5% (15/200), respectively. Almost every second HPV 16 genotype is oncogenically expressed (48.6%; 51/105), and it was detected in 29.7% (51/172) HPV-DNA-positive samples. The oncogenic activity of HPV 31 was detected in approximately every fifth (19.2%; 33/172) HPV-DNA-positive sample. Regarding the oncogenic activity of the remaining tested genotypes, HPV 33 and HPV 51 were detected in roughly every tenth HPV-DNA-positive sample (Table 6). The results of expressing E6 and E7 HR HPV oncogenes were expressed through the dispersion of the obtained Ct values. The oncogenic activity of HPV 16 is detected by the lowest registered value (Ct = 16) (Supplementary Materials Figure S1).

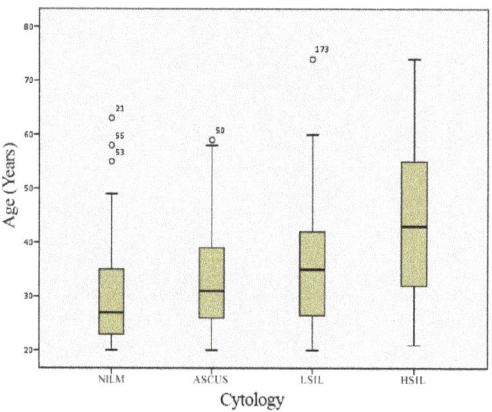

Figure 2. Age-specific analyses of the most prevalent HR HPV DNA in different cytological groups. NILM—negative for an intraepithelial lesion or malignancy; ASCUS—atypical squamous cells of unknown significance; LSIL—low-grade squamous intraepithelial lesions; HSIL—high-grade squamous intraepithelial lesions.

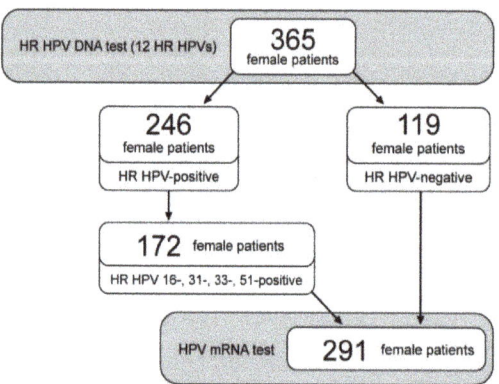

Figure 3. Flowchart presenting the study design. HR—high risk; HPV—human papillomavirus.

3.4. Prevalence of HR HPV Based on E6/E7 mRNA HPV Expression in Different Cytological Groups

The expression of the E6 and E7 genes as indicators of the oncogenic activity of HR HPV 16, 31, 33, and 51 was analyzed concerning cytological findings. The oncogenic activity of the tested genotypes increases with the severity of the cervical intraepithelial lesion. A statistically significant difference in E6/E7 mRNA HPV expression among the various cytological groups was observed (χ^2 test; χ^2 = 108.623; $p < 0.001$). E6/E7 mRNA HPVs are the most prevalent in patients with HSIL cytological findings (88.9%). In the group of patients with LSIL cytological findings, it was demonstrated in a lower percentage

(60%). A two-fold lower prevalence is observed in patients with ASCUS (29.4%). Oncogene activity in women with normal cytological findings is present in 10.9% of samples (Table 7). Subsequently, the E6/E7 mRNA distribution of HR-HPV-DNA-positive samples according to genotype and cytological groups was analyzed. E6/E7 mRNA HR HPV 16 is the most represented in patients with HSIL cytological findings (64.2%), while in the other groups of cytological findings, it was demonstrated in a lower percentage (3.4–22.7%). A statistically significant difference was found in the number of positive findings of E6/E7 mRNA HR HPV 16 concerning the cytological status (χ^2 test; χ^2 = 46.881; $p < 0.001$). This result singled out the HR HPV 16 genotype for further analyses. The presence of E6/E7 mRNA HR HPV 31 was the least detected in HSIL (7.5%) compared to other cytological groups (22.7–26.1%). The distribution of the oncogenic activity of the remaining genotypes (HR HPV 33 and 51) is approximately the same across different cytological groups and remains at a low level (2.2–11.4%) (Table 7).

Table 6. Analyses of E6/E7 mRNA HPV 16, 31, 33, and 51 in cervical samples.

E6/E7 mRNA HPV Genotypes		Genotypes n (%)	HR HPV 16, 31, 33, 51 Cervical Samples (n = 291)		E6/E7 mRNA HR HPV/Most Prevalent HR-HPV-DNA-Positive Samples (%)	E6/E7 mRNA HR HPV Positive/HR-HPV-DNA-Positive (%)
			Positive n (%)	Negative n (%)		
HPV 16	+	51 (25.5)	51 (48.6)	0 (0.0)	29.7 (51/172)	48.5 (51/105)
	−	149 (74.5)	54 (51.4)	186 (63.9)		
	Total:	200 (100)	105 (36.1)	186 (63.9)		
HPV 31	+	33 (16.5)	33 (70.2)	0 (0.0)	19.2 (33/172)	70.2 (33/47)
	−	167 (83.5)	14 (29.8)	244 (83.8)		
	Total:	200 (100)	47 (16.2)	244 (83.8)		
HPV 33	+	16 (8.0)	16 (66.7)	0 (0.0)	9.3 (16/172)	66.7 (16/24)
	−	184 (92.0)	8 (33.3)	267 (91.8)		
	Total:	200 (100)	24 (8.2)	267 (91.8)		
HPV 51	+	15 (7.5)	15 (62.5)	0 (0.0)	8.7 (15/172)	62.5 (15/24)
	−	185 (92.5)	9 (37.5)	267 (91.8)		
	Total:	200 (100)	24 (8.2)	267 (91.8)		
Total E6/E7 mRNA genotypes	+		115 (57.5)	0 (0.0)	66.9 (115/172)	57.5 (115/200)
	−		85 (42.5)	119 (100)		

Table 7. Distribution of E6/E7 mRNA HR HPV according to cytology.

E6/E7 mRNA HPV Genotypes		Cytology				Total n (%)	χ^2	p
		NILM n (%)	ASCUS n (%)	LSIL n (%)	HSIL n (%)			
HPV 16	+	1 (3.4)	6 (13.0)	10 (22.7)	34 (64.2)	51 (29.7)	46.881	0.000 ***
	−	28 (96.6)	40 (87.0)	34 (77.3)	19 (35.8)	121 (70.3)		
	Total:	29 (100)	46 (100)	44 (100)	53 (100)	172 (100)		
HPV 31	+	7 (24.1)	12 (26.1)	10 (22.7)	4 (7.5)	33 (19.2)	6.858	0.077
	−	22 (75.9)	34 (73.9)	34 (77.3)	49 (92.5)	139 (80.8)		
	Total:	29 (100)	46 (100)	44 (100)	53 (100)	172 (100)		
HPV 33	+	3 (10.3)	3 (6.5)	5 (11.4)	5 (9.4)	16 (9.3)	0.682	0.878
	−	26 (89.7)	43 (93.5)	39 (88.6)	48 (90.6)	156 (90.7)		
	Total:	29 (100)	46 (100)	44 (100)	53 (100)	172 (100)		
HPV 51	+	3 (10.3)	1 (2.2)	5 (11.4)	6 (11.3)	15 (8.7)	-	-
	−	26 (89.7)	45 (97.8)	39 (88.6)	47 (88.7)	157 (91.3)		
	Total:	29 (100)	46 (100)	44 (100)	53 (100)	172 (100)		

Table 7. Cont.

E6/E7 mRNA HPV Genotypes		Cytology				Total n (%)	χ^2	p
		NILM n (%)	ASCUS n (%)	LSIL n (%)	HSIL n (%)			
		Cervical samples						
E6/E7 mRNA HPVs	+	13 (10.9)	20 (29.4)	30 (60.0)	48 (88.9)	111 (38.1)	108.623	0.000 ***
	-	106 (89.1)	48 (70.6)	20 (40.0)	6 (11.1)	180 (61.9)		
	Total:	119 (100)	68 (100)	50 (100)	54 (100)	291 (100)		

*** $p < 0.001$. NILM—negative for intraepithelial lesion or malignancy; ASCUS—atypical squamous cells of unknown significance; LSIL—low-grade squamous intraepithelial lesions; HSIL—high-grade squamous intraepithelial lesions.

The analyses of the oncogenic activity of multiple HR HPV infections are presented by frequencies. The overall oncogenic activity, including both single and multiple HR HPV infections detected using the E6/E7 mRNA HR HPV test, increases with the degree of cervical lesion severity (60–100%). The oncogenic activity detected in single-genotype infections (20.0–85.7%) is higher compared to the oncogenic activity of multiple genotypes (0–40%) (Table 8).

Table 8. Analysis of the oncogenic activity of multiple infections of the most prevalent HR HPV.

Cytology	HR HPV DNA	f1	Multiple E6/E7 mRNA HR HPV	f2	Single E6/E7 mRNA HR HPV	f3	Multiple E6/E7 mRNA HR HPV * (%)	Single E6/E7 mRNA HR HPV ** (%)	Total Oncogenic Activity
NILM	16, 31	1	-	0	-	0	40.0	20.0	60.0
	16, 51	1	-	0	51	1			
	31, 33	2	31, 33	1	-	0			
	31, 51	1	31, 51	1	-	0			
	Total:	5	Total:	2	Total:	1			
ASCUS	16, 31	6	-	0	16	1	22.2	44.4	66.6
					31	3			
	16, 51	1	-	0	-	0			
	31, 33	1	31, 33	1	-	0			
	31, 51	1	31, 51	1	-	0			
	Total:	9	Total:	2	Total:	4			
LSIL	16, 31	3	-	0	16	1	0.0	83.3	83.3
					31	2			
	16, 31, 33	1	-	0	33	1			
	16, 51	2	-	0	51	1			
	Total:	6	Total:	0	Total:	5			
HSIL	16, 31	3	16, 31	1	16	1	14.3	85.7	100
					31	1			
	16, 33	2	-	0	16	1			
					33	1			
	16, 51	2	-	0	16	1			
					51	1			
	Total:	7	Total:	1	Total:	6			

* (f2/f1) × 100; ** (f3/f1) × 100; NILM—negative for an intraepithelial lesion or malignancy; ASCUS—atypical squamous cells of unknown significance; LSIL—low-grade squamous intraepithelial lesions; HSIL—high-grade squamous intraepithelial lesions.

3.5. Prevalence of E6/E7 mRNA HR HPV Expression According to Age

The results were categorized according to age categories (≤30, 31–44, ≥45 years) to analyze the prevalence of E6/E7 mRNA HPV in the specific age groups. The lowest percent of E6/E7 mRNA HR HPV 16 was detected in the younger group and the highest percent was detected in patients over 44 years. A statistically significant difference was observed in patients with E6/E7 mRNA HR HPV 16 expression (χ^2 test; $\chi^2 = 7.331$; $p = 0.026$), wherein individuals with positive E6/E7 mRNA HPV results were older than the others. The detection of E6/E7 mRNA HR HPV 31 and 33 decreases with the increasing age of the patient, while E6/E7 mRNA HR HPV 51 increases (Table 9).

Table 9. Analyses of E6/E7 mRNA HPVs according to age.

E6/E7 mRNA HR HPV		Age (years)			Total	χ^2	p
		≤30	31–44	≥45			
		n (%)	n (%)	n (%)	n (%)		
HPV 16	+	13 (19.1)	20 (32.3)	18 (42.9)	51 (29.7)	7.331	0.026 *
	−	55 (80.9)	42 (67.7)	24 (57.1)	121 (70.3)		
	Total:	68 (100)	62 (100)	42 (100)	172 (100)		
HPV 31	+	16 (23.5)	10 (16.1)	7 (16.7)	33 (19.2)	1.373	0.503
	−	52 (76.5)	52 (83.9)	35 (83.3)	139 (80.8)		
	Total:	68 (100)	62 (100)	42 (100)	172 (100)		
HPV 33	+	7 (10.3)	6 (9.7)	3 (7.1)	16 (9.3)	0.322	0.851
	−	61 (89.7)	56 (90.3)	39 (92.9)	156 (90.7)		
	Total:	68 (100)	62 (100)	42 (100)	172 (100)		
HPV 51	+	3 (4.4)	5 (8.1)	7 (16.7)	15 (8.7)	4.951	0.084
	−	65 (95.6)	57 (91.9)	35 (83.3)	157 (91.3)		
	Total:	68 (100)	62 (100)	42 (100)	172 (100)		

* $p < 0.05$.

3.6. Comparison of Tests for the Detection of HR HPV Genotypes and Their Oncogenic Activity

The comparison of tests for the detection of the most prevalent HR HPV genotypes and their oncogenic activity revealed that the presence of the HR HPV genotypes is higher than the presence of the oncogenic activity of the genotypes in younger women (≤30 years), similar in middle-aged women (31–44 years), and lower in women 45 years and older. The prevalence of oncogenic activity of the HPV genotypes increases with the severity of the cervical intraepithelial lesion. Compared to the prevalence of the examined HR HPV genotypes, the same parameter is lower in women with normal and undefined cytological findings, approximately the same in low-grade lesions, and significantly higher in high-grade lesions (Figure 4).

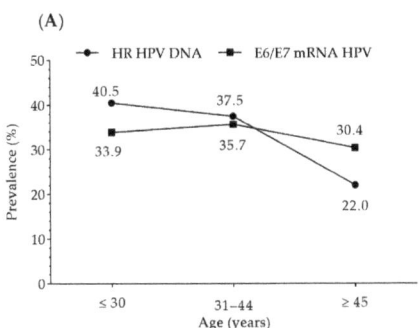
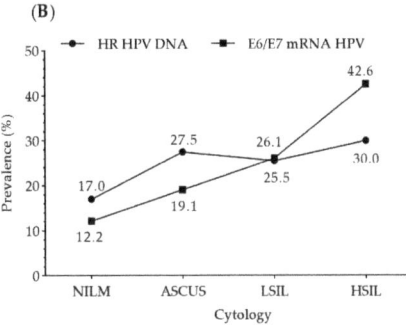

Figure 4. Prevalence of the most prevalent HR HPVs DNA and achieved oncogenic activity according to age (**A**) and cytology (**B**). NILM—negative for an intraepithelial lesion or malignancy; ASCUS—atypical squamous cells of unknown significance; LSIL—low-grade squamous intraepithelial lesions; HSIL—high-grade squamous intraepithelial lesions.

The calculated clinical characteristics of the DNA and E6/E7 mRNA HR HPV tests are shown in Table 10. The sensitivity and NPV of both tests were increased with the severity of the cervical intraepithelial lesion, with the HR HPV DNA test showing a statistically significantly higher level (67.6–98.2%). The specificity of the E6/E7 mRNA HR HPV test (89.1%) is statistically significantly higher than the HR HPV DNA test (75.6%). The PPV of the HR HPV DNA test is approximately the same for all types of cytological findings (60.3–64.6%), while for the mRNA HR HPV test, it increases with the degree of the cervical intraepithelial lesion (69.8–78.7%) and it is statistically significantly higher (Table 10).

Table 10. Clinical characteristics of HR HPV DNA and E6/E7 mRNA HPV tests.

Test	Cytology	Sensitivity (%)	CI (95%)	Specificity (%)	CI (95%)	PPV (%)	CI (95%)	NPV (%)	CI (95%)
HPV DNA	ASCUS	67.6 ***	55.2–78.5	75.6	66.9–83.0	61.3	49.4–72.4	80.4 *	71.8–87.3
	LSIL	88.0 **	75.7–95.5	75.6	66.9–83.0	60.3	48.1–71.6	93.8 *	86.9–97.7
	HSIL	98.2	90.1–100	75.6	66.9–83.0	64.6	53.3–74.9	98.9	94.0–100
E6/E7 mRNA HPV	ASCUS	29.4	19.0–41.7	89.1 **	82.0–94.0	60.6	42.1–77.1	68.8	60.9–76.0
	LSIL	60.0	45.2–73.6	89.1 **	82.0–94.0	69.8 ***	53.9–82.8	84.1	76.6–90.0
	HSIL	88.9	77.4–95.8	89.1 **	82.0–94.0	78.7 ***	66.3–88.1	94.6	88.7–98.0

* $p < 0.05$; ** $p < 0.005$; *** $p < 0.001$. CI (95%)—95% confidence interval; PPV—positive predictive value; NPV—negative predictive value; NILM—negative for intraepithelial lesion or malignancy; ASCUS—atypical squamous cells of unknown significance; LSIL—low-grade squamous intraepithelial lesions; HSIL—high-grade squamous intraepithelial lesions.

To quantify the diagnostic capabilities of the E6/E7 mRNA HPV test and evaluate its significance, an ROC curve was used to assess the assays for detecting HSIL. The area determined by the ROC curve (AUC) of E6/E7 mRNA HR HPV is 0.812 (CI (95%): 0.752–0.871), while the area under the ROC curve formed by the parameters of the HR HPV DNA test is 0.740 (CI (95%): 0.680–0.799) (Table 11, Figure 5).

Table 11. Performance of E6/E7 mRNA HR HPV and HR HPV DNA tests in HSIL.

HSIL	AUC ± SE	p	CI (95%)
E6/E7 mRNA HR HPV	0.812 ± 0.031	0.000 ***	0.752–0.871
HR HPV DNA	0.740 ± 0.030	0.000 ***	0.680–0.799

AUC—area under the ROC curve; SE—standard error; *** $p < 0.001$; CI (95%)—95% confidence intervals.

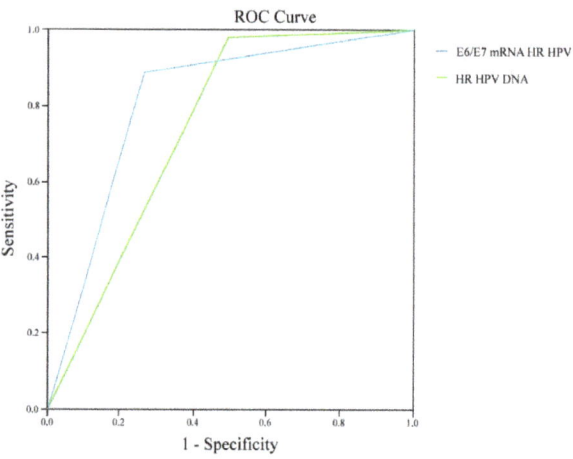

Figure 5. ROC curve of HR HPV and E6/E7 HR HPV tests in HSIL.

The relationships between the oncogenic activity of all of the tested HPVs and previously singled out HPV 16 vs. the cytological results were analyzed using Spearman's (ρ) correlation (Figure 6). There is a statistically significant positive moderate correlation between the presence of HPV 16 oncogenic activity and cytological status (Spearman's correlation; ρ = 0.494; $p < 0.001$) (Figure 6A). The oncogenic activity of the tested HPV genotypes is associated with a strong statistically significant positive correlation with the degree of cervical intraepithelial lesion severity (Spearman's correlation; ρ = 0.594; $p < 0.001$) (Figure 6B).

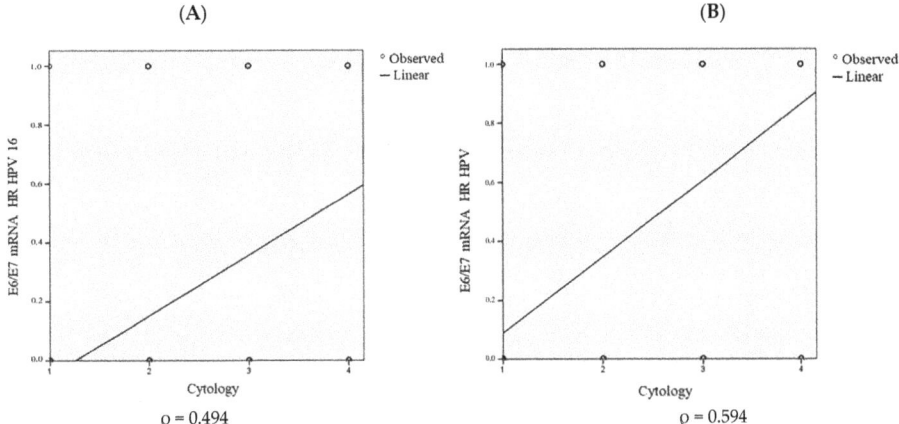

Figure 6. Correlation between the oncogenic activity of the HPV 16 genotype and cytology (**A**) and overall HPVs' oncogenic activity and cytology (**B**). NILM (1), ASCUS (2), LSIL (3), HSIL (4), and Spearman's correlation coefficient (ρ).

Univariate multinomial logistic regression examined the individual factors (the HR HPV DNA 16, the oncogenic activity of all of the tested HR HPVs, the oncogenic activity of the HR HPV 16 genotype, and the age category) that indicated an increased probability of developing HSIL (Supplementary Materials Tables S1–S4).

For the influence of HR HPV 16 on the probability of HSIL, a statistically significant predictive value was determined in the NILM and LSIL cytological groups. Patients with the confirmed presence of the HPV 16 genotype through a DNA test have a higher probability of being diagnosed with HSIL than NILM (3.8-fold), while they will have a 2.6-fold higher probability of being diagnosed with HSIL compared to the probability of being diagnosed with LSIL (Supplementary Materials Table S1).

The influence of the oncogenic activity of all tested of the HR HPV genotypes (E6/E7 mRNA HR HPVs) on diagnosing high-grade lesions of the cervical epithelium has a statistically significant prediction found in all cytological groups, NILM, ASCUS, and LSIL. If patients have confirmed indicators of oncogenic activity, they will have an almost seven-fold higher probability of being diagnosed with HSIL compared to the probability of being diagnosed with NILM. The same patients have a 19-fold higher probability of being diagnosed with HSIL compared to the probability of detecting ASCUS and a 5-fold higher probability of detecting HSIL compared to LSIL (Supplementary Materials Table S2).

E6/E7 mRNA HR HPV 16 is an indicator for diagnosing HSIL, and a statistically significant predictive value was determined for all types of cytological findings, NILM, ASCUS, and LSIL. In a patient with confirmed HPV 16 oncogenic transcripts, the probability of diagnosing HSIL is 50-fold higher than the probability of diagnosing NILM. Patients with a positive result of E6/E7 mRNAs HR HPV 16 are 12-fold more likely to be diagnosed with HSIL compared to the detection of ASCUS, while in patients with the same result, the probability of detection of HSIL is 6-fold higher than the probability of detection of LSIL (Supplementary Materials Table S3).

A statistically significant predictive value for the age category was determined in all cytological groups, NILM, ASCUS, and LSIL. The probability of detecting HSIL concerning normal results in HR-HPV-positive patients is 6.3-fold higher if they are ≥45 years of age than women under 30. A similar prediction for the detection of HSIL was shown concerning ASCUS (6.5-fold). Patients from the oldest age category have a 3.4-fold higher probability of detecting HSIL concerning LSIL than the youngest (Supplementary Materials Table S4).

The predictive model contains four independent variables: HR HPV DNA 16, E6/E7 mRNA HR HPVs, E6/E7 mRNA HR HPV 16, and age category. The HSIL lesion, as a representative of a high degree of cervical atypia, represented a dependent variable concerning all of the analyzed relevant factors. Multivariate logistic regression analysis was applied to all of the analyzed factors to construct a predictive model and named the most relevant predictors for the development of HSIL (Table 12).

Table 12. Analysis of the mutual influence of relevant factors for HSIL development.

	HSIL		OR	CI (95%)	p
NILM	HR HPV DNA 16	+ −	1.627 1.00 [a]	0.351–7.531	0.534
	E6/E7 mRNA HR HPV	+ −	3.989 1.00 [a]	0.843–18.882	0.081
	E6/E7 mRNA HR HPV 16	+ −	19.099 1.00 [a]	1.539–236.983	0.022 *
	Age (years)	≤30 31–44 ≥45	1.00 [a] 5.382 6.654	 1.360–21.296 1.665–26.598	 0.016 * 0.007 **
ASCUS	HR HPV DNA 16	+ −	0.957 1.00 [a]	0.230–3.988	0.952
	E6/E7 mRNA HR HPV	+ −	3.910 1.00 [a]	0.906–16.871	0.068
	E6/E7 mRNA HR HPV 16	+ −	6.384 1.00 [a]	1.215–33.545	0.029 *
	Age (years)	≤30 31–44 ≥45	1.00 [a] 1.401 8.738	 0.469–4.182 2.147–35.568	 0.546 0.002 **
LSIL	HR HPV DNA 16	+ −	1.009 1.00 [a]	0.243–4.192	0.990
	E6/E7 mRNA HR HPV	+ −	1.636 1.00 [a]	0.377–7.102	0.511
	E6/E7 mRNA HR HPV 16	+ −	5.099 1.00 [a]	1.091–23.832	0.038 *
	Age (years)	≤30 31–44 ≥45	1.00 [a] 1.362 3.719	 0.464–3.992 1.161–11.920	 0.574 0.027 *

OR—Odds ratio; [a]—reference; CI (95%)—95% confidence interval; * $p < 0.05$; ** $p < 0.01$; NILM–negative for intraepithelial lesion or malignancy; ASCUS–atypical squamous cells of unknown significance; LSIL–low-grade squamous intraepithelial lesions; HSIL–high-grade squamous intraepithelial lesions.

Analyzing the mutual influence of the examined relevant factors for diagnosing HSIL compared to the probability of diagnosing a normal cytological finding, the strongest statistically significant predictor was determined to be the oncogenic activity of the HPV 16 genotype. If it is detected, the probability of diagnosing HSIL concerning the probability of diagnosing normal results increases 19-fold (OR = 19.10; CI (95%): 1.54–236.98;

$p = 0.022$). A statistically significant but almost three-fold weaker predictor for the detection of HSIL compared to NILM is the patient belonging to the oldest age category (OR = 6.65; CI (95%): 1.66–26.60; $p = 0.007$), while female patients from the age category 31–44 years have a slightly lower statistically significant probability (OR = 5.38; CI (95%): 1.36–21.30; $p = 0.016$) for the detection of the same lesion. The age category was determined as the strongest statistically significant predictor by analyzing the mutual influence of relevant factors for diagnosing HSIL concerning the probability of detecting ASCUS. HR HPV DNA-positive patients belonging to the oldest age category ($\geq$45 years) have an 8.7-fold higher probability of being diagnosed with HSIL compared to the probability of being diagnosed with ASCUS compared to patients belonging to the younger age category (OR = 8.74; CI (95%): 2.15–35.57; $p = 0.002$). Female patients with the proven oncogenic activity of HPV 16 have a probability of detecting HSIL 6.4-fold higher compared to the probability of being diagnosed with ASCUS (OR = 6.38; CI (95%): 1.22–33.54; $p = 0.029$). By analyzing the mutual influence of relevant factors for diagnosing HSIL concerning the probability of detection of LSIL, the strongest statistically significant predictor was determined to be the oncogenic activity of HPV 16 (OR = 5.10; CI (95%): 1.09–23.83; $p = 0.038$), while weaker statistically significant predictability is shown by the patient's belonging to a specific age category. Female patients belonging to the oldest age category ($\geq$45 years) have a 3.7-fold greater probability of detecting an HSIL change compared to the detection of LSIL compared to the younger age category ($\leq$30 years) (OR = 3.72; CI (95 %): 1.16–11.92; $p = 0.027$) (Table 12).

4. Discussion

Persistent infection caused by HR HPV is the leading risk factor for developing cervical intraepithelial lesions and cervical cancer (reviewed in [20]). Many countries have introduced screening programs based on the cytomorphological examination of cervical samples using the PAP test during the last 60 years to reduce the morbidity and mortality caused by cervical cancer. However, this procedure has shown less than optimal sensitivity (50%) and high inter- and intra-individual variability [21,22]. HPV DNA detection and genotyping provide an efficient screening method and enable risk stratification. However, just proving the presence of the HPV genome in a cervical epithelium does not provide insight into the type of infection. It does not answer whether there is a transient or persistent infection in which the virus is actively multiplying and in which there is a high risk of cancer developing (reviewed in [23]). It was established that cervical carcinogenesis is strongly associated with the HPV-caused infection in which the transcription of E6 and E7 HR HPV oncogenes occurs, with the consequent increase of their mRNA and protein levels. For this reason, the detection of E6 and E7 mRNA of HR HPVs can serve as a promising biomarker of their persistence and oncogenic activity (reviewed in [23]), which could enable a better assessment of the progression to high-grade cervical intraepithelial lesions and, in this regard, significantly influence the algorithm for monitoring patients (reviewed in [18,23,24]).

In our study, 365 female patient samples from Serbia were tested for the twelve HR HPV genotypes. It should be emphasized that the study has limitations. Used HPV tests are non-validated according to European Guidelines for use in primary screening (Meijer HPV test criteria) or according to the VALidation of HPV GENoyping Tests (VALGENT) protocols [25]. The commercial molecular HPV test was chosen for research according to Serbia's general requirements for molecular diagnostics and the limited research expenses. From the total number of tested samples, 246 (67.4%) samples were positive for at least one of the 12 tested HR genotypes. These results agree with previous studies in the same area and European countries, where a high prevalence of HPV was registered. Studies in Serbia have reported that the presence of HR HPV infections range from 50% to 79% of women [26,27]. In the countries of our region, such as Croatia, a similar prevalence was shown (59%) [28] and in Bulgaria (61%) [29], while a slightly lower prevalence was registered in Italy (53%) [30]. Contrarily, a low prevalence of HPV infection was registered in Western and North European countries. Some of them are Great Britain (20.6%), Sweden (9.7%), and the Netherlands (3.8%) [7].

HPV genotype 16 (38%) emerged as the most frequently detected genotype in the study group, in concordance with previous reports [26,27]. The presence of HPV 16 is more often present (76%) in high-grade lesions compared to lower-grade lesions of the cervical epithelium. Studies on the HPV 16 genotype's prevalence concerning cytological findings confirm these results (reviewed in [6]). The following frequencies also represented the Alpha-9 genotype, HPV 31 (17%) and HPV 33 (9%). A meta-analysis study on five continents shows that HPV 31 is especially frequent in Europe [31]. The results of this research indicate that the frequency of the HPV 31 genotype statistically significantly decreases with the progression of the intraepithelial lesion. The decreasing trend of the same genotype's presence according to the degree of severity of the cytological lesion, more precisely, a lower prevalence in cancers compared to precancerous lesions, is observed in research from other studies [32–34]. Like HPV 31, a prevalence decrease of HPV 33 in HSIL compared to normal cytology was also registered in this research. Globally, HPV 33 ranks fourth in frequency and is responsible for 4.2% of all registered cervical cancers [6]. The surprising fact is a markedly high prevalence (9%) of the Alpha-5 genotype HPV 51 in our research. In the context of the causative agents of cervical cancer, HPV 51 is not included in the top ten most frequent HPV genotypes registered worldwide [6]. However, the detection of this genotype within this research, as well as previous studies from our region [26] and certain European countries [35–41], places it among the first four most prevalent genotypes detected in precancerous lesions of the cervix. Since HPV vaccines do not protect against all oncogenic HPVs, such as HPV 51, a complete understanding of its oncogenic activity is particularly significant [42]. The remaining tested genotypes (HR HPV 52, 56, 45, 18, 59, 58, 39, and 35) were present in a low percentage which is in concordance with previous reports [26]. Although HPV 18 is considered to be responsible for 15% of invasive cervical cancers, it is essential to note that its prevalence is similar to some studies from neighboring countries [29,43,44]; we found that in our area, HPV 18 was present at a lower percentage. Its frequency (3.6%) was 10-fold lower than that of HPV 16 (Figure 1). The HPV vaccine was introduced in over half of the WHO member countries in 2020 [5]. There is scientific data from numerous countries that have implemented HPV vaccines in their routine immunization programs on decreasing the burden of cervical HPV infections and precancers [45]. According to our data, using the nine-valent vaccine could prevent more than 80% of the cervical precancerous lesions identified in this study.

The presence of HR HPVs determined further examination of their oncogenic potential. In our study, the expression of E6/E7 mRNA HR HPV was identified in 67% of the HPV-positive samples (Table 6). The percentage of expression of the E6 and E7 HPV-examined HR HPVs is proportional to the degree of severity of the cervical lesion (Table 7). It can be observed that approximately every tenth HPV-infected woman (11%) with normal cytological findings is infected with an oncogenically expressed HPV. At the same time, in HSIL, this relationship is the opposite. Namely, the absence of indicators of HPV oncogenic activity is detected in approximately every tenth woman with HSIL status (11.1%). An undoubted trend in E6/E7 mRNA HR HPV positivity with increasing cytology severity has been observed in the data of studies conducted in different regions of the world [46–50]. In agreement with the report of Argyri et al. (2013) and according to the mRNA test, E6/E7 expression was prevalent in 9.1% of women with normal cytology, similar to our study [51]. However, other previously published data indicated the prevalence of those transcripts in a lower proportion of women with normal cytology findings than our study (0%) [52].

In our study, HPV 16 constituted 29.7%, followed by genotype 31 (19.2%), genotype 33 (9.3%), and genotype 51 (8.7%). The results showed that approximately every second HPV 16 genotype is oncogenically expressed (48.6%). Our data agree with the results reported in other studies. Rossi et al. (2017) observed a positivity rate for E6/E7 mRNA HR HPV, ranging from 58% to 77% in HPV-DNA-positive women [50]. A study by Tüney et al. (2017) in Turkey registered 55.6% E6/E7 mRNA HR HPVs, where HPV genotype 16 constituted

57.8% [24]; similar to that, Bruno et al. (2018) found that the HPV 16 genotype was the most oncogenetically active [46]. As confirmed in this research, it is also stated by several other authors that the transcription product HPV 16 is most often detected, which indicates that the tendency of expression of the essential oncogenes of this genotype is significantly higher compared to the other examined genotypes [24,53,54], which gives it the status of the HPV with the most carcinogenic potential [55]. The oncogenic activity of HPV 31 was detected in approximately every fifth (19.2%) HPV-DNA-positive sample. Contrary to HPV 16, the opposite trend is observed with the degree of cervical lesion severity. It can be assumed that the negative transcriptional status of E6 and E7 oncogenes is more prevalent due to the presence of an episomal form of the virus or an established transcriptional control that enables the spontaneous elimination of infection. Within this research, the results of E6/E7 mRNA HPV 51 detection are approximately the same as those of HPV 33. The distribution of oncogenic activity of these two genotypes is approximately the same across cytological groups and remains at a low level (2.2–11.4%) (Table 7). Other studies have registered different percentage ranges of transcriptional detection of oncogenes of a particular genotype (HPV 33), from its absence [52] to complete expression of 100% [55]. The reason for those differences can be explained by the variations in their number in the total sample [55]. Furthermore, the total oncogenic activity increases with the degree of cervical lesion severity (60–100%). The oncogenic activity of individual genotypes (20–86%) is higher than that of multiple genotypes (0–40%) in the same type of lesion and increases with the degree of its severity (Table 8). These data are supported by the literature. Each of the detected genotypes is considered to have an independent mechanism of action in oncogenesis [56–59], which supports the hypothesis that different cells being infected with different viral genotypes rather than their intracellular coexistence is possible [60].

To analyze the oncogenic activity of the four most frequently diagnosed HR HPVs related to the age categories, a statistically significantly higher prevalence of positive E6/E7 mRNA HPV 16 findings was observed in the older age groups (Table 9). In agreement with this result, studies have shown that E6 and E7 mRNA HR HPV detection is significantly higher after 30 years [48,61]. The same result is supported by population-based cohort studies, which state that the majority of young women have an asymptomatic HPV infection which, thanks to the immune response, acquires transitory status [49,62].

The growing interest in molecular diagnostics methods has led various authors to compare the characteristics of the HPV DNA test with the mRNA test, evaluating the diagnostic accuracy in identifying high-grade cervical lesions. Our data showed that the specificity (89%) and PPV (70–79%) of the mRNA test are statistically significantly higher, while the same test has a statistically significantly lower sensitivity than the HPV DNA test. These results agree with the statements of different authors, who emphasized slightly lower values of the sensitivity of the mRNA test compared to the sensitivity of the HPV DNA test. At the same time, the specificity is expressed at a higher level [48,49] (reviewed in [63]). In contrast, others suggest that the sensitivity is similar and that its application would significantly improve the assay's specificity characteristics [49]. Studies evaluating the reliability of the mRNA assay showed heterogeneous findings (reviewed in [32]). The meta-analysis results indicated that the obtained sensitivity value ranged from 41% to 95%, while the registered specificity was 42–97% (reviewed in [64]). The observed difference is explained by the heterogeneous participation of cervical pathology [64] and methodological quality in different studies, which highlights the limitations in the general interpretation of these test characteristics [32]. Although the results are presented broadly, they maintain a unique trend and suggest that the mRNA test over the HPV DNA test improves specificity [64]. By comparing the clinical characteristics of the test, it can be concluded that the detection of E6 and E7 mRNA HR HPV compared to HPV DNA represents a much better marker for more accurate screening of high-grade cellular atypia of the cervix (reviewed in [32]), which make it an appropriate tool for the secondary screening of cervical cancer [47,64].

In our study, the results of the ROC curve analysis indicated that the probability of detecting HPV infection with the mRNA test (81%, AUC = 0.812) in patients with high-grade lesions is higher than the possibility of diagnosing them with the HPV DNA test (74%, AUC = 0.740). The obtained results are in line with the other studies emphasizing the potential usefulness of this test. Sun et al. (2021) also found higher AUC values for the mRNA assay compared to the DNA HPV (0.929 vs. 0.833) [65], while according to Yao et al. (2017), the clinically relevant portion of the AUC of mRNA was 0.721 [66].

According to the previously established degree of influence on diagnosing HSIL, relevant factors were selected in our research. Factors that represent an increased risk for more severe cervical changes were gradually examined (the HPV 16 genotype, the total oncogenic activity of all of the tested HPV genotypes, the HPV 16 oncogenic activity, and the age category of the patient).

Firstly, the HPV-DNA-16-positive results have a statistically significant predictive value for diagnosing HSIL (Table S1). In the same context, the study of Bruno et al. (2018) stated that the presence of the HPV 16 genotype was associated with a five-fold higher risk of developing a high-grade lesion compared to women with the presence of another HPV genotype [46]. Similarly, the data from a recent study indicate that type-specific HPV persistence predicted high-grade lesions, with HPV 16 being the most common type [67].

Secondly, the oncogenic activity of all of the tested HR HPVs has a statistically significant predictive value for diagnosing HSIL (Table S2). The obtained results support the statements related to the research on the importance of oncogenic activity, which show that the detection of E6 and E7 mRNA HR HPV could have a prognostic value in monitoring the development of carcinogenesis [68,69]. The results of the study by Fontecha et al. (2016) [55] showed that in the highest percentage of E6 and E7 mRNA HPV-positive women, the progression of the lesion is diagnosed over time (53%), followed by the persistence of abnormal cytological findings (42%), while regression was recorded in 10-fold lower cases (4%).

Furthermore, in patients with positive results of indicators of the oncogenic activity of HPV 16, a statistically significantly higher probability of diagnosing a high-grade lesion was determined in all types of cytological groups (Table S3). According to the previous insights into the published statements, one of the few prospective follow-up studies that dealt with the predictive value of E6 and E7 mRNA HPV 16 indicated that through the detection of this biomarker, it is possible to identify 87.5% of the HPV infections that progressed. In this case, the risk of progression of negative cytology and low-grade cervical lesions was 10-fold higher than that detected in mRNA-negative women during a follow-up period of 35 months [70]. This is supported by the results of Johansson et al. (2015), which indicated that the absence of E6/E7 mRNA HPV demonstrated a high negative predictive value for the future development of high-grade lesions of the cervix among HR-HPV-DNA-positive women with ASCUS and LSIL [68].

Within the results of this research, a statistically significant final model with all of the predictors was constructed, which shows the strength of the potential of the examined factors, that is, biomarkers for diagnosing precancerous lesions in women with HR HPV infection. Looking at each cytological group individually, two independent variables made a statistically significant contribution to the model and were thus named as the strongest predictors. These are the oncogenic activities of HR HPV 16 and the age category ($\geq$45 years). It is known that the presence of HPV infection is confirmed in all age categories. However, belonging to a particular age group is a determinant significantly associated with the risk of acquiring this infection, depicting the peak in prevalence, which generally takes place around 20–25 years of age. For lesions to progress to more severe forms of cervical disease, a period of 5–14 years is necessary, during which the infection persists and the process of oncogenesis takes place [71]; the results of this research confirm the stated findings. In the examined women, the age category ($\geq$45 years) is a statistically significant prognostic factor for diagnosing HSIL in all of the cytological groups (Tables 12 and S4). Loopik et al. (2020) [58] indicated that the risk of progression of an existing high-grade lesion increases with age, i.e., in women over 50, the risk of developing cervical cancer increases by seven fold. In addition, the risk of developing cervical abnormalities and the need to use an mRNA test in the diagnostic protocol of HPV-DNA-positive postmenopausal women with normal cytology is emphasized by Asciutto et al. (2020) [72].

5. Conclusions

In summary, this study describes the detection rates of the most common HR HPVs (16, 31, 33, and 51) and E6/E7 mRNA HR HPV expression in 365 Serbian women who showed normal and abnormal cytological findings. Those HR HPV genotypes are oncogenically active in more than half of the examined cases, and the detected oncogenic activity has predictive potential in diagnosing high-grade cervical intraepithelial lesions. According to the constructed predictive model, the oncogenic activity of HPV 16 and age are risk factors with the strongest predictive values for developing those lesions. Thus, our data indicate that mRNA testing may be more relevant than HPV DNA for assessing lesion grade and diagnosing and monitoring women at risk of progressive cervical disease. This way, the mRNA test as a tool for better risk stratification of HPV infection could overcome unnecessary examinations, increased costs, and patient anxiety. However, further follow-up studies are needed to determine the clinical utility of the mRNA HR HPV test.

Supplementary Materials: The following supporting information can be downloaded at: https://www.mdpi.com/article/10.3390/diagnostics13050917/s1. Figure S1: Dispersion of Ct values of E6/E7 mRNA HR HPVs. Table S1: Analysis of HR HPV DNA 16's influence on the diagnosis of HSIL; Table S2: Analysis of total E6/E7 mRNA HR HPV's influence on the diagnosis of HSIL; Table S3: Analysis of E6/E7 mRNA HR HPV 16's influence on the diagnosis of HSIL; Table S4: Analysis of the influence of age on the diagnosis of HSIL.

Author Contributions: Conceptualization, N.N., V.G. and V.P; methodology, N.N., N.S., A.M. and T.P.; validation, N.N., N.S. and B.B.; formal analysis, N.N., N.S., M.S. and B.B.; investigation, N.N., A.M., N.S. and B.B.; data curation, N.N., V.G., N.S., D.M. and M.S.; writing—original draft preparation, N.N., B.B. and V.P.; writing—review and editing, V.P., T.P. and A.M.; supervision, V.P. and A.M. All authors have read and agreed to the published version of the manuscript.

Funding: This research received no external funding.

Institutional Review Board Statement: The study was conducted in accordance with the Declaration of Helsinki and approved by the Committee for the Ethics of Clinical Trials on Humans of the Faculty of Medicine of the University of Novi Sad (number: 01-39/136/1, date 2 March 2017) and the Ethics Committee of the Institute of Public Health of Vojvodina (number: 01-252/3, date 13 February 2017).

Informed Consent Statement: All of the women provided written consent for the use of the biological specimens for research purposes.

Data Availability Statement: The data that support the findings of this study are available from the corresponding author upon reasonable request.

Acknowledgments: The authors are grateful to the personnel of the Department of Gynecology, Community Health Centre Novi Sad, Serbia, and the Oncology Institute of Vojvodina, Serbia, for their contribution to this study.

Conflicts of Interest: The authors declare no conflict of interest.

References

1. Araldi, R.P.; Muro, S.; Assaf, R.; De Carvalho, R.F.; Caldas, M.A.; de Carvalho, R.; de Souza, J.M.; Magnelli, R.F.; Grando, D.; Roperto, F.P.; et al. Papillomaviruses: A Systematic Review. *Genet. Mol. Biol.* **2017**, *21*, 1–21. [CrossRef] [PubMed]
2. Gheit, T. Mucosal and Cutaneous Human Papillomavirus Infections and Cancer Biology. *Front. Oncol.* **2019**, *9*, 355. [CrossRef] [PubMed]
3. Mehta, K.; Laimins, L. High-Risk Human Papillomaviruses and DNA Repair. In *Viruses and Human Cancer: From Basic Science to Clinical Prevention (Recent Results in Cancer Research)*; Wu, T.-C., Chang, M.-H., Jeang, K.-T., Eds.; Springer Nature: Cham, Switzerland, 2021; pp. 141–155. ISBN 9783030573614.

4. Sung, H.; Ferlay, J.; Siegel, R.L.; Laversanne, M.; Soerjomataram, I.; Jemal, A.; Bray, F. Global Cancer Statistics 2020: GLOBOCAN Estimates of Incidence and Mortality Worldwide for 36 Cancers in 185 Countries. *CA. Cancer J. Clin.* **2021**, *71*, 209–249. [CrossRef]
5. Rancic, N.K.; Miljkovic, P.M.; Deljanin, Z.M.; Marinkov-Zivkovic, E.M.; Stamenkovic, B.N.; Bojanovic, M.R.; Jovanovic, M.M.; Miljkovic, D.P.; Stankovic, S.M.; Otasevic, S.A. Knowledge about HPV Infection and the HPV Vaccine among Parents in Southeastern Serbia. *Medicina* **2022**, *58*, 1697. [CrossRef]
6. Bruni, L.; Albero, G.; Serrano, B.; Mena, M.; Collado, J.; Gómez, D.; Muñoz, J.; Bosch, F.; de Sanjosé, S. Human Papillomavirus and Related Diseases in Serbia. Available online: https://hpvcentre.net/statistics/reports/SRB.pdf (accessed on 22 January 2022).
7. Bruni, L.; Albero, G.; Serrano, B.; Mena, M.; Collado, J.; Gómez, D.; Muñoz, J.; Bosch, F.; de Sanjosé, S. Human Papillomavirus and Related Diseases in the World. Available online: https://hpvcentre.net/statistics/reports/XWX.pdf (accessed on 22 January 2022).
8. Rosenblum, H.G.; Lewis, R.M.; Gargano, J.W.; Querec, T.D.; Unger, E.R.; Markowitz, L.E. Declines in Prevalence of Human Papillomavirus Vaccine-Type Infection Among Females after Introduction of Vaccine—United States, 2003–2018. *MMWR Surveill. Summ.* **2021**, *70*, 415–420. [CrossRef]
9. Lee, L.Y.; Garland, S.M. Human Papillomavirus Vaccination: The Population Impact. *F1000Research* **2017**, *6*, 866. [CrossRef]
10. Bouvard, V.; Baan, R.; Straif, K.; Grosse, Y.; Secretan, B.; El Ghissassi, F.; Benbrahim-Tallaa, L.; Guha, N.; Freeman, C.; Galichet, L.; et al. A Review of Human Carcinogens–Part B: Biological Agents. *Lancet Oncol.* **2009**, *10*, 321–322. [CrossRef]
11. Egawa, N.; Doorbar, J. The Low-Risk Papillomaviruses. *Virus Res.* **2017**, *231*, 119–127. [CrossRef]
12. Wang, S.S.; Hildesheim, A. Chapter 5: Viral and Host Factors in Human Papillomavirus Persistence and Progression. *J. Natl. Cancer Inst. Monogr.* **2003**, *2003*, 35–40. [CrossRef]
13. McBride, A.A. Mechanisms and Strategies of Papillomavirus Replication. *Biol. Chem.* **2017**, *398*, 919–927. [CrossRef]
14. Williams, V.M.; Filippova, M.; Soto, U.; Duerksen-Hughes, P.J. HPV-DNA Integration and Carcinogenesis: Putative Roles for Inflammation and Oxidative Stress. *Future Virol.* **2011**, *6*, 45–57. [CrossRef]
15. Fernandes, J.V.; de Medeiros Fernandes, T.A.A. Human Papillomavirus: Biology and Pathogenesis. In *Human Papillomavirus and Related Diseases—From Bench to Bedside—A Clinical Perspective*; Broeck, D.D., Vanden, Eds.; InTech Europe: Rijeka, Croatia, 2012; pp. 3–40. ISBN 978-953-307-860-1.
16. Münger, K.; Howley, P.M. Human Papillomavirus Immortalization and Transformation Functions. *Virus Res.* **2002**, *89*, 213–228. [CrossRef] [PubMed]
17. Wentzensen, N.; Arbyn, M.; Berkhof, J.; Bower, M.; Canfell, K.; Einstein, M.; Farley, C.; Monsonego, J.; Franceschi, S. Eurogin 2016 Roadmap: How HPV Knowledge Is Changing Screening Practice. *Int. J. Cancer* **2017**, *140*, 2192–2200. [CrossRef] [PubMed]
18. Burger, E.A.; Kornør, H.; Klemp, M.; Lauvrak, V.; Kristiansen, I.S. HPV MRNA Tests for the Detection of Cervical Intraepithelial Neoplasia: A Systematic Review. *Gynecol. Oncol.* **2011**, *120*, 430–438. [CrossRef]
19. Lindh, M.; Görander, S.; Andersson, E.; Horal, P.; Mattsby-Balzer, I.; Ryd, W. Real-Time Taqman PCR Targeting 14 Human Papilloma Virus Types. *J. Clin. Virol.* **2007**, *40*, 321–324. [CrossRef] [PubMed]
20. Moscicki, A.B.; Ma, Y.; Wibbelsman, C.; Darragh, T.M.; Powers, A.; Farhat, S.; Shiboski, S. Rate of and Risks for Regression of Cervical Intraepithelial Neoplasia 2 in Adolescents and Young Women. *Obstet. Gynecol.* **2010**, *116*, 1373–1380. [CrossRef]
21. Boulet, G.A.V.; Horvath, C.A.J.; Berghmans, S.; Bogers, J. Human Papillomavirus in Cervical Cancer Screening: Important Role as Biomarker. *Cancer Epidemiol. Biomarkers Prev.* **2008**, *17*, 810–817. [CrossRef]
22. Wright, T.C. Cervical Cancer Screening in the 21st Century: Is It Time to Retire the Pap Smear? *Clin. Obstet. Gynecol.* **2007**, *50*, 313–323. [CrossRef]
23. Derbie, A.; Mekonnen, D.; Woldeamanuel, Y.; Van Ostade, X.; Abebe, T. HPV E6/E7 MRNA Test for the Detection of High Grade Cervical Intraepithelial Neoplasia (CIN2+): A Systematic Review. *Infect. Agent. Cancer* **2020**, *15*, 9. [CrossRef]
24. Tüney, İ.; Altay, A.; Ergünay, K.; Önder, S.Ç.; Usubütün, A.; Salman, M.C.; Bozdayi, G.; Karabulut, E.; Badur, O.S.; Yüce, K.; et al. Hpv Types and E6/E7 MRNA Expression in Cervical Samples from Turkish Women with Abnormal Cytology in Ankara, Turkey. *Turkish J. Med. Sci.* **2017**, *47*, 194–200. [CrossRef]
25. Poljak, M.; Oštrbenk Valenčak, A.; Gimpelj Domjanič, G.; Xu, L.; Arbyn, M. Commercially Available Molecular Tests for Human Papillomaviruses: A Global Overview. *Clin. Microbiol. Infect.* **2020**, *26*, 1144–1150. [CrossRef] [PubMed]
26. Kovacevic, G.; Nikolic, N.; Jovanovic-Galovic, A.; Hrnjakovic-Cvjetkovic, I.; Vuleta, D.; Patic, A.; Radovanov, J.; Milosevic, V. Frequency of Twelve Carcinogenic Human Papilloma Virus Types among Women from the South Backa Region, Vojvodina, Serbia. *Turkish J. Med. Sci.* **2016**, *46*, 97–104. [CrossRef] [PubMed]
27. Kovacevic, G.; Milosevic, V.; Nikolic, N.; Patic, A.; Dopudj, N.; Radovanov, J.; Cvjetkovic, I.H.; Petrovic, V.; Petrovic, M. The Prevalence of 30 HPV Genotypes Detected by EUROArray HPV in Cervical Samples among Unvaccinated Women from Vojvodina Province, Serbia. *PLoS ONE* **2021**, *16*, e0249134. [CrossRef] [PubMed]
28. Milutin-Gašperov, N.; Sabol, I.; Halec, G.; Matovina, M.; Grce, M. Retrospective Study of the Prevalence of High-Risk Human Papillomaviruses among Croatian Women. *Coll. Antropol.* **2007**, *31*, 89–96.
29. Grozdanov, P.; Zlatkov, V.; Ganchev, G.; Karagiosov, I.; Toncheva, D.; Galabov, A.S. HPV Prevalence and Type Distribution in Women with Normal or Abnormal Pap Smear in Bulgaria. *J. Med. Virol.* **2014**, *86*, 1905–1910. [CrossRef]
30. Schettino, M.T.; De Franciscis, P.; Schiattarella, A.; La Manna, V.; Della Gala, A.; Caprio, F.; Tammaro, C.; Ammaturo, F.P.; Guler, T.; Yenigün, E.H. Prevalence of HPV Genotypes in South Europe: Comparisons between an Italian and a Turkish Unvaccinated Population. *J. Environ. Public Health* **2019**, *2019*, 8769535. [CrossRef]

31. Bruni, L.; Diaz, M.; Castellsagué, X.; Ferrer, E.; Bosch, F.X.; De Sanjosé, S. Cervical Human Papillomavirus Prevalence in 5 Continents: Meta-Analysis of 1 Million Women with Normal Cytological Findings. *J. Infect. Dis.* **2010**, *202*, 1789–1799. [CrossRef]
32. Sabol, I.; Gašperov, N.M.; Matovina, M.; Božinovic, K.; Grubišic, G.; Fistonic, I.; Belci, D.; Alemany, L.; Džebro, S.; Dominis, M.; et al. Cervical HPV Type-Specific Pre-Vaccination Prevalence and Age Distribution in Croatia. *PLoS ONE* **2017**, *12*, e0180480. [CrossRef]
33. Guan, P.; Howell-Jones, R.; Li, N.; Bruni, L.; De Sanjosé, S.; Franceschi, S.; Clifford, G.M. Human Papillomavirus Types in 115,789 HPV-Positive Women: A Meta-Analysis from Cervical Infection to Cancer. *Int. J. Cancer* **2012**, *131*, 2349–2359. [CrossRef]
34. Karadža, M.; Lepej, S.Ž.; Planinić, A.; Grgić, I.; Ćorušić, A.; Planinić, P.; Ćorić, M.; Hošnjak, L.; Komloš, K.F.; Poljak, M.; et al. Distribution of Human Papillomavirus Genotypes in Women with High-Grade Cervical Intraepithelial Lesions and Cervical Carcinoma and Analysis of Human Papillomavirus-16 Genomic Variants. *Croat. Med. J.* **2021**, *62*, 68–79. [CrossRef]
35. Bowden, S.J.; Fiander, A.N.; Hibbitts, S. HPV 51: A Candidate for Type-Replacement Following Vaccination? *medRxiv* **2021**. [CrossRef]
36. Schmitt, M.; Depuydt, C.; Benoy, I.; Bogers, J.; Antoine, J.; Arbyn, M.; Pawlita, M. Prevalence and Viral Load of 51 Genital Human Papillomavirus Types and Three Subtypes. *Int. J. Cancer* **2013**, *132*, 2395–2403. [CrossRef]
37. Yuce, K.; Pinar, A.; Salman, M.C.; Alp, A.; Sayal, B.; Dogan, S.; Hascelik, G. Detection and Genotyping of Cervical HPV with Simultaneous Cervical Cytology in Turkish Women: A Hospital-Based Study. *Arch. Gynecol. Obstet.* **2012**, *286*, 203–208. [CrossRef]
38. Mollers, M.; Boot Hein, J.; Vriend Henrike, J.; King Audrey, J.; van den Broek Ingrid, V.F.; van Bergen Jan, E.A.M.; Brink Antoinette, A.T.P.; Wolffs Petra, F.G.; Hoebe Christian, J.P.A.; Meijer Chris, J.L.M.; et al. Prevalence, Incidence and Persistence of Genital HPV Infections in a Large Cohort of Sexually Active Young Women in the Netherlands. *Vaccine* **2013**, *31*, 394–401. [CrossRef] [PubMed]
39. Piana, A.; Sotgiu, G.; Cocuzza, C.; Musumeci, R.; Marras, V.; Pischedda, S.; Deidda, S.; Muresu, E.; Castiglia, P. High HPV-51 Prevalence in Invasive Cervical Cancers: Results of a Pre-Immunization Survey in North Sardinia, Italy. *PLoS ONE* **2013**, *8*, 6–11. [CrossRef]
40. Dalgo Aguilar, P.; Loján González, C.; Córdova Rodríguez, A.; Acurio Paéz, K.; Arévalo, A.P.; Bobokova, J. Prevalence of High-Risk Genotypes of Human Papillomavirus: Women Diagnosed with Premalignant and Malignant Pap Smear Tests in Southern Ecuador. *Infect. Dis. Obstet. Gynecol.* **2017**, *2017*, 12–14. [CrossRef] [PubMed]
41. Tang, S.; Liao, Y.; Hu, Y.; Shen, H.; Wan, Y.; Wu, Y. HPV Prevalence and Genotype Distribution Among Women From Hengyang District of Hunan Province, China. *Front. Public Heal.* **2021**, *9*, 1346. [CrossRef] [PubMed]
42. Sladič, M.; Taneska, P.; Cvjetićanin, B.; Velikonja, M.; Smrkolj, V.; Smrkolj, Š. Cervical Intraepithelial Neoplasia Grade 3 in a HPV-Vaccinated Patient: A Case Report. *Medicina* **2022**, *58*, 339. [CrossRef] [PubMed]
43. Učakar, V.; Poljak, M.; Klavs, I. Pre-Vaccination Prevalence and Distribution of High-Risk Human Papillomavirus (HPV) Types in Slovenian Women: A Cervical Cancer Screening Based Study. *Vaccine* **2012**, *30*, 116–120. [CrossRef]
44. Ursu, R.; Onofriescu, M.; Nemescu, D.; Iancu, L.S. HPV Prevalence and Type Distribution in Women with or without Cervical Lesions in the Northeast Region of Romania. *Virol. J.* **2011**, *8*, 558. [CrossRef]
45. Oliveira, C.R.; Niccolai, L.M. Monitoring HPV Vaccine Impact on Cervical Disease: Status and Future Directions for the Era of Cervical Cancer Elimination. *Prev. Med.* **2021**, *144*, 106363. [CrossRef] [PubMed]
46. Bruno, M.T.; Ferrara, M.; Fava, V.; Rapisarda, A.; Coco, A. HPV Genotype Determination and E6/E7 MRNA Detection for Management of HPV Positive Women. *Virol. J.* **2018**, *15*, 52. [CrossRef] [PubMed]
47. Pan, D.; Zhang, C.Q.; Liang, Q.L.; Hong, X.C. An Efficient Method That Combines the ThinPrep Cytologic Test with E6/E7 MRNA Testing for Cervical Cancer Screening. *Cancer Manag. Res.* **2019**, *11*, 4773–4780. [CrossRef] [PubMed]
48. Pruski, D.; Millert-Kalinska, S.; Lewek, A.; Kedzia, W. Sensitivity and Specificity of HR HPV E6/E7 MRNA Test in Detecting Cervical Squamous Intraepithelial Lesion and Cervical Cancer. *Ginekol. Pol.* **2019**, *90*, 66–71. [CrossRef] [PubMed]
49. Wang, J.; Xu, X. The Diagnostic Value of HPV E6/E7 MRNA Test in Young Women with Cervical Squamous Intraepithelial Lesion: A Retrospective Analysis. Research Square. *Res. Sq.* **2021**, *4*, 1–14. [CrossRef]
50. Rossi, P.G.; Bisanzi, S.; Allia, E.; Mongia, A.; Carozzi, F.; Gillio-Tos, A.; De Marco, L.; Ronco, G.; Gustinucci, D.; Del Mistro, A.; et al. Determinants of Viral Oncogene E6-E7 MRNA Overexpression in a Population- Based Large Sample of Women Infected by High-Risk Human Papillomavirus Types. *J. Clin. Microbiol.* **2017**, *55*, 1056–1065. [CrossRef]
51. Argyri, E.; Tsimplaki, E.; Daskalopoulou, D.; Stravopodis, D.J.; Kouikoglou, O.; Terzakis, E.; Panotopoulou, E. E6/E7 MRNA Expression of High-Risk HPV Types in 849 Greek Women. *Anticancer Res.* **2013**, *33*, 4007–4012.
52. Baron, C.; Henry, M.; Tamalet, C.; Villeret, J.; Richet, H.; Carcopino, X. Relationship Between HPV 16, 18, 31, 33, 45 DNA Detection and Quantitation and E6/E7 MRNA Detection Among a Series of Cervical Specimens With Various Degrees of Histological Lesions. *J. Med. Virol.* **2015**, *87*, 1389–1396. [CrossRef]
53. Dabeski, D.; Duvlis, S.; Basheska, N.; Antovska, V.; Stojovski, M.; Trajanova, M.; Dimitrov, G.; Dabeski, A.; Gureva-Gjorgievska, N. Comparison Between HPV DNA Testing and HPV E6/E7 MRNA Testing in Women with Squamous Cell Abnormalities of the Uterine Cervix. *Prilozi* **2019**, *40*, 51–58. [CrossRef]
54. Salimović-Bešić, I.; Tomić-Čiča, A.; Smailji, A.; Hukić, M. Comparison of the Detection of HPV-16, 18, 31, 33, and 45 by Type-Specific DNA- and E6/E7 MRNA-Based Assays of HPV DNA Positive Women with Abnormal Pap Smears. *J. Virol. Methods* **2013**, *194*, 222–228. [CrossRef]
55. Fontecha, N.; Basaras, M.; Hernáez, S.; Andía, D.; Cisterna, R. Assessment of Human Papillomavirus E6/E7 Oncogene Expression as Cervical Disease Biomarker. *BMC Cancer* **2016**, *16*, 852. [CrossRef]

56. Quint, W.; Jenkins, D.; Molijn, A.; Struijk, L.; Van De Sandt, M.; Doorbar, J.; Mols, J.; Van Hoof, C.; Hardt, K.; Struyf, F.; et al. One Virus, One Lesion—Individual Components of CIN Lesions Contain a Specific HPV Type. *J. Pathol.* **2012**, *227*, 62–71. [CrossRef] [PubMed]
57. van den Heuvel, C.N.A.M.; Loopik, D.L.; Ebisch, R.M.F.; Elmelik, D.; Andralojc, K.M.; Huynen, M.; Bulten, J.; Bekkers, R.L.M.; Massuger, L.F.A.G.; Melchers, W.J.G.; et al. RNA-Based High-Risk HPV Genotyping and Identification of High-Risk HPV Transcriptional Activity in Cervical Tissues. *Mod. Pathol.* **2020**, *33*, 748–757. [CrossRef] [PubMed]
58. Loopik, D.L.; IntHout, J.; Ebisch, R.M.F.; Melchers, W.J.G.; Massuger, L.F.A.G.; Siebers, A.G.; Bekkers, R.L.M. The Risk of Cervical Cancer after Cervical Intraepithelial Neoplasia Grade 3: A Population-Based Cohort Study with 80,442 Women. *Gynecol. Oncol.* **2020**, *157*, 195–201. [CrossRef] [PubMed]
59. Bruno, M.T.; Scalia, G.; Cassaro, N.; Boemi, S. Multiple HPV 16 Infection with Two Strains: A Possible Marker of Neoplastic Progression. *BMC Cancer* **2020**, *20*, 444. [CrossRef] [PubMed]
60. Soto-De Leon, S.; Camargo, M.; Sanchez, R.; Munoz, M.; Perez-Prados, A.; Purroy, A.; Patarroyo, M.E.; Patarroyo, M.A. Distribution Patterns of Infection with Multiple Types of Human Papillomaviruses and Their Association with Risk Factors. *PLoS ONE* **2011**, *6*, e14705. [CrossRef]
61. Wang, H.Y.; Lee, D.; Park, S.; Kim, G.; Kim, S.; Han, L.; Yubo, R.; Li, Y.; Park, K.H.; Lee, H. Diagnostic Performance of HPV E6/E7 MRNA and HPV DNA Assays for the Detection and Screening of Oncogenic Human Papillomavirus Infection among Woman with Cervical Lesions in China. *Asian Pacific J. Cancer Prev.* **2015**, *16*, 7633–7640. [CrossRef]
62. Mittal, S.; Basu, P.; Muwonge, R.; Banerjee, D.; Ghosh, I.; Sengupta, M.M.; Das, P.; Dey, P.; Mandal, R.; Panda, C.; et al. Risk of High-Grade Precancerous Lesions and Invasive Cancers in High-Risk HPV-Positive Women with Normal Cervix or CIN 1 at Baseline—A Population-Based Cohort Study. *Int. J. Cancer* **2017**, *140*, 1850–1859. [CrossRef]
63. Zorzi, M.; Del Mistro, A.; Giorgi Rossi, P.; Laurino, L.; Battagello, J.; Lorio, M.; Soldà, M.; Martinotti Gabellotti, E.; Maran, M.; Dal Cin, A.; et al. Risk of CIN2 or More Severe Lesions after Negative HPV-MRNA E6/E7 Overexpression Assay and after Negative HPV-DNA Test: Concurrent Cohorts with a 5-Year Follow-Up. *Int. J. Cancer* **2020**, *146*, 3114–3123. [CrossRef]
64. Macedo, A.C.L.; Gonçalves, J.C.N.; Bavaresco, D.V.; Grande, A.J.; Chiaramonte Silva, N.; Rosa, M.I. Accuracy of MRNA HPV Tests for Triage of Precursor Lesions and Cervical Cancer: A Systematic Review and Meta-Analysis. *J. Oncol.* **2019**, *2019*, 6935030. [CrossRef]
65. Sun, J.; Yue, Y.; Li, R.; Sun, Q.; Hu, C.; Ge, X.; Guan, Q. Detection of HPV E6/E7 MRNA in the Diagnosis of Cervical Cancer and Precancerous Lesions after Kidney Transplantation. *Am. J. Transl. Res.* **2021**, *13*, 7312–7317. [PubMed]
66. Yao, Y.L.; Tian, Q.F.; Cheng, B.; Cheng, Y.F.; Ye, J.; Lu, W.G. Human Papillomavirus (HPV) E6/E7 MRNA Detection in Cervical Exfoliated Cells: A Potential Triage for HPV-Positive Women. *J. Zhejiang Univ. Sci. B* **2017**, *18*, 256–262. [CrossRef] [PubMed]
67. Sahlgren, H.; Elfström, K.M.; Lamin, H.; Carlsten-Thor, A.; Eklund, C.; Dillner, J.; Elfgren, K. Colposcopic and Histopathologic Evaluation of Women with HPV Persistence Exiting an Organized Screening Program. *Am. J. Obstet. Gynecol.* **2020**, *222*, 253.e1–253.e8. [CrossRef] [PubMed]
68. Johansson, H.; Bjelkenkrantz, K.; Darlin, L.; Dilllner, J.; Forslund, O. Presence of High-Risk HPV MRNA in Relation to Future High-Grade Lesions among High-Risk HPV DNA Positive Women with Minor Cytological Abnormalities. *PLoS ONE* **2015**, *10*, e0124460. [CrossRef] [PubMed]
69. Liu, S.; Minaguchi, T.; Lachkar, B.; Zhang, S.; Xu, C.; Tenjimbayashi, Y.; Shikama, A.; Tasaka, N.; Akiyama, A.; Sakurai, M.; et al. Separate Analysis of Human Papillomavirus E6 and E7 Messenger RNAs to Predict Cervical Neoplasia Progression. *PLoS ONE* **2018**, *13*, 6–17. [CrossRef] [PubMed]
70. Martí, P.; Marimón, L.; Glickman, A.; Henere, C.; Saco, A.; Rakislova, N.; Torné, A.; Ordi, J.; Del Pino, M. Usefulness of E7 Mrna in Hpv16-Positive Women to Predict the Risk of Progression to Hsil/Cin^{2+}. *Diagnostics* **2021**, *11*, 1634. [CrossRef]
71. de Sanjosé, S.; Brotons, M.; Pavón, M.A. The Natural History of Human Papillomavirus Infection. *Best Pract. Res. Clin. Obstet. Gynaecol.* **2018**, *47*, 2–13. [CrossRef]
72. Asciutto, K.C.; Borgfeldt, C.; Forslund, O. 14-Type HPV MRNA Test in Triage of HPV DNA-Positive Postmenopausal Women with Normal Cytology. *BMC Cancer* **2020**, *20*, 1025. [CrossRef]

Disclaimer/Publisher's Note: The statements, opinions and data contained in all publications are solely those of the individual author(s) and contributor(s) and not of MDPI and/or the editor(s). MDPI and/or the editor(s) disclaim responsibility for any injury to people or property resulting from any ideas, methods, instructions or products referred to in the content.

HPV Tests Comparison in the Detection and Follow-Up after Surgical Treatment of CIN2+ Lesions

Fabio Bottari [1,2,*], Anna Daniela Iacobone [2,3], Davide Radice [4], Eleonora Petra Preti [3], Mario Preti [5], Dorella Franchi [3], Sara Boveri [6], Maria Teresa Sandri [7] and Rita Passerini [1]

1. Division of Laboratory Medicine, European Institute of Oncology IRCCS, 20139 Milan, Italy
2. Department of Biomedical Sciences, University of Sassari, 07100 Sassari, Italy
3. Preventive Gynecology Unit, European Institute of Oncology IRCCS, 20139 Milan, Italy
4. Division of Epidemiology and Biostatistics, European Institute of Oncology IRCCS, 20139 Milan, Italy
5. Department of Surgical Sciences, University of Torino, 10124 Torino, Italy
6. Scientific Directorate, IRCCS Policlinico San Donato, 20097 San Donato, Italy
7. Bianalisi Laboratory, Carate Brianza, 20841 Carate Brianza, Italy
* Correspondence: fabio.bottari@ieo.it; Fax: +39-0294379237

Abstract: Background: HPV tests differ for technology, targets, and information on genotyping of high risk (HR) HPV. In this study, we evaluated the performance of 6 HPV DNA tests and one mRNA test in the detection of cervical intraepithelial lesions (CIN) and as a test-of-cure in the follow-up after surgical conservative treatment. Methods: One hundred seventy-two women referred to the European Institute of Oncology, Milan, for surgical treatment of pre-neoplastic cervical lesions, were enrolled in this study (IEO S544) from January 2011 to June 2015. For all women, a cervical sample was taken before treatment (baseline) and at the first follow-up visit (range 3 to 9 months): on these samples Qiagen Hybrid Capture 2 (HC2), Roche Linear Array HPV Test (Linear Array), Roche Cobas 4800 HPV test (Cobas), Abbott RealTime High Risk HPV test (RT), BD Onclarity HPV assay (Onclarity), Seegene Anyplex II HPV HR Detection (Anyplex), and Hologic Aptima HPV Assay (Aptima) histology and cytology were performed at baseline, and the same tests and cytology were performed at follow-up. Results: At baseline 158/172 (92%), histologies were CIN2+, and 150/172 (87%) women were recruited at follow-up. Assuming HC2 as a comparator, the concordance of HPV tests ranges from 91% to 95% at baseline and from 76% to 100% at follow-up (PABAK ranging from 0.81 to 0.90 at baseline and PABAK ranging from 0.53 to 1 at follow-up). All HPV showed a very good sensitivity in CIN2+ detection at baseline, more than 92%, and a very good specificity at follow-up, more than 89%. Conclusions: HPV tests showed a good concordance with HC2 and a very good and comparable sensitivity in CIN2+ detection. Hence, an HPV test represents a valid option as test-of-cure in order to monitor patients treated for CIN2+ lesions during follow-up.

Keywords: HPV; cervical intraepithelial neoplasia; follow-up; real time PCR; genotyping; concordance

1. Introduction

High-risk (HR) human papillomavirus (HPV) persistent infection has been widely recognized as the main causal risk factor for the development of cervical intraepithelial neoplasia (CIN) and progression to cervical cancer [1,2].

Nowadays, an increasing number of HPV tests, which differ for technology, targets, and genotyping [3], is available for HPV detection. Unfortunately, few of these have been studied and even less validated for screening [4].

The threshold of validated HR-HPV tests is CIN2+ detection because this is the clinical target for screening. However, HPV tests have been employed not only for screening, but also as a triage test and test-of-cure for follow-up of women treated for precancerous lesions.

If many studies are not present in previous literature regarding HPV tests in the screening setting, even less is known about their use in the follow-up after surgical treatment [5]. The objectives of post-treatment follow-up testing are to confirm that treatment was effective, to identify recurrence early, and to reassure women. Therefore, looking for the persistence of the same HPV genotype identified at baseline would be helpful for stratifying the risk of CIN recurrence, also known as "treatment failure" [6,7].

The aim of the present study is to evaluate and to compare the performance of six HPV DNA tests and one HPV mRNA test from liquid-based cervical cytology samples, for the detection of CIN2+ at baseline and as "test-of-cure" during post-treatment follow-up. The secondary objective of the study is to determine the sensitivity and the specificity of different HPV tests in the settings of screening and post-treatment follow-up.

2. Patients and Methods

2.1. Population

All women aged between 25–61 years, scheduled to be conservatively treated for CIN2+ at the European Institute of Oncology (IEO), Milan, from January 2011 to June 2015, were enrolled. "Conservative treatment" included excisional procedures, such as Loop Electro-Excision Procedure (LEEP) and laser conization, and ablative procedures, such as laser vaporization, in cases of ectocervical lesion and no evidence of ICC at pre-treatment colposcopic-guided biopsies. The study was approved by the Institutional Ethical Committee (IEO S544 study), and informed consent was obtained from all women at enrollment. A ThinPrep PreservCyt (Hologic, Inc. Bedford, MA, USA) cervical sample was collected in all patients before treatment and at the first follow-up visit planned at 6 ± 3 months after surgical treatment, in order to perform cytology, Qiagen Hybrid Capture 2 (HC2) and Roche Linear Array HPV Test (Linear Array). Roche Cobas® 4800 HPV Test (Cobas), Abbott RealTime High Risk HPV (RT), BD Onclarity HPV Assay (Onclarity), and Seegene Anyplex II HPV HR (Anyplex) test were carried out on a left-over aliquot. Hologic APTIMA mRNA assay (Aptima) has been performed placing an aliquot of Thin Prep sample in the Aptima storage liquid upon arrival in the laboratory. The results of histology at baseline and at relapse, when occurred, were available for all patients. Principal characteristics of all HPV tests are detailed in Table 1.

Table 1. HPV test features.

Test	Company	Method	HPV TARGET	TARGET Region	16	18	31	33	35	39	45	51	52	56	58	59	66	68	Validation References
Hybrid Capture II	Qiagen	Hybridization and signal amplification	DNA	Whole genome	•	•	•	•	•	•	•	•	•	•	•	•	•	•	Gold standard, NTCC study
Linear Array HPV Test	Roche	PCR and oligonucleotide hybridization	DNA	L1	•	•	•	•	•	•	•	•	•	•	•	•	•	•	[8]
Cobas 4800 HPV Test	Roche	Real Time PCR	DNA	L1	•	•	•	•	•	•	•	•	•	•	•	•	•	•	[9], ATHENA study
RealTime High Risk HPV Test	Abbott	Real Time PCR	DNA	L1	•	•	•	•	•	•	•	•	•	•	•	•	•	•	[10]
Onclarity HPV Assay	BD	Real Time PCR	DNA	E6 E7	•	•	•	•	•	•	•	•	•	•	•	•	•	•	[11]
Anyplex II HPV HR Test	Seegene	TOCE Real Time PCR	DNA	L1	•	•	•	•	•	•	•	•	•	•	•	•	•	•	[12]
APTIMA mRNA assay	Hologic	Transcription-Mediated Amplification	mRNA	E6 E7	•	•	•	•	•	•	•	•	•	•	•	•	•	•	[13]
in pool																			
in small pool																			

2.2. Hybrid Capture 2

Qiagen HC2 test is a sandwich capture molecular hybridization assay: it is a signal amplification detection method based on chemiluminescence that detects 13 HR HPV types: HPV 16, 18, 31, 33, 35, 39, 45, 51, 52, 56, 58, 59, and 68. The DNA:RNA hybrids are captured on a microplate, and the emitted light is measured in a luminometer as relative light units (RLU). Samples were considered as positive if the ratio RLU/cut-off was >1.0 (equivalent to 5000 copies/reaction). All samples with RLU between 1 and 2.5 should be retested, as requested in package insert instructions.

2.3. Linear Array

The Roche Diagnostics Linear Array test uses biotinylated PGMY09/11 consensus primers to amplify a 450-bp region of the L1 gene. It is capable of detecting 37 HPV genotypes: HPV6, 11, 16, 18, 26, 31, 33, 35, 39, 40, 42, 45, 51, 52, 53, 54, 55, 56, 58, 59, 61, 62, 64, 66, 67, 68, 69, 70, 71, 72, 73 (MM9), 81, 82 (MM4), 83 (MM7), 84 (MM8), IS39 e CP6108. The denatured PCR products were then hybridized to an array strip containing immobilized oligonucleotide probes. The results were visually interpreted by using the provided reference guide according to manufacturer's protocol by two independent operators, and the results were compared to reach the final one.

2.4. Cobas 4800 HPV Test

Cobas is a real-time PCR-based test able to detect HR-HPV genotypes: HPV 16 and 18 are reported as single genotypes, as well as a group of 12 other HR-HPV types (31, 33, 35, 39, 45, 51, 52, 56, 58, 59, 66, and 68) are reported as HR positive readout. This fully automated test detects the same genotypes of HC2, which have been classified as HR by (the International Agency for Research on Cancer (IARC)), and in addition HPV66, and includes an internal control (B-globin) as the marker of sample adequacy.

2.5. Real Time HR HPV

The Abbott RealTime HR HPV test (Abbott, Wiesbaden, Germany) is a qualitative real-time PCR for the detection of DNA from 12 HR-HPV genotypes (16, 18, 31, 33, 35, 39, 45, 51, 52, 56, 58, 59, 66, and 68), and includes an internal control (B-globin) as the marker of sample adequacy. Even an RT test is able to provide the identified genotype: for HPV 16 and 18 as single and for other HR genotypes in the pool, respectively.

2.6. Onclarity

The BD Onclarity HPV Assay detects 14 HR-HPV genotypes and co-amplifies a beta-globin internal control (IC) that acts as processing control. The primers for the 14 HPV genotypes are designed to target a region of 79–137 bases in the E6/E7 genome, whereas the IC primers amplify a 75 base region in the human beta-globin gene. The assay consists of three PCR assay tubes (G1, G2, and G3) and four optical channels for the detection of the 14 HR-HPV genotypes (16, 18, 31, 45, 51, 52) as single infections and the remaining eight genotypes in three groups (33/58, 56/59/66, 35/39/68) and the IC.

2.7. Anyplex II

The Seegene Anyplex II HPV HR test simultaneously detects 14 HR-HPV genotypes (HPV 16, 18, 31, 33, 35, 39, 45, 51, 52, 56, 58, 59, 66, and 68), and co-amplifies a beta-globin internal control (IC), which acts as processing control in only one real-time PCR reaction based on TOCE (tagging oligonucleotide cleavage and extension) technology. In case of positivity, Anyplex also provides the information of semi-quantitative viral load level of amplification, which can be measured repeatedly at 30, 40, and 50 cycles during the PCR process.

2.8. Aptima

The APTIMA HPV Assay searches for E6/E7 HR-HPV mRNA by three main steps, which take place in a single tube: target capture, target amplification through amplification mediated by the transcription (Transcription-Mediated Amplification, or TMA), and detection of amplification products (amplicons) by Hybridization Protection dosage Assay. The assay incorporates an internal control for the capture, amplification, and detection of nucleic acid, as well as any operator or instrumentation errors.

2.9. Cytology

The physician-collected ThinPrep PreservCyt cervical specimens were processed in the ThinPrep 2000 machine (Cytyc Corporation, Boxborough, Mass). All liquid-based cytology slides were stained according to the Pap method and all cytologic diagnosis were performed by trained specialist biotechnicians, following automated Focal Point evaluation of all slides. In case of abnormal cytology, a dedicated pathologist from the Cytology Unit of IEO reviewed cytology slides to confirm diagnosis. Results were reported according to the 2001 Bethesda Reporting System.

2.10. Histology

All histological diagnoses were made on a colposcopic-guided biopsy of the transformation zone alone or with endocervical curettage or on excision surgical specimens, by dedicated gynecological pathologists working at the Division of Pathology of IEO.

2.11. Statistical Methods

Patients' characteristics were summarized by count and percent or mean and standard deviation (SD) for categorical and continuous variables, respectively. HPV test agreement, at both baseline and at follow-up, were estimated by the proportion of concordant cases. In order to take into account the low prevalence of negative and positive cases at baseline and at follow-up, respectively, concordance was estimated by the prevalence-adjusted and bias-adjusted kappa (PABAK) [14] statistic. Point estimates were tabulated alongside 95% confidence interval and the significance of the agreement between each HPV test with the HC2 test was determined by using the McNemar test. Sensitivity and specificity of each test at baseline and at follow-up were plotted in a forest-like plot for all patients and tabulated for the CIN2+ patients only. All tests were two-tailed and considered significant at the 5% level. The HC2 test was used as the reference test. All analyses were conducted using SAS 9.4 (N.C, Cary) and STATA (StataCorp. 2021. *Stata Statistical Software: Release 17*. College Station, TX, USA: StataCorp LLC).

3. Results

One hundred and seventy-two women scheduled to be conservatively treated with LEEP or laser conization or laser vaporization for CIN2+ were enrolled. The main characteristics of the study population at baseline are listed in Table 2.

Not all HPV tests were performed at baseline and follow-up due to lack of supply of reagents. Histological diagnosis on surgical specimens at baseline confirmed a CIN2+ lesion in 158 (91.9%) patients. Only histology confirmed samples were included in the final analysis.

Table 2. Patients' Characteristics at Baseline.

Characteristic	Level	Statistic [a]
Age, years		39.0 (7.8) [b]
Histology	CIN 1	14 (8.1)
	CIN 2+	158 (91.9)
HC2	Negative	12 (7.0)
	Positive	160 (93.0)
Cytology	Negative	6 (3.5)
	ASCUS	6 (3.5)
	LSIL	18 (10.5)
	HSIL/ASC-H	107 (62.2)
	AGC	2 (1.2)
	SCC	7 (4.1)
	missing	26 (15.1)

[a] Statistics are: Mean (SD) for Age, N (%) otherwise; SD = Standard Deviation; [b] min = 25, max = 61 years.

Overall, 150 patients were recruited at post-treatment follow-up, but only 118 in a time range between 3 and 6 months. Twenty-two patients (12.8%) were lost to follow-up and 32 (21.3%) were excluded due to incorrect timing of test-of-cure. Assuming HC2 as comparator, all HPV tests employed showed a good degree of comparison at both baseline (PABAK ranging from 0.81 to 0.90) and follow-up (PABAK ranging from 0.53 to 1). The concordance between different HPV tests and HC2 ranges from 91% to 95% at baseline and from 76% to 100% at follow-up, respectively, as shown in Tables 3 and 4.

Table 3. HPV Test Results at Baseline Compared to Hc2 (Reference).

HPV Test		HC2, N (col %) [a]		PABAK (95% CI)	p-Value [b]	Agreement % (95% CI)
		Negative	Positive			
Abbott	Negative	8 (72.7)	3 (2.9)	0.90		95%
	Positive	3 (27.3)	100 (97.1)	(0.81, 0.98)	1.00	(88.9, 98.0)
Roche	Negative	3 (60.0)	3 (4.3)	0.87		93%
	Positive	2 (40.0)	67 (95.7)	(0.75, 0.98)	1.00	(85.1, 97.8)
Aptima	Negative	8 (66.7)	12 (7.6)	0.81		91%
	Positive	4 (33.3)	147 (92.5)	(0.73, 0.90)	0.08	(85.3, 94.6)
Linear Array	Negative	6 (54.6)	9 (5.7)	0.84		92%
	Positive	5 (45.4)	150 (94.3)	(0.75, 0.91)	0.42	(86.6, 95.4)
BD Onclarity	Negative	6 (66.7)	7 (4.9)	0.87		93%
	Positive	3 (33.3)	136 (95.1)	(0.79, 0.95)	0.34	(88.2, 96.8)
Seegene	Negative	4 (40.0)	4 (2.8)	0.87		93%
	Positive	6 (60.0)	137 (97.2)	(0.79, 0.95)	0.75	(88.2, 96.8)

[a] Column percent on non-missing counts; [b] McNemar test exact p-Values. PABAK = Prevalence and Bias adjusted Kappa; 95%CI = 95% Confidence Interval.

Table 4. HPV Test Results at Follow-Up [a] Compared to Hc2 (Reference).

HPV Test		HC2, N (col %) [b]		PABAK (95% CI)	p-Value [c]	Agreement % (95% CI)
		Negative	Positive			
Abbott	Negative	43 (97.7)	7 (25.9)	0.78		89%
	Positive	1 (2.3)	20 (74.1)	(0.63, 0.92)	0.07	(79.0, 95.0)
Roche	Negative	28 (100)	0	1.00		100%
	Positive	0	16 (100)	(1.00, 1.00)	1.00	(92.0, 100)
Aptima	Negative	52 (98.1)	7 (21.2)	0.81		88%
	Positive	1 (1.9)	26 (78.8)	(0.69, 0.94)	0.07	(80.1, 93.1)
Linear Array	Negative	36 (100)	8 (24.2)	0.77		88%
	Positive	0	25 (75.8)	(0.62, 0.92)	0.008	(78.4, 94.9)
BD Onclarity	Negative	63 (95.5)	16 (47.1)	0.62		81%
	Positive	3 (4.6)	18 (52.9)	(0.47, 0.77)	0.004	(71.9, 88.2)
Seegene	Negative	57 (89.1)	16 (48.5)	0.53		76%
	Positive	7 (10.9)	17 (51.5)	(0.36, 0.70)	0.09	(66.6, 84.3)

[a] N = 118 patients with first visit at 3–6 months, median f.u. days = 108, (min = 90, max = 179) [b] Column percent on non-missing counts; [c] McNemar test; PABAK = Prevalence and Bias adjusted Kappa; 95%CI = 95% Confidence Interval.

Sensitivity and specificity of all employed tests for CIN2+ at baseline and at follow-up, compared to HC2, are summarized in Figures 1 and 2. All HPV tests showed a very good sensitivity in detecting CIN2+ at baseline, more than 92%, and a very good specificity at follow-up, more than 89%.

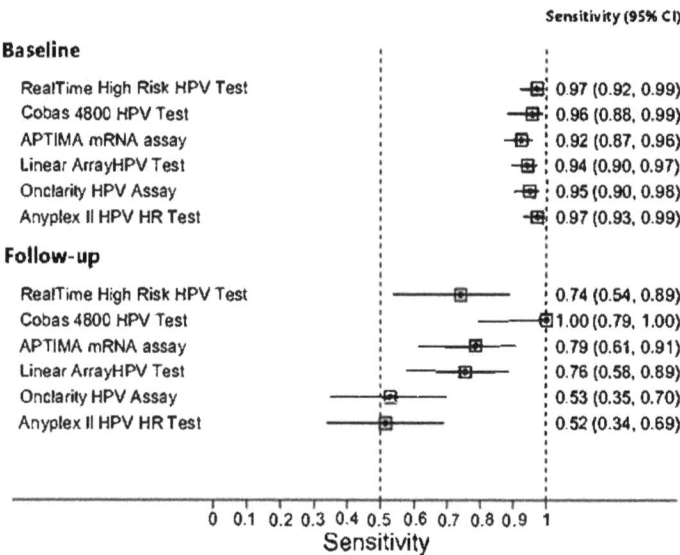

Figure 1. Sensitivity for CIN2+ at baseline and at follow-up.

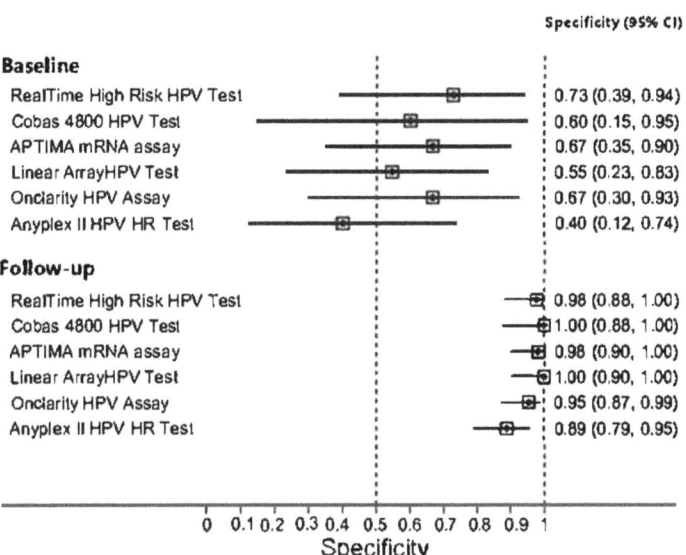

Figure 2. Specificity of all employed tests for CIN2+ at baseline and at follow-up.

4. Discussion

The results of our study showed a very good concordance among different HPV tests performed in liquid-based cervical samples from a group of women with high prevalence of preneoplastic cervical disease. The confidence intervals of these concordances overlap, further demonstrating the similarities of these HPV tests in performance. These data are in agreement with previous studies summarized in the 2020 list of human papillomavirus assays suitable for primary cervical cancer screening, published by Arbyn et al. (Arbyn et al., 2021). All HPV tests employed at baseline and follow-up have been validated according to Meijer's guidelines [9–13]. As requested by validation guidelines (Meijer's guidelines or Valgent protocol), the relative sensitivity and specificity must be high to be considered "validated". Only LA is a test not fully validated according to Meijer's guidelines, due to the additional search for low-risk (LR) HPV genotypes and the high sensitivity that does not correlate with CIN2+. However, data regarding positivity for LR-HPV have not been included in our analysis. Moreover, LA is a test previously validated according to Valgent protocol [8].

Since validations have been usually performed in the screening setting, these data are only indicative for baseline. In the present analysis, we focused on comparing tests' performance not only at baseline, but also at the post-treatment follow-up. Interestingly, our data showed comparable performance of the tests in terms of sensitivity and specificity at both baseline and test-of-cure.

Due to the setting of samples, which show a high prevalence of positive at baseline and negative at follow-up, respectively, sensitivities were found to be higher at baseline and lower at follow-up. On the contrary, specificities are notably higher at follow-up than at baseline. Due to the low prevalence of HPV after treatment, we chose the prevalence and bias adjusted kappa, instead of either the simple or the weighted kappa, to estimate the HPV tests' agreement.

However, all tests perform similarly at baseline and follow-up. Although Cobas seems to show better performance than other tests, these data might suffer from a bias related to the smaller number of samples that have been tested with the Cobas method.

A negative HPV result at follow-up provides a good negative predictive value. Indeed, we found only a case of disease recurrence in the cohort of patients with a post-treatment negative HPV test result, for any validated HPV test. In this patient, cytology was HSIL at follow-up and only LA revealed the presence of HPV18 and 73 at baseline, with the persistence of HPV 73 at relapse. Actually, LR HPV genotypes are not detected by validated HPV tests.

Furthermore, HPV tests that provide partial or extended genotyping showed comparable results.

The Aptima test, which detects HPV mRNA, showed no particular advantages in terms of sensitivity or specificity: the test performances are in line with other tests that detect HPV DNA.

Strengths of the present study include the type of population (women with only confirmed CIN2 + histology) and the timing of test-of-cure that was performed at 6 ± 3 months, as also suggested by the most recent guidelines from the Italian Group for Cervical Cancer Screening (GISCi) [15]. On the contrary, the main limit consists in the impossibility of performing all HPV tests in all samples.

In conclusion, our results demonstrate that validated HPV tests produce comparable results, and this cannot be extended to non-validated tests without proven evidence. Thus, only the use of validated HPV DNA or RNA tests is strongly recommended in both screening and test-of-cure settings. Moreover, HPV genotyping could be helpful in post-treatment management, by identifying women at higher risk of CIN2+ recurrence, due to the persistence of the same HPV genotype, and reassuring women who may present new HPV genotype infection after surgical treatment.

Author Contributions: F.B., A.D.I. and D.R. collected, analyzed data, and drafted the manuscript. E.P.P., M.P., D.F. and R.P. revised and edited the manuscript. M.T.S. and S.B. conceived the project. F.B., R.P. and A.D.I. participated in the coordination of the study and manuscript modification. All authors have read and agreed to the published version of the manuscript.

Funding: The funding for this study was provided by HPV test companies that supplied free kits for the assays. The Funder had the right to read and comment upon the manuscript, but without editorial rights, nor any role in the final interpretation of the data.

Institutional Review Board Statement: The study was conducted according to the guidelines of the Declaration of Helsinki, and approved by the Institutional Review Board of the European Institute of Oncology, Milan, Italy (protocol IEO S544/210, date of approval: 26 May 2010).

Informed Consent Statement: Informed consent was obtained from all women at the entry of the study.

Data Availability Statement: The data presented in this study are available on request from the corresponding author. The data are not publicly available due to patients' privacy restrictions. The data are safely stored in a private database of the European Institute of Oncology, Milan, Italy.

Acknowledgments: We are grateful to all HPV test manufacturing companies that supported the study, providing free kits to perform the tests. This work was partially supported by the Italian Ministry of Health with Ricerca Corrente and 5×1000 funds.

Conflicts of Interest: The authors declare no conflict of interest. None of the authors received financial support or funding for this work.

Abbreviations and Acronyms

HPV =	Human Papillomavirus
CIN =	Cervical intraepithelial neoplasia
HR =	High risk
LR =	Low risk
IEO =	European Institute of Oncology
LBC =	Liquid based cytology
LSIL =	Low grade squamous intraepithelial lesion
HSIL =	High grade squamous intraepithelial lesion

PCR = Polymerase chain reaction
HC2 = Qiagen Hybrid Capture 2
PABAK = Prevalence-Adjusted and Bias-Adjusted Kappa

References

1. Zur Hausen, H. Papillomaviruses in the causation of human cancers—A brief historical account. *Virology* **2009**, *384*, 260–265. [CrossRef] [PubMed]
2. Kjær, S.K.; Frederiksen, K.; Munk, C.; Iftner, T. Long-term absolute risk of cervical intraepithelial neoplasia grade 3 or worse following human papillomavirus infection: Role of persistence. *J. Natl. Cancer Inst.* **2010**, *102*, 1478–1488. [CrossRef] [PubMed]
3. Poljak, M.; Oštrbenk Valenčak, A.; Gimpelj Domjanič, G.; Xu, L.; Arbyn, M. Commercially available molecular tests for human papillomaviruses: A global overview. *Clin. Microbiol. Infect.* **2020**, *26*, 1144–1150. [CrossRef] [PubMed]
4. Arbyn, M.; Simon, M.; Peeters, E.; Xu, L.; Meijer, C.J.L.M.; Berkhof, J.; Cuschieri, K.; Bonde, J.; Ostrbenk Vanlencak, A.; Zhao, F.H.; et al. 2020 list of human papillomavirus assays suitable for primary cervical cancer screening. *Clin. Microbiol. Infect.* **2021**, *27*, 1083–1095. [CrossRef] [PubMed]
5. Mariani, L.; Sandri, M.T.; Preti, M.; Origoni, M.; Costa, S.; Cristoforoni, P.; Bottari, F.; Sideri, M. HPV-Testing in Follow-up of Patients Treated for CIN2+ Lesions. *J. Cancer* **2016**, *7*, 107–114. [CrossRef] [PubMed]
6. Bottari, F.; Iacobone, A.D.; Passerini, R.; Preti, E.P.; Sandri, M.T.; Cocuzza, C.E.; Gary, D.S.; Andrews, J.C. Human Papillomavirus Genotyping Compared with a Qualitative High-Risk Human Papillomavirus Test After Treatment of High-Grade Cervical Intraepithelial Neoplasia: A Systematic Review. *Obstet. Gynecol.* **2019**, *134*, 452–462. [CrossRef] [PubMed]
7. Iacobone, A.D.; Radice, D.; Sandri, M.T.; Preti, E.P.; Guerrieri, M.E.; Vidal Urbinati, A.M.; Pino, I.; Franchi, D.; Passerini, R.; Bottari, F. Human Papillomavirus Same Genotype Persistence and Risk of Cervical Intraepithelial Neoplasia2+ Recurrence. *Cancers* **2021**, *13*, 3664. [CrossRef] [PubMed]
8. Xu, L.; Ostrbenk, A.; Poljak, M.; Arbyn, M. Assessment of the Roche linear array HPV genotyping test within the VALGENT framework. *J. Clin. Virol.* **2018**, *98*, 37–42. [CrossRef] [PubMed]
9. Heideman, D.A.M.; Hesselink, A.T.; Berkhof, J.; Van Kemenade, F.; Melchers, W.J.G.; Daalmeijer, N.F.; Verkuijten, M.; Meijer, C.J.L.M.; Snijders, P.J.F. Clinical validation of the cobas(R)4800 HPV test for cervical screening purposes. *J. Clin. Microbiol.* **2011**, *49*, 3983–3985. [CrossRef] [PubMed]
10. Carozzi, F.M.; Burroni, E.; Bisanzi, S.; Puliti, D.; Confortini, M.; Giorgi Rossi, P.; Sani, C.; Scalisi, A.; Chini, F. Comparison of clinical performance of Abbott RealTime high risk HPV test with that of Hybrid Capture 2 assay in a screening setting. *J. Clin. Microbiol.* **2011**, *49*, 1446e51. [CrossRef] [PubMed]
11. Ejegod, D.; Bottari, F.; Pedersen, H.; Sandri, M.T.; Bonde, J. The BD onclarity HPV assay on SurePath collected samples meets the international guidelines for human papillomavirus test requirements for cervical screening. *J. Clin. Microbiol.* **2016**, *54*, 2267–2272. [CrossRef] [PubMed]
12. Hesselink, A.T.; Sahli, R.; Berkhof, J.; Snijders, P.J.; van der Salm, M.L.; Agard, D.; Bleeker, M.C.; Heideman, D.A. Clinical validation of Anyplex II HPV HR detection according to the guidelines for HPV test requirements for cervical cancer screening. *J. Clin. Virol.* **2016**, *76*, 36–39. [CrossRef] [PubMed]
13. Heideman, D.A.; Hesselink, A.T.; Van Kemenade, F.J.; Iftner, T.; Berkhof, J.; Topal, F.; Agard, D.; Meijer, C.J.; Snijders, P.J. The APTIMA HPV assay fulfills the cross-sectional clinical and reproducibility criteria of international guidelines for HPV test requirements for cervical screening. *J. Clin. Microbiol.* **2013**, *51*, 3653–3657. [CrossRef] [PubMed]
14. Byrt, T.; Bishop, J.; Carlin, J.B. Bias, prevalence and kappa. *J. Clin. Epidemiol.* **1993**, *46*, 423–429. [CrossRef]
15. Ruano, Y.; Torrents, M.; Ferrer, F.J. Human papillomavirus combined with cytology and margin status identifies patients at risk for recurrence after conization for high-grade cervical intraepithelial neoplasia. *Eur. J. Gynaecol. Oncol.* **2015**, *36*, 245–251. [PubMed]

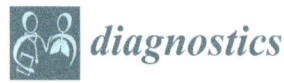

Article

Vaginosonography versus MRI in Pre-Treatment Evaluation of Early-Stage Cervical Cancer: An Old Tool for a New Precision Approach?

Ailyn M. Vidal Urbinati [1,2,*], Ida Pino [1], Anna D. Iacobone [1,2], Davide Radice [3], Giulia Azzalini [1,4], Maria E. Guerrieri [1], Eleonora P. Preti [1], Silvia Martella [1] and Dorella Franchi [1]

1 Preventive Gynecology Unit, European Institute of Oncology IRCCS, 20141 Milan, Italy
2 Department of Biomedical Sciences, University of Sassari, 07100 Sassari, Italy
3 Division of Epidemiology and Biostatistics, European Institute of Oncology IRCCS, 20141 Milan, Italy
4 Obstetrics and Gynecology Specialization School, University of Udine, 33100 Udine, Italy
* Correspondence: ailyn.vidalurbinati@ieo.it; Tel.: +39-02-57-489-120; Fax: +39-02-94379243

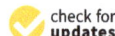

Citation: Vidal Urbinati, A.M.; Pino, I.; Iacobone, A.D.; Radice, D.; Azzalini, G.; Guerrieri, M.E.; Preti, E.P.; Martella, S.; Franchi, D. Vaginosonography versus MRI in Pre-Treatment Evaluation of Early-Stage Cervical Cancer: An Old Tool for a New Precision Approach?. *Diagnostics* 2022, 12, 2904. https://doi.org/10.3390/diagnostics12122904

Academic Editor: Ralph P. Mason

Received: 20 October 2022
Accepted: 21 November 2022
Published: 22 November 2022

Publisher's Note: MDPI stays neutral with regard to jurisdictional claims in published maps and institutional affiliations.

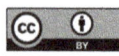

Copyright: © 2022 by the authors. Licensee MDPI, Basel, Switzerland. This article is an open access article distributed under the terms and conditions of the Creative Commons Attribution (CC BY) license (https://creativecommons.org/licenses/by/4.0/).

Abstract: This study aims to analyze the sensitivity of vaginosonography (VGS) and magnetic resonance imaging (MRI) in the preoperative local evaluation of early-stage cervical cancers and to assess their accuracy in the detection of tumors, size of the lesions and stromal invasion by comparing them with the final histopathology report. This single-center study included 56 consecutive patients with cervical cancer who underwent VGS and MRI from November 2012 to January 2021. VGS significantly overestimated the lesion size by 2.7 mm ($p = 0.002$), and MRI underestimated it by 1.9 mm ($p = 0.11$). Both MRI and VGS had a good concordance with the pathology report (Cohen's kappa of 0.73 and 0.81, respectively). However, MRI had a false-negative rate (38.1%) that was greater than VGS (0%) in cases of cervical tumor size <2 cm. We found a good concordance between histology and VGS in the stromal infiltration assessment, with 89% sensitivity (95% CI 0.44–0.83) and 89% specificity (95% CI 0.52–0.86). VGS is a simple, inexpensive, widely available, and fast execution method that can complement ultrasound in particular cases and show a good correlation with MRI in the assessment of tumor dimensions, with a better performance in detecting small tumors (<2 cm).

Keywords: vaginosonography; transvaginal ultrasound; cervical cancer; MRI and gynecological oncology diagnosis

1. Introduction

Cervical cancer is one of the leading causes of morbidity and mortality in women, representing the second most common cancer in developing countries and the fourth worldwide [1].

Although a pelvic examination continues to be the first approach to detecting cervical cancer, the 2018 FIGO classification has updated the cancer staging, highlighting the central role of imaging. In fact, imaging techniques allow a better definition of the tumor size, parametrial invasion, extension to the pelvic wall or adjacent organs, and lymph node involvement [2].

Many diagnostic methods are used in clinical practice; their use depends on availability, cost, and the expertise of clinicians and radiologists. Although magnetic resonance imaging (MRI) is considered the main technique to assess tumor size and parametrial extension [3–6], transvaginal ultrasound (TVUS) or transrectal ultrasound (TRUS) can provide comparable information (especially if performed by expert examiners) while being more widely available, faster, and cheaper [4,7–10]. Moreover, the sonographic appearance of cervical lesions seems to predict the histopathological subtype: hypoechogenicity is associated with squamous cell carcinoma in 73% of cases, while isoechogenicity suggests an adenocarcinoma in 68% of women [11]. The role of imaging in assessing vaginal invasion is less clear, as several false-negative and false-positive results have been reported for large tumors that spread to the upper vagina [2,8]. Several sonographic and anatomical factors may reduce the performance of ultrasound techniques in the detection of vaginal and distal cervix lesions, such as similar echogenicity and collapsed vaginal walls [9,11,12].

Vaginosonography (VGS) is a technique first described by Dessole et al. in 2003 [13] that combines TVUS with the vaginal instillation of saline solution or ultrasound gel. It is used to evaluate local disorders of the cervix and vagina, such as benign or malignant lesions, malformations, and infiltrating endometriosis. The acoustic window created by the passive distention of the vaginal walls allows a better analysis of the anatomical structures, making the ultrasound evaluation easier, especially in the detection of exophytic early-stage cervical cancers [13–15].

Our study aims to analyze the sensitivity of VGS and MRI in the preoperative local evaluation of early-stage cervical cancers and to assess their accuracy in the detection of tumor presence, size of the lesion, and stromal invasion by comparing them with the final histopathology report.

2. Materials and Methods

We enrolled 81 consecutive women diagnosed with cervical cancer by clinical examination and referred to the European Institute of Oncology from November 2012 to January 2021. All patients underwent diagnostic evaluation, including a cervical biopsy or a pathological review of the original slides if the initial diagnosis was made at a different institution. All tumors were staged according to the FIGO (2018) criteria using vaginal and rectal examinations, standard chest and abdominal computed tomography (CT), TVUS or TRUS, and MRI. Twenty-five patients were excluded either because they received non-surgical treatments [12] or their FIGO stage was above IB2 [13]. Data from 56 patients were analyzed in the study. We included only the patients that underwent both VGS and MRI, whose surgical specimen was available within 30 days from the imaging evaluation, and that had early FIGO stages ($\leq$IB2).

The results of MRI and VGS were compared with the pathology report. If the MRI scan was performed outside the European Institute of Oncology, an internal gynecological oncology radiologist reviewed the images.

All patients underwent both TVUS and VGS. The scans were performed by two experienced ultrasound examiners with 25 and 15 years of experience in ultrasound for gynecologic oncology (D.F. and A.M.V.U.), respectively. The examiners were blinded to the MRI results.

All women were examined in the lithotomy position with an empty bladder using high-end ultrasound equipment, with the frequency of the vaginal probes varying between 5.0 and 9.0 MHz. Ultrasonographic images were acquired according to a standardized time gray-scale examination technique.

The VGS procedure consists of four steps: (1) a 5.3 Fr sonohysterography catheter is inserted into the vagina by an assistant; then, (2) the probe is inserted by the operator; (3) the assistant closes the vaginal channel by narrowing the major labia; (4) approximately 60 cc of room temperature saline solution is instilled while the ultrasound is performed.

The following parameters were evaluated by VGS and TVUS: tumor presence, maximum diameter of the tumor, parametrial and fornix infiltration, vaginal involvement, stromal invasion, anterior and posterior septum involvement, and blood flow of the lesion. The blood flow was assessed by a color Doppler score based on the intensity of the color signal with the following value ranges: (1) no flow, (2) minimal flow, (3) moderate flow, and (4) high vascular flow.

A dedicated pathologist, highly experienced in gynecologic cancers, assessed the specimens and described the size and extent of the tumor, histology type, grading, stromal invasion, minimum free thickness, and maximum deep infiltration.

Approval was obtained from the ethics committee of the European Institute of Oncology (UID 2731), and all patients signed an informed consent form.

3. Statistical Analysis

Patients' characteristics were summarized either by count and percent or mean and standard deviation (SD) for categorical and continuous variables, respectively. Methods agreement was estimated using Cohen's kappa coefficient and Lin's correlation. Lesion size (maximum diameter) differences between VGS and MRI with respect to histology were summarized by mean, SD, and 95% confidence intervals (95% CI) and compared using Bland–Altman and Passing–Bablok regression methods. All method comparisons considered histology as the gold standard. Cross-tabulation of the categorical variables was tested for significance using Fisher's exact test; the mean comparison was made using the unpaired t-test. All tests were two-tailed and considered significant at the 5% level. All analyses were done using SAS 9.4 (NC, Cary) and STATA (StataCorp., College Station, Texas, USA, 2021. Stata Statistical Software: Release 17. College Station, TX: StataCorp LLC).

4. Results

The demographic and clinicopathological characteristics of the 56 patients included in the study and their previous treatments are reported in Table 1. The median age was 39.1 years (range 24–72), and the population was mainly Italian (92.9%). In total, 23 cancers (41%) were squamous cell carcinomas, 23 (41%) adenocarcinomas, and 10 other histotypes (18%), including 4 adenosquamous tumors, 3 clear cell variants, 2 neuroendocrine carcinomas, and 1 adenoid basal carcinoma. Invasive cervical cancer tumors were confirmed in 55 patients, while no residual tumor was found in one case. None of our patients reported any discomfort during the procedure.

Forty-two (75%) lesions were described as highly vascularized (color score 4—CS 4), 12 (21.4%) as moderately vascularized (CS 3), and 2 (3.6%) as minimally vascularized. We did not find any correlation between vascularization and histotype, but we found a statistically significant correlation between vascularization and the largest dimension of the lesion, with a mean of 26.9 mm in CS 4 and 12.4 mm in CS 3 ($p < 0.001$).

Out of the six patients with prior conization and residual disease, MRI detected the lesion only in three cases, while VGS detected all six cases. In Figure 1, it is possible to observe one of these cases.

Squamous tumors were predominantly hypoechoic (14/23; 60.1%), while adenocarcinomas were mainly hyperechoic (16/23; 69.5%) ($p = 0.005$). Figure 2 shows an example of two echogenicities, with and without VGS.

When the stromal infiltration was analyzed, there was a good concordance between histology and VGS, with a sensitivity of 89% (95% CI 0.44–0.83), a specificity of 89% (95% CI 0.52–0.86), and a Cohen's kappa of 0.78. When the stromal invasion was >2/3, the histological exam identified five of six (83.3%) cases with positive lymph nodes (6), while VGS predicted four cases (66.6%).

Although we did not compare the fornix infiltration to the gold standard because of the early stage of the tumors, we observed eight false-positive cases of fornix infiltration with MRI and two with VGS, with a specificity of 85.7% and 96.4% and a negative predictive value (NPV) of 88.9% and 100%, respectively.

VGS significantly overestimated the lesion size by 2.7 mm compared to the gold standard. On the other hand, MRI underestimated it by 1.9 mm (Table 2). Figure 3 is an example of the small difference in lesion size by the methods compared with the final specimen.

Table 1. Patients' characteristics and treatments, N = 56.

Characteristic	Level	Statistics [a]
Country of origin	Italian	49 (87.5)
	Other EU	4 (7.1)
	Non-EU	3 (5.4)
FIGO Stage	IA1	2 (3.6)
	IB1	45 (80.4)
	IB2	9 (16.1)
Pre-conization		6 (10.7)
Pre- NACHT [b]		4 (7.1)
Stromal invasion	<2/3	29 (51.8)
	>2/3	27 (48.2)
Echogenicity	Isoechogenic	8 (14.3)
	Hypoechogenic	21 (37.5)
	Hyperechogenic	25 (44.6)
	Mixed	2 (3.6)
Score PD	2	2 (3.6)
	3	12 (21.4)
	4	42 (75.0)
Intervention	Hysterectomy rad	43 (76.8)
	Conization	8 (14.3)
	NACHT + Hysterectomy rad	3 (5.4)
	LA + NACHT + Conization	2 (3.6)
Histology	Adenocarcinoma	23 (41.1)
	SCC	23 (41.1)
	Other [c]	10 (17.8)
Grading	G1	2 (3.6)
	G2	21 (37.5)
	G3	33 (58.9)
Lymph node status	pN0	50 (89.3)
	pN1	6 (10.7)
Age [d], years		38.8 (8.9)
Maximum diameter of the lesion (mm) by method	Histology	23.4 (11.2)
	VGS	26.1 (9.8)
	MRI [e]	21.5 (12.5)
Minimum free thickness (mm) [f]		7.0 (4.3)
Maximum infiltration depth (mm) [e]		8.2 (5.9)

[a] Statistics are: N (%) for categorical variables, mean (SD) otherwise; SD = standard deviation; [b] NACHT = neoadjuvant chemotherapy; [c] adenosquamous N = 4, clear cell spinocellular variant N = 3, adenoid basal carcinoma N = 1, large cell neuroendocrine carcinoma N = 2; [d] min = 24, max = 72; [e] N = 49; [f] N = 54. VGS = vaginosonography; SCC = squamous cells carcinoma; MRI = magnetic resonance imaging.

Table 2. Maximum diameter (mm) methods comparison with histology (gold standard) and summary statistics.

Method	N	Mean (SD)	95% CI	p-Value [a]
Histology	56	23.4 (11.2)	(20.4, 26.4)	-
VGS	56	26.1 (9.8)	(23.5, 28.7)	-
MRI	56	21.5 (12.5)	(18.2, 24.9)	-
Bias VGS—Histology [b]	56	2.7 (6.3)	(1.1, 4.4)	0.002
Bias MRI—Histology [c]	56	−1.9 (8.5)	(−4.2, 0.4)	0.11

[a] Two-sided paired t-test: lower limit of agreement: [b] −9.5 mm, [c] −18.8 mm; cases under limit: [b] N = 2 (3.6%), [c] N = 1 (1.8%); upper limit of agreement: [b] 15.0 mm, [c] 15.1 mm; cases over limit: [b] N = 3 (5.4%), [c] N = 2 (3.6%).

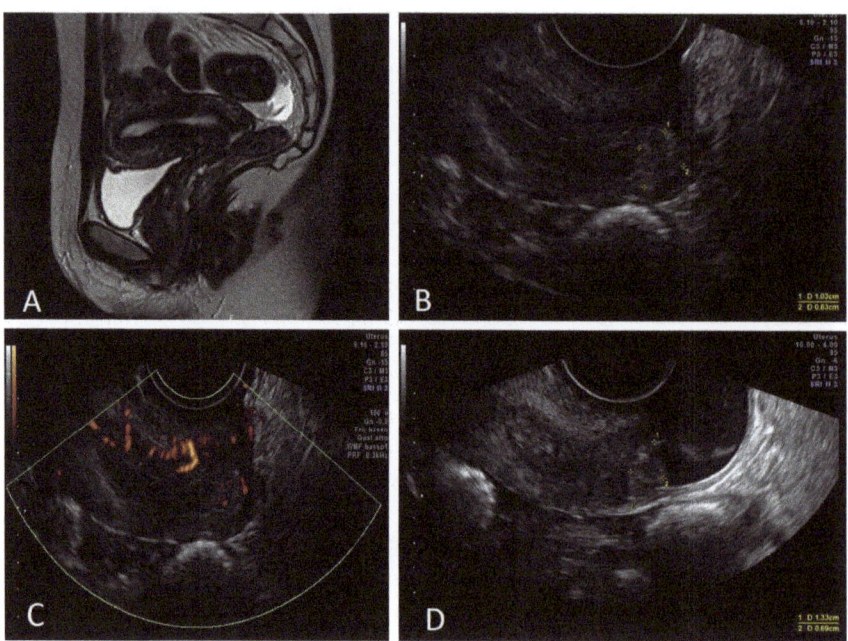

Figure 1. Small tumor after conization. (**A**) Not detectable disease by MRI. (**B**) Detectable disease by TVUS, measuring 10.3 × 8.3 mm. (**C**) Lesion vascularization by power Doppler. (**D**) Disease detectable by VGS, measuring 13.3 × 6.9 mm.

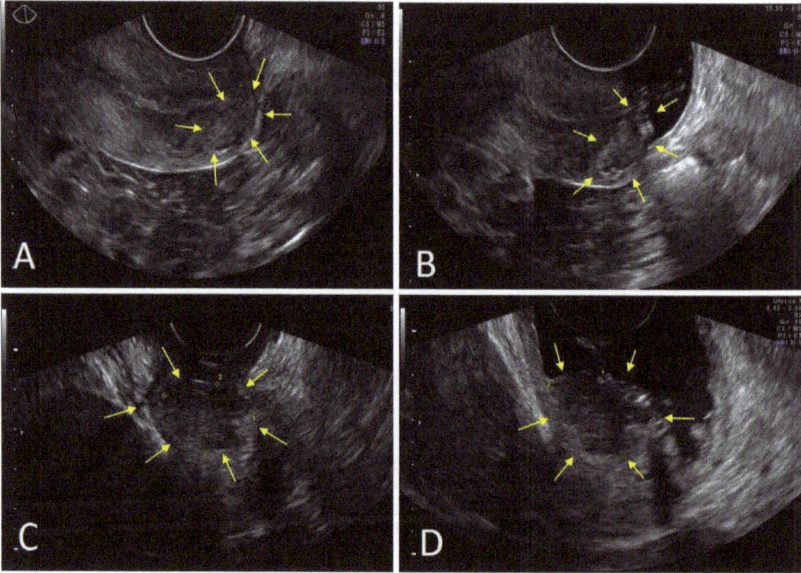

Figure 2. Echogenicity by TVUS and VGS. (**A**) Small adenocarcinoma (arrows) at TVUS; (**B**) the same tumor at VGS, with better definitions of the margins and more hyperechoic echogenicity (arrows). (**C**) Squamous tumors (arrows) at TVUS; (**D**) the same tumor at VGS, with better definitions of the margins and more hypoechoic echogenicity (arrows).

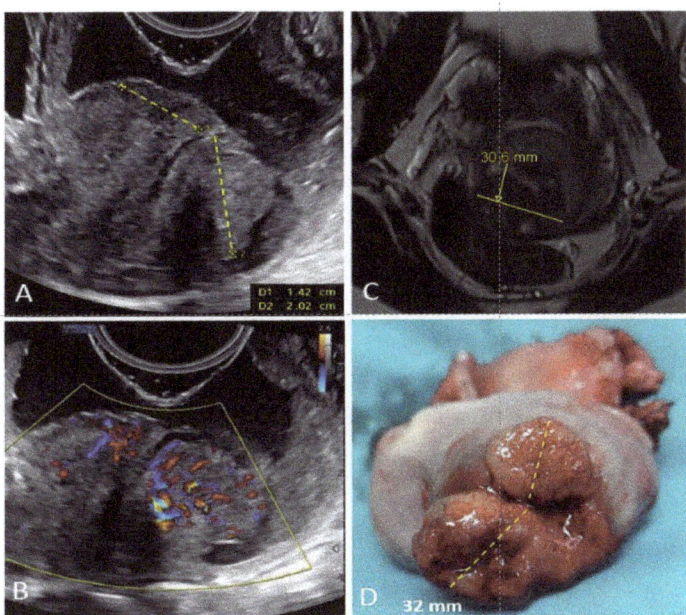

Figure 3. Dimensions with both techniques compared with final histology. VGS image of IB2 N+ squamous tumor (**A,B**), MRI (**C**), and macroscopic appearance (**D**).

When comparing the size of the lesions, both MRI and VGS had a good concordance with the pathology report (Table 3), showing a Cohen's kappa of 0.73 and 0.81, respectively. If the tumor was <2 cm, VGS identified 16 cases, while MRI identified 18 cases out of 21. However, in the latter group, MRI missed eight cases whose dimensions were recorded as 0 mm (Figure 2D), corresponding to a false-negative rate of 38.1% (95% CI: 18.1–61.6%). This explains the apparently higher sensitivity of MRI with respect to VGS for tumors smaller than 2 cm (Figure 4).

Table 3. Methods comparison with the gold standard by tumor size (maximum diameter, mm).

Method	Size (mm)	Size (mm) by Histology N (col %)		Cohen's Kappa (95% CI)	p-Value [a]
		<20 N = 21	≥20 N = 35		
VGS	<20	16 (76.2)	2 (5.7)	0.73	
	≥20	5 (23.8)	33 (94.3)	(0.54, 0.91)	0.26
MRI	<20	18 (85.7)	2 (5.7)	0.81	
	≥20	3 (14.3)	33 (94.3)	(0.65, 0.97)	0.65

[a] McNemar's test.

Figure 5A shows the Bland–Altman plot of the maximum diameters in VGS and histopathology, while Figure 5B shows the diameter in MRI and histopathology. Visual inspection of the scatterplots suggests a good distribution of the data with both methods. The magnitude of the differences did not change with the mean of the two measurements. Overall, Figure 5C,D show no differences despite the diameter of the tumors, except for the cluster of eight tumors missed by the MRI (Figure 5B,D). Lin's correlation was strong for VGS (0.8) and moderate for MRI (0.7).

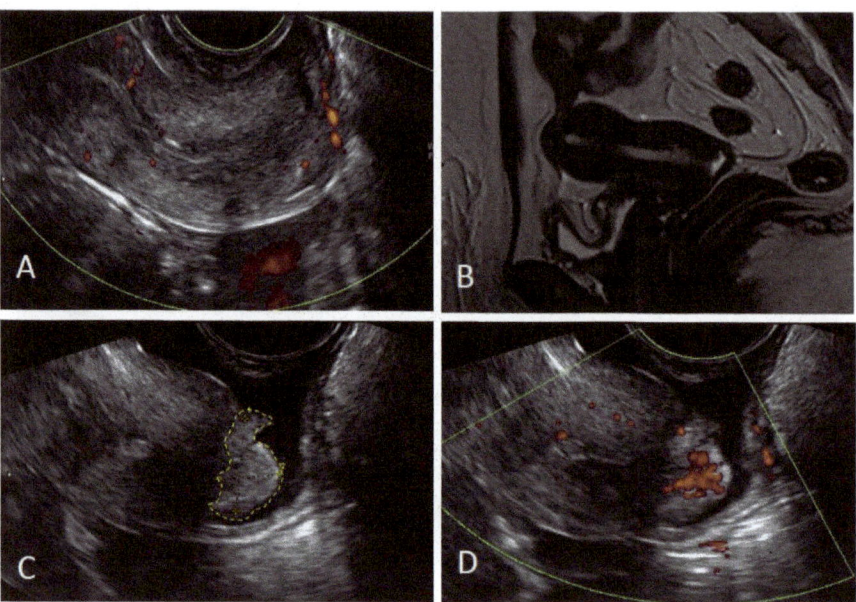

Figure 4. Detection of small tumors with VGS. (**A**,**B**) Small tumor not detectable at TVUS and MRI; (**C**,**D**) the same tumor detected by adding VGS and PD.

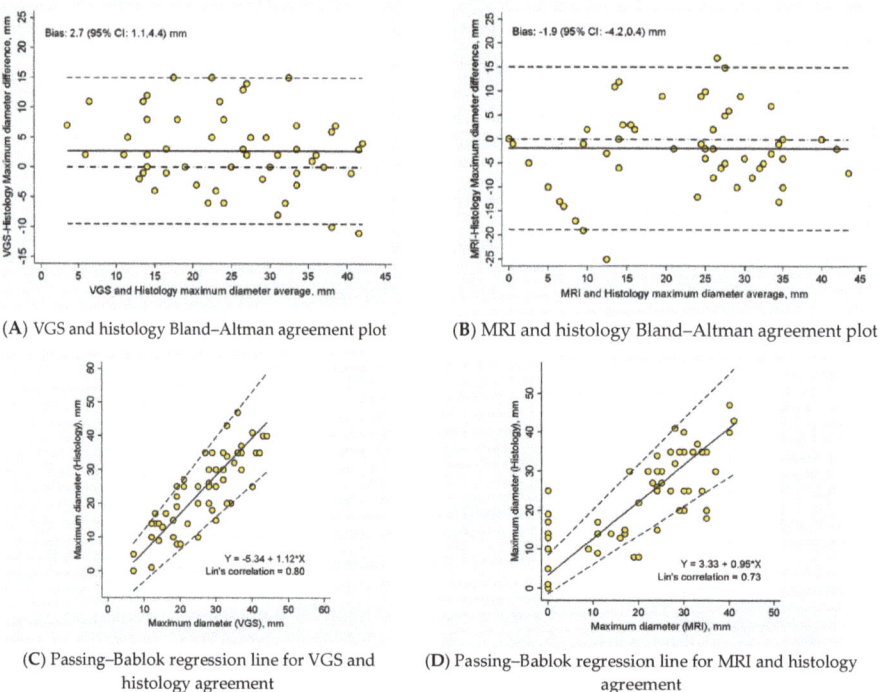

(**A**) VGS and histology Bland–Altman agreement plot

(**B**) MRI and histology Bland–Altman agreement plot

(**C**) Passing–Bablok regression line for VGS and histology agreement

(**D**) Passing–Bablok regression line for MRI and histology agreement

Figure 5. Bland–Altman plot of both methods compared with the gold standard.

5. Discussion

The role of ultrasound in the pre-treatment evaluation of cervical cancer is well established [2,16–18]. However, some factors hinder the ultrasound evaluation of some tumor characteristics, such as lesion margins (especially the small exophytic ones), fornix involvement, and vascular patterns [9,11,19].

To the best of our knowledge, this is the first study that investigates the accuracy of VGS in the assessment of early-stage cervical cancer. VGS is an inexpensive and well-tolerated ultrasound technique that can increase the image quality of cervical tumors. The acoustic windows created by saline solution results in a distance of the probe to the lesion, the distension of vaginal walls, and the exclusion of hindering factors, including vaginal collapse, bleeding, and/or mucus secretions.

Compared to histology (used as the gold standard), VGS and MRI assess the dimension of the lesion with similar accuracy. However, we found that VGS tended to overestimate the dimensions, whereas MRI underestimated them. Previous studies have reported that ultrasounds overestimate tumor dimensions [7,17]. Despite avoiding confounding factors, such as adjacent normal tissues, by using liquid distension in order to create an acoustic window, our data showed that the small difference between VGS and histology was statistically significant, while the difference between MRI and histology was not. Even if overestimating the tumor size could be better than underestimating it in oncological cases, it may compromise the opportunity for fertility-sparing surgery in selected patients.

The value of Lin's concordance in the assessment of the lesion dimensions was better between VGS and histology than MRI and histology. This is because MRI did not detect some small tumors, recorded as 0 mm in our study. Indeed, when the tumor was <2 cm, MRI was not able to identify 38.1% of the tumors. Therefore, the real detection rate of MRI was 47% (10 out of 21) versus 76.1% of VGS (16 out of 21). Hence, VGS is more sensitive than MRI in identifying small lesions. Prior studies did not find that TVUS was better than MRI in the detection of lesions <2 cm [9,20]. Only one previous study showed that TRUS was superior to MRI in the identification of very small lesions (<1 cm) [7].

As our study focuses on early-stage cervical cancers, we have limited data on fornix infiltration. Nevertheless, we found that VGS was more sensitive than MRI in excluding fornix infiltration, with an NPV of 100% and 88.9%, respectively. Recently, similar results have been reported by comparing the accuracy of histology to TVUS, MRI, and clinical examination under anesthesia [21]. TVUS can be a good method to exclude but not to predict vaginal infiltration, which is often overestimated. Probably, VGS could play a role in the assessment of more advanced stages of cervical cancer with vaginal involvement.

We confirmed that different histotypes have different echogenicities, as demonstrated in a previous report [11]. Epstein et al. found that the echogenicity/histotype correlation was statistically significant, with a hypoechoic pattern in the squamous tumor cells and an isoechoic pattern in adenocarcinoma tumor cells. In our study, squamous tumor cells were predominantly hypoechoic, while the adenocarcinoma tumor cells were hyperechoic. These differences could be explained by the changes in the echogenicity of surrounding tissues due to the acoustic windows placed between the ultrasound probe and the tumor.

As observed in previous studies [7,9,11,22], almost all tumors analyzed presented moderate or intense vascularization (96.4%). The power Doppler can be useful in the assessment of the presence and borders of the tumor, especially when the echogenicity does not help. Only two adenocarcinomas were poorly vascularized. These two cases did not present any other special characteristic; both tumors were >15 mm, and the patients did not receive prior therapy nor conization; one tumor showed > 2/3 stromal invasion and the other <2/3 stromal invasion.

Stromal infiltration is another interesting issue. Some studies reported that comparing ultrasound and MRI results with the final histology report led to high false-positive rates [8,17,18], and a prospective multicenter study found that the subjective assessment of TVUS or TRUS was better than objective measurements at predicting deep stromal invasion in patients with cervical cancer [23]. In our study, we observed a good concordance between

VGS and histology (89%), with a low false-positive rate (11%). The comparison between MRI and VGS for stromal invasion was not possible because MRI data were not available in all cases.

It is a well-known matter that the incidence of lymph node metastasis in cervical cancer depends on the stage: 2% in IA2, 14–36% in IB, 38–51% in IIA, and 47% in IIB (14). Stromal infiltration is one of the independent factors identified for the risk of lymph node metastases in patients with cervical cancers, along with age, tumor size, lymph vascular space invasion, histological grade, and type [23,24]. In our series, we found six patients (11%) with lymph node metastasis; all cases were FIGO stage IB. In these patients, the stromal invasion was >2/3 in five patients out of six at the histology of cervical specimens. VGS correctly identified four out of five tumor cases with stromal invasion >2/3. The only discordant patient had a not-usual histotype of cervical cancer (adenoid basal carcinoma), with an extension of 17 mm.

6. Conclusions

VGS is a simple, inexpensive, widely available, and fast execution method that can complement ultrasound in particular cases. To our knowledge, this is the first study that has evaluated the diagnostic accuracy of VGS and MRI in cancer and compared it with the final histology. Our results show a good correlation between VGS and MRI in the assessment of tumor dimensions, highlighting the better performance of VGS in detecting small tumors (<2 cm) and in predicting the absence of fornix infiltration as it shows higher sensitivity.

Moreover, the acoustic windows created between the ultrasound probe and the tumor can improve the study of the echogenicity of squamous tumors and adenocarcinomas by emphasizing the hyperechogenicity of the latter. There was a very good concordance between stromal invasion predicted by VGS and histology, which is an independent factor for the risk of lymph node involvement.

However, VGS has some limitations: despite its widespread availability, it is an operator-dependent technique, and this can limit its application to centers with highly qualified examiners.

Future studies are needed to assess the use of VGS in patients with advanced tumor stages, especially the ability to correctly identify patients with vaginal spread and septal infiltration.

Author Contributions: A.M.V.U.: supervision, conceptualization, methodology, formal analysis, writing—original draft, visualization, supervision, writing—review and editing; I.P.: data curation, investigation, visualization, formal analysis, writing; A.D.I.: methodology, formal analysis, writing—review; D.R.: statistical analysis; G.A.: methodology, formal analysis, writing; M.E.G.: data curation, investigation; E.P.P.: visualization, data curation; S.M.: data curation, methodology, investigation; D.F.: conceptualization, methodology, writing—review and editing. All authors have read and agreed to the published version of the manuscript.

Funding: This research did not receive any specific grant from funding agencies in the public, commercial, or not-for-profit sectors.

Institutional Review Board Statement: The study was conducted according to the guidelines of the Declaration of Helsinki and approved by the Institutional Review Board of the European Institute of Oncology (protocol code UID 2731, approved on 6 September 2021).

Informed Consent Statement: All patients signed a formal consent form for the use of their data for scientific purposes.

Data Availability Statement: Not applicable.

Acknowledgments: This work was partially supported by the Italian Ministry of Health with Ricerca Corrente and 5 × 1000 funds.

Conflicts of Interest: The authors declare that they have no conflict of interest.

References

1. Sung, H.; Ferlay, J.; Siegel, R.L.; Laversanne, M.; Soerjomataram, I.; Jemal, A.; Bray, F. Global Cancer Statistics 2020: GLOBOCAN Estimates of Incidence and Mortality Worldwide for 36 Cancers in 185 Countries. *CA Cancer J. Clin.* **2021**, *71*, 209–249. [CrossRef] [PubMed]
2. Bhatla, N.; Aoki, D.; Sharma, D.N.; Sankaranarayanan, R. Cancer of the cervix uteri. *Int. J. Gynecol. Obs.* **2018**, *143* (Suppl. l.2), 22–36. [CrossRef] [PubMed]
3. Hricak, H.; Gatsonis, C.; Chi, D.S.; Amendola, M.A.; Brandt, K.; Schwartz, L.H.; Koelliker, S.; Siegelman, E.S.; Brown, J.J.; McGhee, R.B., Jr.; et al. Role of imaging in pretreatment evaluation of early invasive cervical cancer: Results of the intergroup study American College of Radiology Imaging Network 6651-Gynecologic Oncology Group 183. *J. Clin. Oncol.* **2005**, *23*, 9329–9337. [CrossRef] [PubMed]
4. Fischerova, D.; Cibula, D. Ultrasound in Gynecological Cancer: Is It Time for Re-evaluation of Its Uses? *Curr. Oncol. Rep.* **2015**, *17*, 28. [CrossRef]
5. Bipat, S.; Glas, A.S.; Van Der Velden, J.; Zwinderman, A.H.; Bossuyt, P.M.M.; Stoker, J. Computed tomography and magnetic resonance imaging in staging of uterine cervical carcinoma: A systematic review. *Gynecol. Oncol.* **2003**, *91*, 59–66. [CrossRef]
6. Patel-Lippmann, K.; Robbins, J.B.; Barroilhet, L.; Anderson, B.; Sadowski, E.A.; Boyum, J. MR Imaging of Cervical Cancer. *Magn. Reson. Imaging Clin. N. Am.* **2017**, *25*, 635–649. [CrossRef]
7. Fischerová, D.; Cibula, D.; Stenhova, H.; Vondrichova, H.; Calda, P.; Zikan, M.; Freitag, P.; Slama, J.; Dundr, P.; Belacek, J. Transrectal ultrasound and magnetic resonance imaging in staging of early cervical cancer. *Int. J. Gynecol. Cancer* **2008**, *18*, 766–772. [CrossRef]
8. Testa, A.C.; Ludovisi, M.; Manfredi, R.; Zannoni, G.; Gui, B.; Basso, D.; Di Legge, A.; Licameli, A.; Di Bidino, R.; Scambia, G.; et al. Transvaginal ultrasonography and magnetic resonance imaging for assessment of presence, size and extent of invasive cervical cancer. *Ultrasound Obstet. Gynecol.* **2009**, *34*, 335–344. [CrossRef] [PubMed]
9. Epstein, E.; Testa, A.; Gaurilcikas, A.; Di Legge, A.; Ameye, L.; Atstupenaite, V.; Valentini, A.L.; Gui, B.; Wallengren, N.-O.; Pudaric, S.; et al. Early-stage cervical cancer: Tumor delineation by magnetic resonance imaging and ultrasound—A European multicenter trial. *Gynecol. Oncol.* **2013**, *128*, 449–453. [CrossRef]
10. Testa, A.C.; Ferrandina, G.; Moro, F.; Pasciuto, T.; Moruzzi, M.C.; De Blasis, I.; Mascilini, F.; Foti, E.; Autorino, R.; Collarino, A.; et al. PRospective Imaging of CErvical cancer and neoadjuvant treatment (PRICE) study: Role of ultrasound to predict partial response in locally advanced cervical cancer patients undergoing chemoradiation and radical surgery. *Ultrasound Obstet Gynecol.* **2018**, *51*, 684–695. [CrossRef]
11. Epstein, E.; Di Legge, A.; Måsbäck, A.; Lindqvist, P.G.; Kannisto, P.; Testa, A.C. Sonographic characteristics of squamous cell cancer and adenocarcinoma of the uterine cervix. *Ultrasound Obs Gynecol.* **2010**, *36*, 512–516. [CrossRef] [PubMed]
12. Testa, A.C.; Di Legge, A.; De Blasis, I.; Moruzzi, M.C.; Bonatti, M.; Collarino, A.; Rufini, V.; Manfredi, R. Imaging techniques for the evaluation of cervical cancer. *Best Pract. Res. Clin. Obstet. Gynaecol.* **2014**, *28*, 741–768. [CrossRef] [PubMed]
13. Dessole, S.; Farina, M.; Rubattu, G.; Cosmi, E.; Ambrosini, G.; Nardelli, G.B. Sonovaginography is a new technique for assessing rectovaginal endometriosis. *Fertil. Steril.* **2003**, *79*, 1023–1027. [CrossRef]
14. Sibal, M. Gel sonovaginography: A new way of evaluating a variety of local vaginal and cervical disorders. *J. Ultrasound Med.* **2016**, *35*, 2699–2715. [CrossRef] [PubMed]
15. Arezzo, F.; Cormio, G.; La Forgia, D.; Kawosha, A.A.; Mongelli, M.; Putino, C.; Silvestris, E.; Oreste, D.; Lombardi, C.; Cazzato, G.; et al. The Application of Sonovaginography for Implementing Ultrasound Assessment of Endometriosis and Other Gynaecological Diseases. *Diagnostics* **2022**, *12*, 820. [CrossRef]
16. Salvo, G.; Odetto, D.; Saez Perrotta, M.C.; Noll, F.; Perrotta, M.; Pareja, R.; Wernicke, A.; Ramirez, P.T. Measurement of tumor size in early cervical cancer: An ever-evolving paradigm. *Int. J. Gynecol. Cancer* **2020**, *13*, 1215–1223. [CrossRef]
17. Gaurilcikas, A.; Vaitkiene, D.; Cizauskas, A.; Inciura, A.; Svedas, E.; Maciuleviciene, R.; Di Legge, A.; Ferrandina, G.; Testa, A.C.; Valentin, L. Early-stage cervical cancer: Agreement between ultrasound and histopathological findings with regard to tumor size and extent of local disease. *Ultrasound Obstet. Gynecol.* **2011**, *38*, 707–715. [CrossRef]
18. Moloney, F.; Twomey, M.; Hewitt, M.; Barry, J.; Ryan, D.J. Comparison of MRI and high-resolution transvaginal sonography for the local staging of cervical cancer. *J. Clin. Ultrasound* **2015**, *44*, 78–84. [CrossRef]
19. Testa, A.C.; Di Legge, A.; Virgilio, B.; Bonatti, M.; Manfredi, R.; Mirk, P.; Rufini, V. Which imaging technique should we use in the follow up of gynaecological cancer? *Best Pract. Res. Clin. Obstet. Gynaecol.* **2014**, *28*, 769–791. [CrossRef]
20. Goldberg, Y.; Siegler, Y.; Segev, Y.; Mandel, R.; Siegler, E.; Auslander, R.; Lavie, O. The added benefit of transvaginal sonography in the clinical staging of cervical carcinoma. *Acta Obstet. Gynecol. Scand.* **2019**, *99*, 312–316. [CrossRef]
21. Sozzi, G.; Berretta, R.; Fiengo, S.; Ferreri, M.; Giallombardo, V.; Finazzo, F.; Messana, D.; Capozzi, V.A.; Colacurci, N.; Scambia, G.; et al. Integrated pre-surgical diagnostic algorithm to define extent of disease in cervical cancer. *Int. J. Gynecol. Cancer* **2019**, *30*, 16–20. [CrossRef] [PubMed]
22. Alcázar, J.L.; Arribas, S.; Minguez, J.A.; Jurado, M. The Role of Ultrasound in the Assessment of Uterine Cervical Cancer. *J. Obstet. Gynecol. India* **2014**, *64*, 311–316. [CrossRef] [PubMed]

23. Palsdottir, K.; Fischerová, D.; Franchi, D.; Testa, A.C.; Di Legge, A.; Epstein, E. Preoperative prediction of lymph node metastasis and deep stromal invasion in women with invasive cervical cancer: Prospective multicenter study using 2D and 3D ultrasound. *Ultrasound Obstet. Gynecol.* **2015**, *45*, 470–475. [CrossRef] [PubMed]
24. Olthof, E.P.; van der Aa, M.A.; Adam, J.A.; Stalpers, L.J.A.; Wenzel, H.H.B.; van der Velden, J.; Mom, C.H. The role of lymph nodes in cervical cancer: Incidence and identification of lymph node metastases—A literature review. *Int. J. Clin. Oncol.* **2021**, *26*, 1600–1610. [CrossRef] [PubMed]

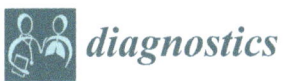

Article

Clinical, Sonographic, and Hysteroscopic Features of Endometrial Carcinoma Diagnosed after Hysterectomy in Patients with a Preoperative Diagnosis of Atypical Hyperplasia: A Single-Center Retrospective Study

Luca Pace [1], Silvia Actis [1,*], Matteo Mancarella [1], Lorenzo Novara [2], Luca Mariani [1], Gaetano Perrini [2], Francesca Govone [1], Alessandra Testi [1], Paola Campisi [3], Annamaria Ferrero [1] and Nicoletta Biglia [1]

1. Gynecology and Obstetrics Unit, Umberto I Hospital, Department of Surgical Sciences, University of Turin, Largo Turati 62, 10128 Turin, Italy
2. Gynecology and Obstetrics Unit, Umberto I Hospital, Largo Turati 62, 10128 Turin, Italy
3. Anatomic Pathology Unit, Umberto I Hospital, Largo Turati 62, 10128 Turin, Italy
* Correspondence: silvia.actis@unito.it

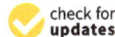

Citation: Pace, L.; Actis, S.; Mancarella, M.; Novara, L.; Mariani, L.; Perrini, G.; Govone, F.; Testi, A.; Campisi, P.; Ferrero, A.; et al. Clinical, Sonographic, and Hysteroscopic Features of Endometrial Carcinoma Diagnosed after Hysterectomy in Patients with a Preoperative Diagnosis of Atypical Hyperplasia: A Single-Center Retrospective Study. *Diagnostics* **2022**, *12*, 3029. https://doi.org/10.3390/diagnostics12123029

Academic Editors: Fabio Bottari and Anna Daniela Iacobone

Received: 31 October 2022
Accepted: 30 November 2022
Published: 2 December 2022

Publisher's Note: MDPI stays neutral with regard to jurisdictional claims in published maps and institutional affiliations.

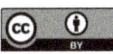

Copyright: © 2022 by the authors. Licensee MDPI, Basel, Switzerland. This article is an open access article distributed under the terms and conditions of the Creative Commons Attribution (CC BY) license (https://creativecommons.org/licenses/by/4.0/).

Abstract: Background: atypical endometrial hyperplasia (AEH) is a precancerous condition implying a high risk of concurrent endometrial cancer (EC), which might be occult and only diagnosed at postoperative histopathological examination after hysterectomy. Our study aimed to investigate potential differences in preoperative clinical, sonographic, and hysteroscopic characteristics in patients with AEH and postoperative diagnosis of EC. Methods: a retrospective single-center study was carried out on a case series of 80 women with AEH undergoing diagnostic workup, including ultrasonography and hysteroscopy, with subsequent hysterectomy. Women with AEH confirmed at the histopathological examination were compared with patients with a postoperative diagnosis of EC. Results: in our population, EC was diagnosed in 53 women, whereas the preoperative diagnosis of AEH was confirmed in 27 cases. At ultrasonography, women with occult EC showed greater endometrial thickness (20.3 mm vs. 10.3 mm, $p\ 0.001$) and size of the endocavitary lesion (maximum diameter 25.2 mm vs. 10.6 mm, $p\ 0.001$), and a higher prevalence of irregular endometrial-myometrial junction (40.5% vs. 6.7%, $p\ 0.022$) and endouterine vascularization at color Doppler (64.2% vs. 34.6%, $p\ 0.017$). At hysteroscopy, patients with occult EC showed a higher prevalence of necrosis (44.2% vs. 4.2%, $p\ 0.001$) and atypical vessels (70.6% vs. 33.3%, $p\ 0.003$), whereas true AEH mainly presented as a protruding intracavitary lesion (77.8% vs. 50.9%, $p\ 0.029$). In EC, subjective assessment by the operator was more frequently indicative of cancer (80.0% vs. 12.5%). No difference was found for clinical variables. Conclusions: occult EC in AEH may exhibit some differences in ultrasonographic and hysteroscopic patterns of presentation compared with real AEH, which could prompt a more significant suspect for the possible presence of concurrent EC at preoperative diagnostic workup.

Keywords: atypical endometrial hyperplasia; endometrial cancer; hysteroscopy; transvaginal ultrasound

1. Introduction

Endometrial hyperplasia (EH) is defined as an irregular proliferation of the endometrial glands leading to an increase in the gland-to-stroma ratio in contrast to proliferative endometrium.

The histological classification of EH has undergone numerous changes over the years, reflecting its diagnostic complexity and making it difficult to compare studies performed with different classifications. In 2014, the World Health Organization (WHO) suggested a dichotomous classification of EH [1], which was accepted by the International Society of Gynecological Pathologists, to reduce the multitude of terms used worldwide. EH has been divided into two groups: non-atypical EH/benign hyperplasia and atypical EH (AEH) or Endometrial Intraepithelial Neoplasia (EIN) according to the presence or absence of atypical cytological features. AEH is a premalignant lesion, with an approximately 30% risk of progression to endometrial carcinoma (EC) [2,3]. The prevalence of concurrent occult EC in patients diagnosed with AEH undergoing hysterectomy approaches 43% [4]. EC is the most common gynecologic cancer in women; it is a more common disease among postmenopausal women, but in the last few years, there has been a rise in the number of EC among premenopausal women [5]. EC is more prevalent in high/intermediate-developed countries [6].

Preoperative diagnostics play a central role in defining the correct treatment course of action and surgical approach of AEH and EC. For instance, although lymph node evaluation remains crucial in the surgical management of endometrial carcinoma, there remain no clear consensus guidelines regarding nodal evaluation in patients with AEH.

Pre-operative identification of factors that may help to stratify a patient's risk of concurrent EC is mandatory to reduce the risk of over- or under-treatment.

Our study aims at evaluating the presence of pre-operative clinical, ultrasonographic, hysteroscopic, and anatomopathological features in patients with a hysteroscopic diagnosis of AEH and a postoperative diagnosis of EC.

2. Materials and Methods

The study was retrospectively conducted on patients who underwent hysterectomy for AEH at the Obstetrics and Gynecology University Department of Mauriziano Umberto I Hospital in Turin from January 2015 to September 2022.

Data were retrieved through a retrospective review of hospital medical records.

The inclusion criteria were women diagnosed with AEH on hysteroscopic endometrial biopsy with a subsequent total hysterectomy and bilateral salpingo-oophorectomy and histopathological examination of the uterus.

The exclusion criteria were the absence of any available report of preoperative ultrasound examination and/or endometrial biopsy, and women who were conservatively managed and/or received medical therapy before surgery.

All patients were referred to our center for diagnostic evaluation, including transvaginal ultrasound (TVUS) and hysteroscopy for abnormal uterine bleeding or after the finding of sonographic anomalies of the endometrium during a routine scan at outpatient clinics. Diagnostic protocol at our center routinely included:

- An interview with the patient to collect anamnestic and clinical data.
- A TVUS performed by an expert highly-trained sonographer (L.M.) with an Affiniti 70 ultrasound machine (Philips, Amsterdam, The Netherlands, 2013) equipped either with a C10-3v Endocavitary Probe with a 3.0–10.0 MHz frequency range; all examinations were performed according to the recommendations of the main international guidelines [7,8].
- A hysteroscopy was performed in an outpatient setting by two highly trained expert operators (A.F. and G.P.) with an endometrial biopsy. All the procedures included vaginoscopy, distension of the uterine cavity with normal saline, diagnostic evaluation of the cervical canal and uterine cavity with visualization of tubal ostia, and targeted biopsy on any suspicious area of the endometrium using a BETTOCCHI® Hysteroscope equipped with bipolar electrode systems [9]. Diagnosis of AEH was made on endometrial specimens according to WHO 2014 criteria [1].

TVUS was always performed at our center before the hysteroscopy assessment.

After the diagnosis, all the patients included in the study underwent a total hysterectomy and bilateral salpingo-oophorectomy according to the management suggested by the main international guidelines [10,11]. Histopathological examination of the uterus was obtained, either confirming AEH or revealing EC.

Data were retrospectively collected about:

- The anamnestic features, including age, body mass index (BMI), parity, menopausal status, the prevalence of diabetes and hypertension, use of hormone replacement therapy or tamoxifen, and symptoms;
- The ultrasound characteristics regarding endometrial thickness and echogenicity, endometrial–myometrial junction, presence of intracavitary fluid, vascularization at color Doppler (CD) study, size and appearance of the lesion, posterior sliding sign, uterine volume calculated by the formula ellipsoid volume [12], and presence of leiomyomas;
- The hysteroscopic reports about the appearance of the lesion (protruding into the uterine cavity vs. superficial anomaly of the endometrium), presence of necrosis or atypical vascular pattern, subjective assessment indicative of carcinoma by the operator, and visualization of tubal ostia;
- The histopathological reports on the endometrial biopsy regarding the presence of endometrial intraepithelial neoplasia, multiple foci of hyperplasia, and endometrial polyp with AEH arising on its surface, and the number of specimens retrieved by the hysteroscopy operator;
- Histopathological reports on the uterus, most notably the presence of endometrial carcinoma and its features according to WHO 2014 classification [13].

Statistical Analysis

The study population was divided into two groups according to the presence or absence of EC at the histopathological examination of the uterus after hysterectomy. The two groups were compared for the variables collected to evaluate potential differences in preoperative features.

Continuous variables were expressed as mean ± standard error (SE), and categorical variables were expressed as n (%). Univariate analysis was performed for continuous variables with a two-tailed t-test for independent samples with unequal variances, and categorical variables with a Fisher's test after checking with the Kolmogorov–Smirnov test that the distribution of our samples did not differ from the normal one. A difference was considered statistically significant when it was associated with a two-tailed $p < 0.05$.

Statistical analyses were performed using SPSS 22.0 (Statistical Package for the Social Sciences) software (IBM Corp. Released 2013. IBM SPSS Statistics for Windows, Version 22.0. Armonk, NY, USA: IBM Corp.).

3. Results

The archiving software (Winsapp vers. 3) of the Pathology Department of Mauriziano Umberto I Hospital was used for patient selection.

Through a search with the query "endometrial hyperplasia" of patients undergoing hysteroscopy, 492 patients with a diagnosis of EH at biopsy were identified.

Of these, 317 were excluded given the diagnosis of EH without atypia. Of the remaining 178, 54 were excluded because they underwent surgery at another center. An additional 32 patients were excluded because a qualitatively inferior and different ultrasound was used compared with the Philips Affiniti 70 model. Two were excluded because of synchronous diagnosis of endometrioid adenocarcinoma of the ovary and inability to establish with certainty the origin of the primary lesion. For seven patients, anamnestic data (abnormal uterine bleeding [AUB], BMI, and comorbidities) could not be found and it was, therefore, decided not to include them in the case series. Our study population included 80 women who were diagnosed with AEH from January 2015 to September 2022 at our center and underwent surgery. Table 1 summarizes the characteristics of this population: most women were post-menopausal (87.0%) with a mean age of 64.9 years; a high prevalence of obesity (45.1%) was seen with a mean BMI 30.7 kg/m^2; and in 67.5% of cases, AUB was reported and prompted diagnostic evaluation. Among the tests performed during the work-up, TVUS highlighted a high prevalence of endometrial thickening as sonographic presentation, with a mean thickness of 16.4 mm which is far above the high-risk cut-off suggested by the literature [7].

Table 1. Characteristics of the study population.

Category	Characteristics	
Clinical features	Age at diagnosis (years) *	64.9 ± 1.1
	BMI (kg/m^2) *	30.7 ± 1.0
	Obesity (%)	32 (45.1)
	Diabetes (%)	16 (21.6)
	Hypertension (%)	40 (54.1)
	Number of VD *	1.2 ± 0.1
	Post-menopausal status (%)	67 (87.0)
	Time between menopause and diagnosis (years)	14.7 ± 1.1
	Use of HRT (%)	0 (0)
	Use of tamoxifene (%)	5 (6.9)
	Presence of AUB (%)	52 (67.5)
Ultrasonography features	Endometrial thickness (mm) *	16.3 ± 1.7
	Non-uniform endometrial echogenicity (%)	10 (12.5)
	Irregular endometrial–myometrial junction (%)	18 (31.6)
	Intracavitary fluid (%)	6 (8.5)
	Intracavitary vascularization at CD (%)	43 (54.4)
	Focal endometrial lesion (%)	24 (37.5)
	Maximum diameter of the lesion (ml) *	22.0 ± 2.5
	Volume of the uterus (cm^3) *	76.4 ± 6.6
	Presence of uterine fibroids (%)	29 (41.4)
Hysteroscopy features	Protruding intracavitary lesion (%)	48 (60)
	Necrosis (%)	24 (31.6)
	Atypical vascularization (%)	44 (58.7)
	Visualization of tubal ostia (%)	80 (100)
	Subjective assessment suggesting cancer (%)	43 (58.1)
	EH on endometrial polyps (%)	41 (52.6)
	EIN (%)	6 (7.7)
	Multiple foci of hyperplasia (%)	30 (42.9)
	Number of endometrial biopsies *	1.7 ± 0.07

BMI, body mass index; VD, vaginal delivery; HRT, hormone replacement therapy; CD, color Doppler; AUB, abnormal uterine bleeding; EH, endometrial hyperplasia; EIN, endometrial intraepithelial neoplasia; patients are classified as obese when their body mass index (BMI) is over 30 kg/m^2. *: data are reported as mean ± standard error.

At the histopathological examination of the uterus after surgery, EC was revealed in 53 women, whereas the preoperative diagnosis of EAH was confirmed in 27 patients (Figure 1).

The cases of malignancy were all represented by EC, with coexistent hyperplasia confirmed in 29 out of 53 women (54.7%). Twenty-eight EC cases were histological grade 1 (52.8%), twenty-three cases were classified as grade 2 (43.4%), two cases as grade 3 (3.8%), and lymphovascular invasion was reported in fifteen patients (28.3%). The endometrial invasion was detected in 44 (83%) of the 53 EC. Most EC patients (34 out of 53 women, 66.0%) were classified as stage Ia according to FIGO classification [14].

The group of patients with a postoperative diagnosis of EC was compared with the group of women for whom the diagnosis of AEH was confirmed to analyze potential differences in the variables relating to preoperative presentation.

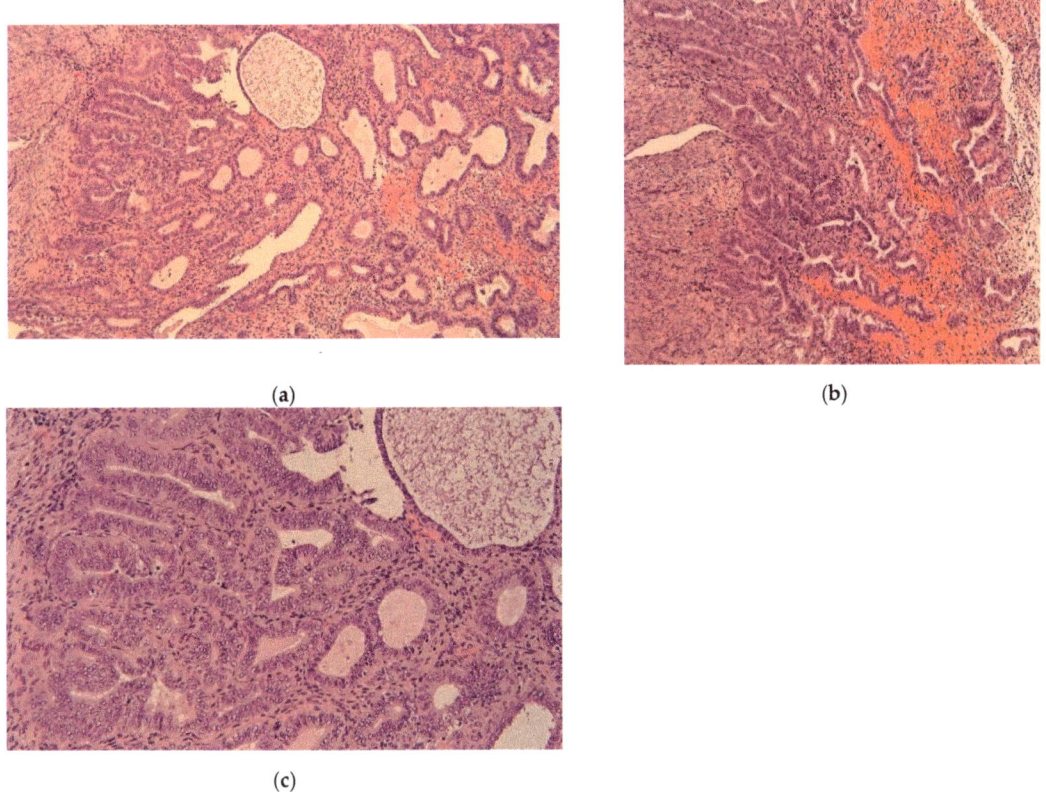

Figure 1. Histopathological images of atypical endometrial hyperplasia (a–c).

Table 2 shows the results regarding the anamnestic features of the two groups, which appeared to be similar without any statistically significant difference, although patients with EC were on average older ($p = 0.09$).

Table 2. Anamnestic features of the study groups.

Variables	Endometrial Hyperplasia (N = 27)	Endometrial Carcinoma (N = 53)	p [§]
Age at diagnosis (years) *	62.3 ± 1.8	66.2 ± 1.4	0.09
BMI (kg/m^2) *	29.3 ± 1.5	31.4 ± 1.2	0.29
Obesity (%)	11 (47.8)	21 (43.8)	0.80
Diabetes (%)	5 (20.8)	11 (22.0)	0.91
Hypertension (%)	11 (45.8)	29 (58)	0.46
Number of VD *	1.1 ± 0.2	1.3 ± 0.2	0.42
Post-menopausal status (%)	23 (88.5)	44 (86.3)	0.79
Time between menopause and diagnosis (years) *	12.6 ± 1.9	15.7 ± 1.4	0.19
Use of HRT (%)	0 (0)	0 (0)	-
Use of tamoxifene (%)	1 (4.0)	4 (8.5)	0.65
Presence of AUB (%)	15 (57.7)	37 (72.5)	0.21

BMI, body mass index; VD, vaginal delivery; HRT, hormone replacement therapy; AUB, abnormal uterine bleeding; patients are classified as obese when their body mass index (BMI) is over 30 kg/m^2. *: data are reported as mean ± standard error. [§]: analysis was carried out with a two-tailed t-test for independent samples with unequal variances for continuous variables, and with Fisher's test for categorical variables.

In Table 3, the main sonographic characteristics of the two groups are shown, highlighting significantly greater endometrial thickness and size of the lesion measured at TVUS for the women with EC. This difference is also relevant in absolute terms, with measures that are on average double the ones reported in AEH patients (notably, 10.3 vs. 20.3 mm for endometrial thickness). Among the other variables, cases of EC showed a significantly higher proportion of irregularity in the appearance of the endometrial–myometrial junction and the presence of endometrial vascularization, expressed by a color score of 2 or higher in the Doppler study.

Table 3. Ultrasound features of the endometrial lesions in the two groups.

Variables	Endometrial Hyperplasia (N = 27)	Endometrial Carcinoma (N = 53)	p §
Endometrial thickness (mm) *	10.3 ± 1.3	20.3 ± 2.4	**0.001**
Non-uniform endometrial echogenicity (%)	2 (7.4)	8 (15.1)	0.48
Irregular endometrial-myometrial junction (%)	1 (6.7)	17 (40.5)	**0.022**
Intracavitary fluid (%)	2 (8.7)	4 (8.3)	0.96
Intracavitary vascularization at CD (%)	9 (34.6)	34 (64.2)	**0.017**
Focal endometrial lesion (%)	8 (44.4)	16 (34.8)	0.57
Maximum diameter of the lesion (mm) *	10.6 ± 2.5	25.2 ± 3.0	**0.001**
Volume of the uterus (cm^3) *	78.5 ± 10.4	75.6 ± 8.3	0.83
Presence of uterine fibroids (%)	6 (27.3)	23 (47.9)	0.12

CD, color Doppler. *: data are reported as mean ± standard error. §: analysis was carried out with a two-tailed t-test for independent samples with unequal variances for continuous variables, and with Fisher's test for categorical variables.

In Tables 4 and 5, findings at hysteroscopy and histopathological examination of endometrial biopsies are shown: among women with EC, a significantly higher prevalence of necrosis (44.2%) and atypical vascularization (70.6%) was reported. In about half of the cases, a surface or nodular growth was described for the lesion. On the contrary, in patients with AEH, the most common presentation was a polypoid lesion protruding into the uterine cavity (77.8%), with a frequent histopathological report of atypical cells in the context of an endometrial polyp (73.1%). It is noteworthy that in 80.0% of cases of endometrial carcinoma, a subjective assessment of malignancy was provided by the operator performing hysteroscopy, whereas this evaluation was reported just in 12.5% of cases of hyperplasia.

Table 4. Hysteroscopic findings in the two groups.

Variables	Endometrial Hyperplasia (N = 27)	Endometrial Carcinoma (N = 53)	p §
Protruding intracavitary lesion (%)	21 (77.8)	27 (50.9)	**0.029**
Necrosis (%)	1 (4.2)	23 (44.2)	**0.001**
Atypical vascularization (%)	8 (33.3)	36 (70.6)	**0.003**
Visualization of tubal ostia (%)	27 (100)	53 (100)	-
Subjective assessment suggesting cancer (%)	3 (12.5)	40 (80.0)	**0.001**

§ analysis was carried out with a two-tailed t-test for independent samples with unequal variances for continuous variables, and with Fisher's test for categorical variables.

Table 5. Histopathologic pre-operative features of the endometrial lesions in the two groups.

Variables	Endometrial Hyperplasia (N = 27)	Endometrial Carcinoma (N = 53)	p §
EH on endometrial polyp (%)	19 (73.1)	22 (42.3)	**0.016**
Multiple foci of hyperplasia (%)	11 (44.0)	19 (42.2)	0.86
Number of endometrial biopsies *	1.7 ± 0.1	1.7 ± 0.1	0.94

EH, endometrial hyperplasia; EIN, endometrial intraepithelial neoplasia. *: data are reported as mean ± standard error. §: analysis carried out with a two-tailed t-test for independent samples with unequal variances for continuous variables, and with Fisher's test for categorical variables.

4. Discussion

The present study analyzed several pre-operative factors, including patient characteristics and ultrasonographic, hysteroscopic, and anatomopathological features in patients pre-operatively diagnosed with AEH.

No statistically significant factor suggestive of concomitant EC could be identified regarding the anamnestic data analyzed. Obesity, diabetes, and hypertension were found to be similarly prevalent in both groups under analysis. This is in agreement with the literature, where the above risk factors are common in both diseases, and no medical comorbidities appear to be associated with concurrent EC in patients pre-operatively diagnosed with AEH [3,15].

In the present study, women with EC were on average of older age compared with real AEH, although no statistically significant difference was detected ($p = 0.09$). In the literature, older age seems predictive of concurrent EC at the time of hysterectomy for AEH [3,15]. The non-significance of the result in our study could be related to the low sample size.

Among ultrasonographic features, it appears that a thickened endometrial stripe, a greater diameter of the lesion, an interrupted endometrial–myometrial junction, and a high vascular density at CD was associated with increased odds of EC.

Results on endometrial thickness are consistent with prior data from Vetter et al. [3] on a retrospective case series of 169 patients, and from Abt et al. [16] on 378 patients. Both retrospective studies demonstrated that among patients with a preoperative diagnosis of AEH, those with preoperative endometrial stripe $\geq$ 20 mm were more likely to have concurrent EC. According to a prospective study on 2216 patients with AUB by the International Endometrial Tumor Analysis (IETA), endometrial thickness predictive for AEH is attested at 10.1 mm, while a mean endometrial thickness of 16 mm looks predictive for the EC [17]. The relevance and reproducibility of different studies of this finding should be applied in clinical practice by suggesting that endometrial thickness might be used as one preoperative determinant (Figure 2).

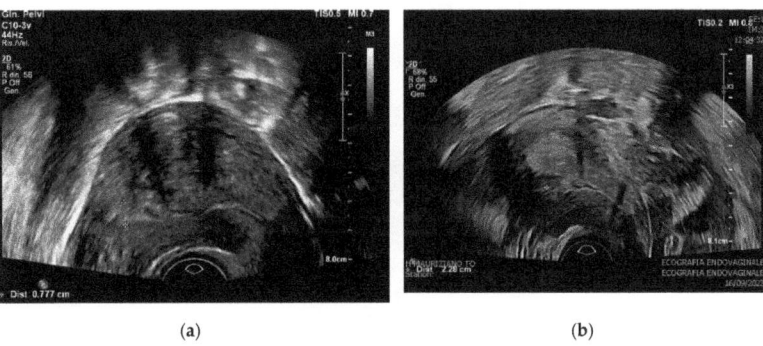

(a)   (b)

Figure 2. Transvaginal ultrasound (TVUS), endometrial thickness of two patients with a preoperative di-agnosis of atypical endometrial hyperplasia (AEH). (a) TVUS: 7.7 mm of endometrial thickness with a posterior leiomyoma of the uterus, postoperative diagnosis of AEH. (b) TVUS: 22.8 mm of en-dometrial thickness, postoperative diagnosis of endometrial cancer pT1a G2.

In our study, a greater ultrasonography diameter of the lesion appears to be strongly correlated with the presence of occult EC. This finding is not well investigated in the literature. A retrospective study on 250 patients which analyzed the diagnostic value of endometrial volume under 3D ultrasound acquisition in endometrial lesions demonstrated that the endometrial volume was bigger in the EC group [18].

Regarding the ultrasound assessment of the vascularization of the lesion, although this is a remarkably operator-dependent finding, it has been reported in the literature that flow characteristics such as resistance (RI), pulsatility (PI), and peak systolic velocity (PSV) can also help in the differential diagnosis [19].

In the present study, a significant difference was reported for the presence of intracavitary vascularization in the Doppler study, since 64.2% of cases of EC were described as color score 2 or higher at ultrasonography. This result is consistent with the prospective study by Van Den Bosh [20] where a highly vascularized pattern of presentation with a color score of 3 or 4 at CD has been attributed to 65% of EC.

In the prospective study by Van Den Bosh on 2216 patients, a regular endometrial–myometrial junction at ultrasonography is reported in 65% of AEH, very similar compared with EC in which endometrial–myometrial junction is described as irregular in 42% of cases [20]. In our study, 93.3% of AEH showed regular endometrial–myometrial junction, while only one case (6.3%) had an altered endometrial–myometrial junction. The regular endometrial–myometrial junction at ultrasonography appears in a much lower percentage of EC (40%), in which altered junction was described as irregular in 60% of cases. This result can be analyzed considering the postoperative histologic results; in fact, in our case series, 83% of EC showed endometrial invasion. This data is not available in the previously mentioned study, so we cannot assess inhomogeneity in the case series. Furthermore, this variable is an extremely subjective, highly operator-dependent assessment.

Hysteroscopy is considered the gold standard to diagnose endometrial lesions that are clinically or sonographically suspected. Hysteroscopy is a sensitive and specific method to identify coexisting endometrial carcinoma in patients with an AEH diagnosis [21]. Standard hysteroscopy has better results than curette for aspirated endometrial sampling, such as Vabra sampling, which often fails to correctly diagnose endometrial polyps, as the samples have often insufficient endometrial mucosa [22]. That is, the visual assessment of the endometrial cavity reduces blind sampling. Even other poor sensitivity endometrial sampling techniques, such as dilation and curettage, cannot be considered reliable. One of the main advantages of hysteroscopy is the possibility to have a subjective evaluation of the endometrial pattern [23]. It is, therefore, necessary to perform a visual hysteroscopy, as a direct view of the lesion and its relationship to the uterine cavity is necessary for proper assessment (Figure 3).

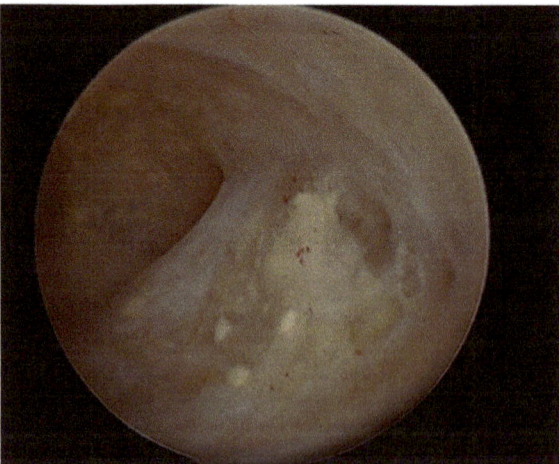

Figure 3. Hysteroscopic image of atypical endometrial hyperplasia (AEH).

As for the hysteroscopic phase of preoperative diagnostics in our case series, the presence of necrosis and an atypical vascularization proved to be strongly indicative of EC.

Necrosis at hysteroscopic evaluation in our study has been much more frequently detected in occult EC than in AEH at postoperative assessment (44.2% vs. 4.2%). This is consistent with the literature where necrosis has been included in many hysteroscopic scores for the diagnosis of suspected EC [23].

Atypical vascularization (Figure 4) in our case series, was more frequently found in the case of occult EC (70.6%) compared with AEH (33.3%). Atypical vascularization usually includes the finding of abnormal vessel sprouts, tortuous vessels, vessel loops, branching with angles over 90°, narrowing of vessels, a disorganized network, and an overall irregular distribution with an area with dense vessels, varying with an area without vessels [23]. The abnormal vascularization has been reported to be suggestive of malignant neoplastic lesions of the endometrium, but this finding appears to have been derived from large retrospective cohorts and not from randomized controlled trials [24]. However, a simple increased vascular density must be combined with other parameters in the diagnosis of cancer [25].

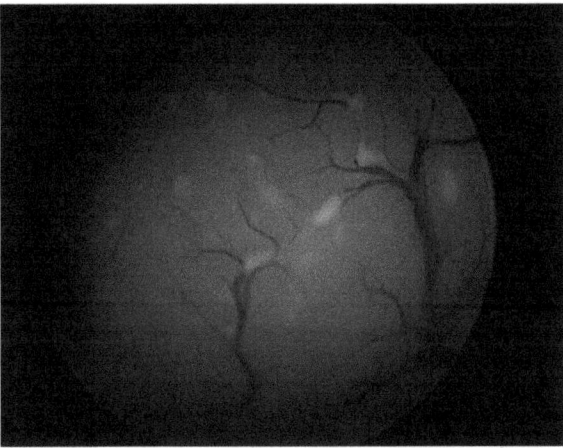

Figure 4. Atypical vascularization at hysteroscopic evaluation.

The finding of a protruding intracavitary lesion, on the other hand, seems to be more frequent in the case of AEH. This result is consistent with evidence from the literature in which it appears that the hysteroscopic finding of a polyp only rarely correlates with the presence of hyperplasia (about 2% of the cases), and subsequently of a cancerous polyp [22].

The sensitivity and specificity of hysteroscopic subjective assessment in determining the risk of adenocarcinoma have been investigated in numerous studies. The major limitation of this parameter is that it is the result of the subjective evaluation of numerous parameters that are not strictly determined. As a result, hysteroscopic subjective assessment emerges with a wide heterogeneity among different studies. Despite this point, subjective assessment is a valuable tool in the hands of an experienced clinician [15,26,27]. In our case series, subjective assessment ensured superior performance to that found in the literature, with 80% of EC correctly identified by the expert clinician's report as high-risk lesions.

To standardize the subjective assessment reports, a structured hysteroscopic score based on lesion surface, necrosis, and vessels has been suggested [23]. Considering the relevance of subjective assessment in the diagnostic procedure of AEH, the definition of standardized and shared criteria for use by experienced operators appears to be a necessary development to improve the diagnostic definition of these lesions.

One of the most controversial issues in the field of endometrial carcinoma is the selection of patients for lymph node staging to avert the risk of understaging. In this regard, preoperative diagnosis of adenocarcinoma is crucial in establishing the correct diagnostic and therapeutic course. Several studies have demonstrated that routine sentinel lymph node biopsy (SLNB) in all patients with AEH has limited benefit and is not cost-effective [28–30] given the high prevalence of low-grade and early-stage disease in this category. For AEH and early-stage low-grade EC, a comprehensive surgical staging with lymph node assessment via lymphadenectomy or SLNB would result in overtreatment [31]. Yet, 12% of patients with a pre-operative misdiagnosis of AEH show post-operative histology of EC at a more advanced stage or mid- to high grade. This latter population might benefit from lymph node assessment to guide adjuvant treatment [3].

In our case series, almost 34% of the EC had FIGO stage greater than or equal to IB (20.4% of all lesions), and 23% showed lymphovascular invasion.

The histological features of EC in patients with a previous diagnosis of AEH are remarkably heterogeneous in the literature. Myometrial invasion varies from 30 to 90% depending on the case series, while about 10% of cases show lymphovascular invasion [4,26].

This finding underscores the complexity of the histologic evaluation of hysteroscopic biopsy specimens and the need for accurate ultrasound examination by an experienced operator.

A strength of this study is the fact that demographic, anamnestic, hysteroscopic, and ultrasonographic parameters were evaluated in the same group of patients. Furthermore, the case series presented in our study is one of the largest in the literature to date analyzing all of the above parameters together in a single case series.

The major limitations of this study are the pure retrospective design, which makes it impossible to exclude possible confounding factors, and the fact that some of the variables are strongly based on subjective assessment. Subjective assessment is by its nature operator-dependent and directly influenced by the experience and skills of the operator. As a result, the ultrasound and hysteroscopic evidence of the present study may not widely apply to all centers and may not be universally generalizable. In addition to this, the small sample size may not have allowed additional potentially clinically relevant differences to be identified. Statistical power was not calculated.

Some future insights for improving the preoperative diagnostic definition of AEH can be identified. In any patient with preoperatively diagnosed AEH, the diagnostic evaluation should include both ultrasound and visual hysteroscopy performed by experienced clinicians. To make hysteroscopic parameters more reproducible and reduce the subjectivity of the assessment as much as possible, a consensus between expert operators to define high-risk hysteroscopic characteristics would be necessary. Integration into the diagnostic pathway of a comprehensive score, including both hysteroscopic and sonographic features, may be evaluated in the future. Ultimately, to ensure the best clinical management for high-risk patients with EC-suggestive criteria despite a preoperative diagnosis of AEH, centralized management to specialized EC centers might be suggested.

5. Conclusions

The importance of a detailed preoperative diagnosis of AEH and the difficulty in defining AEH on hysteroscopic biopsy dictate careful evaluation of features associated with the finding of AEH. Occult EC cases diagnosed after hysterectomy for AEH may have some differences at preoperative diagnostic workup compared with confirmed AEH cases. In our study, the endometrial thickness and other ultrasonographic features, such as thickened endometrial stripe, a greater diameter of the lesion, an interrupted endometrial–myometrial junction, and a high vascular density at CD, along with the subjective hysteroscopic assessment by experienced clinicians are elements that can suggest the presence of occult EC in patients with a preoperative histologic diagnosis of AEH.

The results of our study should be prospectively verified on larger and prospective case series. A multicenter prospective study should be conducted based on the prospective use of an inclusive score of standardized clinical, hysteroscopic, and ultrasound features in the preoperative diagnostic pathway. This is also to select a population of patients with a pre-operative misdiagnosis of AEH who might benefit from lymph node assessment to guide adjuvant treatment.

Patients with a pre-operative misdiagnosis of AEH show post-operative histology of EC at a more advanced stage or mid- to high grade. This latter population might benefit from lymph node assessment to guide adjuvant treatment.

Author Contributions: Conceptualization, L.N. and L.P.; methodology, M.M. and L.N.; validation, L.M., G.P. and A.F.; formal analysis, M.M.; investigation, L.P., S.A., F.G. and A.T.; resources, P.C., A.F. and N.B.; data curation, L.P., S.A. and M.M.; writing—original draft preparation, M.M., L.N., L.P. and S.A.; writing—review and editing, L.P. and S.A.; supervision, A.F. and N.B. All authors have read and agreed to the published version of the manuscript.

Funding: This research received no external funding.

Institutional Review Board Statement: The study was conducted per the 1964 Declaration of Helsinki. Since this was a retrospective study with no experimental research on participants, being all the procedures performed as part of the routine care according to international recommendations, exemption from formal approval was granted by the Ethics Committee of our institution when inquired.

Informed Consent Statement: Written informed consent was obtained from all individual participants included in the study. All patients gave their consent to the anonymous use and publication of clinical, instrumental, and photographic data for scientific purposes.

Data Availability Statement: The data presented in this study are available on request from the corresponding author.

Conflicts of Interest: The authors declare no conflict of interest.

References

1. Sobczuk, K.; Sobczuk, A. New classification system of endometrial hyperplasia WHO 2014 and its clinical implications. *Menopausal Rev.* **2017**, *16*, 107–111. [CrossRef]
2. Sanderson, P.A.; Critchley, H.O.; Williams, A.R.; Arends, M.J.; Saunders, P.T. New concepts for an old problem: The diagnosis of endometrial hyperplasia. *Hum. Reprod. Updat.* **2017**, *23*, 232–254. [CrossRef] [PubMed]
3. Vetter, M.H.; Smith, B.; Benedict, J.; Hade, E.M.; Bixel, K.; Copeland, L.J.; Cohn, D.E.; Fowler, J.M.; O'Malley, D.; Salani, R.; et al. Preoperative predictors of endometrial cancer at time of hysterectomy for endometrial intraepithelial neoplasia or complex atypical hyperplasia. *Am. J. Obstet. Gynecol.* **2020**, *222*, 60.e1–60.e7. [CrossRef] [PubMed]
4. Trimble, C.L.; Kauderer, J.; Zaino, R.; Silverberg, S.; Lim, P.C.; Burke, J.J.; Alberts, D.; Curtin, J. Concurrent endometrial carcinoma in women with a biopsy diagnosis of atypical endometrial hyperplasia: A Gynecologic Oncology Group study. *Cancer* **2006**, *106*, 812–819. [CrossRef] [PubMed]
5. Manap, N.A.; Ng, B.K.; Phon, S.E.; Karim, A.K.A.; Lim, P.S.; Fadhil, M. Endometrial Cancer in Pre-Menopausal Women and Younger: Risk Factors and Outcome. *Int. J. Environ. Res. Public Health* **2022**, *19*, 9059. [CrossRef]
6. Ferlay, J.; Colombet, M.; Soerjomataram, I.; Mathers, C.; Parkin, D.M.; Piñeros, M.; Znaor, A.; Bray, F. Estimating the global cancer incidence and mortality in 2018: GLOBOCAN sources and methods. *Int. J. Cancer* **2019**, *144*, 1941–1953. [CrossRef]
7. Leone, F.P.G.; Timmerman, D.; Bourne, T.; Valentin, L.; Epstein, E.; Goldstein, S.R.; Marret, H.; Parsons, A.K.; Gull, B.; Istre, O.; et al. Terms, definitions and measurements to describe the sonographic features of the endometrium and intrauterine lesions: A consensus opinion from the International Endometrial Tumor Analysis (IETA) group. *Ultrasound Obstet. Gynecol.* **2010**, *35*, 103–112. [CrossRef]
8. Van den Bosch, T.; Dueholm, M.; Leone, F.P.; Valentin, L.; Rasmussen, C.K.; Votino, A.; Van Schoubroeck, D.; Landolfo, C.; Installé, A.J.; Guerriero, S.; et al. Terms, definitions and measurements to describe sonographic features of myometrium and uterine masses: A consensus opinion from the Morphological Uterus Sonographic Assessment (MUSA) group. *Ultrasound Obstet. Gynecol.* **2015**, *46*, 284–298. [CrossRef]
9. Carugno, J.; Grimbizis, G.; Franchini, M.; Alonso, L.; Bradley, L.; Campo, R.; Catena, U.; De Angelis, C.; Sardo, A.D.S.; Farrugia, M.; et al. International Consensus Statement for recommended terminology describing hysteroscopic procedures. *Facts Views Vis. Obgyn.* **2021**, *13*, 287–294. [CrossRef]
10. Royal College of Obstetricians and Gynaecologists. *Management of Endometrial Hyperplasia (Green-top Guideline No. 67)*; RCOG/BSGE Joint Guideline | February 2016; Royal College of Obstetricians and Gynaecologists: London, UK, 2016.
11. Parkash, V.; Fadare, O.; Tornos, C.; McCluggage, W.G. Committee Opinion No. 631: Endometrial Intraepithelial Neoplasia. *Obstet. Gynecol.* **2015**, *126*, 897. [CrossRef]
12. Casikar, I.; Mongelli, M.; Reid, S.; Condous, G. Estimation of uterine volume: A comparison between Viewpoint and 3D ultrasound estimation in women undergoing laparoscopic hysterectomy. *Australas. J. Ultrasound Med.* **2015**, *18*, 27–32. [CrossRef] [PubMed]

13. Concin, N.; Creutzberg, C.L.; Vergote, I.; Cibula, D.; Mirza, M.R.; Marnitz, S.; Ledermann, J.A.; Bosse, T.; Chargari, C.; Fagotti, A.; et al. ESGO/ESTRO/ESP Guidelines for the management of patients with endometrial carcinoma. *Int. J. Gynecol. Cancer* **2021**, *478*, 153–190.
14. Koskas, M.; Amant, F.; Mirza, M.R.; Creutzberg, C.L. Cancer of the corpus uteri: 2021 update. *Int. J. Gynecol. Obstet.* **2021**, *155* (Suppl. 1), 45–60. [CrossRef]
15. Touboul, C.; Piel, B.; Koskas, M.; Gonthier, C.; Ballester, M.; Cortez, A.; Daraï, E. Factors predictive of endometrial carcinoma in patients with atypical endometrial hyperplasia on preoperative histology. *Anticancer Res.* **2014**, *34*, 5671–5676.
16. Abt, D.; Macharia, A.; Hacker, M.R.; Baig, R.; Esselen, K.M.; Ducie, J. Endometrial stripe thickness: A preoperative marker to identify patients with endometrial intraepithelial neoplasia who may benefit from sentinel lymph node mapping and biopsy. *Int. J. Gynecol. Cancer* **2022**, *32*, 1091–1097. [CrossRef] [PubMed]
17. Smith-Bindman, R.; Weiss, E.; Feldstein, V. How thick is too thick? When endometrial thickness should prompt biopsy in postmenopausal women without vaginal bleeding. *Ultrasound Obstet. Gynecol.* **2004**, *24*, 558–565. [CrossRef] [PubMed]
18. Liao, Y.M.; Li, Y.; Yu, H.X.; Li, Y.K.; Du, J.H.; Chen, H. Diagnostic value of endometrial volume and flow parameters under 3D ultrasound acquisition in combination with serum CA125 in endometrial lesions. *Taiwan Obstet. Gynecol.* **2021**, *60*, 492–497. [CrossRef]
19. Gharibvand, M.M.; Ahmadzade, A.; Azhine, S. Correlation of color Doppler ultrasound and pathological grading in endometrial carcinoma. *J. Fam. Med. Prim. Care* **2020**, *9*, 5188–5192. [CrossRef]
20. Bosch, T.V.D.; Verbakel, J.Y.; Valentin, L.; Wynants, L.; De Cock, B.; Pascual, M.A.; Leone, F.P.G.; Sladkevicius, P.; Alcazar, J.L.; Votino, A.; et al. Typical ultrasound features of various endometrial pathologies described using International Endometrial Tumor Analysis (IETA) terminology in women with abnormal uterine bleeding. *Ultrasound Obstet. Gynecol.* **2021**, *57*, 164–172. [CrossRef]
21. Garuti, G.; Mirra, M.; Luerti, M. Hysteroscopic view in atypical endometrial hyperplasias: A correlation with pathologic findings on hysterectomy specimens. *J. Minim. Invasive Gynecol.* **2006**, *13*, 325–330. [CrossRef]
22. Daniele, A.; Ferrero, A.; Maggiorotto, F.; Perrini, G.; Volpi, E.; Sismondi, P. Suspecting malignancy in endometrial polyps: Value of hysteroscopy. *Tumori J.* **2013**, *99*, 204–209. [CrossRef] [PubMed]
23. Dueholm, M.; Hjorth, I.M.; Secher, P.; Jørgensen, A.; Ørtoft, G. Structured Hysteroscopic Evaluation of Endometrium in Women With Postmenopausal Bleeding. *J. Minim. Invasive Gynecol.* **2015**, *22*, 1215–1224. [CrossRef] [PubMed]
24. Vitale, S.G.; Riemma, G.; Carugno, J.; Chiofalo, B.; Vilos, G.A.; Cianci, S.; Budak, M.S.; Lasmar, B.P.; Raffone, A.; Kahramanoglu, I. Hysteroscopy in the management of endometrial hyperplasia and cancer in reproductive aged women: New developments and current perspectives. *Transl. Cancer Res.* **2020**, *9*, 7767–7777. [CrossRef] [PubMed]
25. Spadoto-Dias, D.; Dias, F.N.B.; Dias, R.; Nahás-Neto, J.; Nahas, E.; Leite, N.J.; Domingues, M.A.C.; Angela, S.P.B.; Padovani, C.R. Usefulness of clinical, ultrasonographic, hysteroscopic, and immunohistochemical parameters in differentiating endometrial polyps from endometrial cancer. *J. Minim. Invasive Gynecol.* **2014**, *21*, 296–302. [CrossRef]
26. Shutter, J.; Wright, T.C., Jr. Prevalence of underlying adenocarcinoma in women with atypical endometrial hyperplasia. *Int. J. Gynecol. Pathol.* **2005**, *24*, 313–318. [CrossRef] [PubMed]
27. Miller, C.; Bidus, M.A.; Pulcini, J.P.; Maxwell, G.L.; Cosin, J.A.; Rose, G.S. The ability of endometrial biopsies with atypical complex hyperplasia to guide surgical management. *Am. J. Obstet. Gynecol.* **2008**, *199*, 69.e1–69.e4. [CrossRef] [PubMed]
28. Sullivan, M.W.; Philp, L.; Kanbergs, A.N.; Safdar, N.; Oliva, E.; Bregar, A.; del Carmen, M.G.; Eisenhauer, E.L.; Goodman, A.; Muto, M.; et al. Lymph node assessment at the time of hysterectomy has limited clinical utility for patients with pre-cancerous endometrial lesions. *Gynecol. Oncol.* **2021**, *162*, 613–618. [CrossRef]
29. Touhami, O.; Grégoire, J.; Renaud, M.C.; Sebastianelli, A.; Grondin, K.; Plante, M. The utility of sentinel lymph node mapping in the management of endometrial atypical hyperplasia. *Gynecol. Oncol.* **2018**, *148*, 485–490. [CrossRef]
30. Lim, S.L.; Moss, H.A.; Secord, A.A.; Lee, P.S.; Havrilesky, L.J.; Davidson, B.A. Hysterectomy with sentinel lymph node biopsy in the setting of pre-operative diagnosis of endometrial intraepithelial neoplasia: A cost-effectiveness analysis. *Gynecol. Oncol.* **2018**, *151*, 506–512. [CrossRef]
31. ASTEC study group; Kitchener, H.; Swart, A.M.C.; Qian, Q.; Amos, C.; Parmar, M.K.B. Efficacy of systematic pelvic lymphadenectomy in endometrial cancer (MRC ASTEC trial): A randomised studys. *Lancet* **2009**, *373*, 125–136, Erratum in: *Lancet* **2009**, *373*, 1764. [CrossRef]

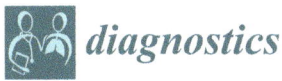

Article

Which Risk Factors and Colposcopic Patterns Are Predictive for High-Grade VAIN? A Retrospective Analysis

Anna Daniela Iacobone [1,2,*], Davide Radice [3], Maria Elena Guerrieri [1], Noemi Spolti [1], Barbara Grossi [1,4], Fabio Bottari [2,5], Sara Boveri [6], Silvia Martella [1], Ailyn Mariela Vidal Urbinati [1], Ida Pino [1], Dorella Franchi [1] and Eleonora Petra Preti [1]

1. Preventive Gynecology Unit, European Institute of Oncology IRCCS, Via Ripamonti 435, 20141 Milan, Italy
2. Department of Biomedical Sciences, University of Sassari, 07100 Sassari, Italy
3. Division of Epidemiology and Biostatistics, European Institute of Oncology, 20141 Milan, Italy
4. Department of Obstetrics and Gynecology, Luigi Sacco Hospital, ASST-Fatebenefratelli-Sacco, University of Milan, 20157 Milan, Italy
5. Division of Laboratory Medicine, European Institute of Oncology IRCCS, 20141 Milan, Italy
6. Laboratory of Biostatistics and Data Management, Scientific Directorate, IRCCS Policlinico San Donato, San Donato Milanese, 20097 Milan, Italy
* Correspondence: annadaniela.iacobone@ieo.it; Tel.: +39-02-57489120

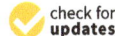

Citation: Iacobone, A.D.; Radice, D.; Guerrieri, M.E.; Spolti, N.; Grossi, B.; Bottari, F.; Boveri, S.; Martella, S.; Vidal Urbinati, A.M.; Pino, I.; et al. Which Risk Factors and Colposcopic Patterns Are Predictive for High-Grade VAIN? A Retrospective Analysis. *Diagnostics* **2023**, *13*, 176. https://doi.org/10.3390/diagnostics13020176

Academic Editor: Dah Ching Ding

Received: 31 October 2022
Revised: 24 December 2022
Accepted: 30 December 2022
Published: 4 January 2023

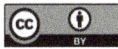

Copyright: © 2023 by the authors. Licensee MDPI, Basel, Switzerland. This article is an open access article distributed under the terms and conditions of the Creative Commons Attribution (CC BY) license (https://creativecommons.org/licenses/by/4.0/).

Abstract: Colposcopic patterns of Vaginal Intraepithelial Neoplasia (VAIN) are not definitively related to histological grade. The aim of the present study was to investigate any correlation between clinical and colposcopic features and the development of high-grade VAIN. Two hundred and fifty-five women diagnosed with VAIN (52 VAIN1, 55 VAIN2 and 148 VAIN3) at the European Institute of Oncology, Milan, Italy, from January 2000 to June 2022, were selected for a retrospective analysis. Multivariate logistic regression was performed to estimate the association of risk factors and colposcopic patterns with VAIN grade. Smoking was associated with the development of VAIN (34.1%, $p = 0.01$). Most women diagnosed with VAIN3 (45.3%, $p = 0.02$) had a previous history of hysterectomy for CIN2+. At multivariate analysis, colposcopic grade G2 (OR = 20.4, 95%CI: 6.67–61.4, $p < 0.001$), papillary lesion (OR = 4.33, 95%CI: 1.79–10.5, $p = 0.001$) and vascularity (OR = 14.4, 95%CI: 1.86–112, $p = 0.01$) were significantly associated with a greater risk of VAIN3. The risk of high-grade VAIN should not be underestimated in women with a history of smoking and previous hysterectomy for CIN2+, especially when colposcopic findings reveal vaginal lesions characterized by grade 2, papillary and vascular patterns. Accurate diagnosis is crucial for an optimal personalized management, based on risk factors, colposcopic patterns and histologic grade of VAIN.

Keywords: high-grade vaginal intraepithelial neoplasia (VAIN); smoking; previous hysterectomy for CIN2+; colposcopic grade; papillary lesion; vascular pattern

1. Introduction

Vaginal Intraepithelial Neoplasia (VAIN) is a rare premalignant lesion of the female lower genital tract, approximately 100-fold less common than cervical squamous intraepithelial lesions [1–3], with an estimated incidence of 0.2–2 per 100,000 women/year [4,5]. The prevalence of VAIN has recently increased due to improvements in screening methods, such as cytology and Human Papillomavirus (HPV) testing [5].

HPV infection is the fundamental etiological factor for the development of VAIN. However, other risk factors have been identified and investigated over time, including young age at first intercourse, a large number of sexual partners, cigarette smoking, immunosuppression, past or concurrent diagnosis of cervical or vulvar preinvasive or invasive lesions, previous hysterectomy for cervical intraepithelial neoplasia (CIN) or cervical cancer, prior radiotherapy, and a history of in utero exposure to diethylstilbestrol [6–8]. Recently, more attention has also been paid to the potential role of the vaginal microbiota, whose composition is influenced by hormonal status and changes during the development and progression of VAIN [9].

According to the depth of vaginal epithelium involved by dysplasia, VAIN is usually classified into grades 1, 2 or 3. The 2014 WHO classification of VAIN replaced the previous three-tiered system and recognizes only two categories: low-grade VAIN (VAIN1 or vaginal low-grade squamous intraepithelial lesion, LSIL) and high-grade VAIN (VAIN2-3 or vaginal high-grade squamous intraepithelial lesion, HSIL) [10,11]. VAIN1 is the result of a transient low-risk (LR) or high-risk (HR) HPV infection, with a high rate of spontaneous regression within 2 years. High-grade VAIN is due to a persistent and transforming HR-HPV infection and has a higher potential for recurrence and progression towards invasive vaginal carcinoma [12]. Since the risk of progression of VAIN2 to invasive cancer is still under discussion and should be intermediate between VAIN1 and VAIN3, some authors still consider VAIN2 as a separate category [13,14].

VAIN mostly occurs in women over 60 years of age, who are commonly asymptomatic but sometimes report vaginal discharge or bleeding [15]. Furthermore, post-menopausal women may be at increased risk of VAIN due to Lactobacillus depletion, overgrowth of anaerobic species and increased frequency of bacterial vaginosis, which have been indicated as agents responsible for delayed HPV clearance and subsequent carcinogenic progression [9,16].

The diagnosis is usually made by colposcopic-guided biopsy of suspicious vaginal lesions. After an abnormal cervical screening test with no lesion identified on the cervix, great attention should be paid to the complete evaluation of the vagina. Vaginal colposcopy is quite challenging, often due to vaginal dystrophy in post-menopausal women. In addition, colposcopic patterns of VAIN are highly heterogeneous and not very specific, thus resulting in a lack of correlation between colposcopy and histology, unlike CIN [17,18]. Nevertheless, few previous studies have investigated the potential link between colposcopic findings and the histopathologic grade of VAIN, in order to improve the predictive role of the colposcopic examination for treatment management [19,20].

The aim of the present study was to identify the potential risk factors for the development of VAIN to evaluate the diagnostic accuracy of colposcopy in relation to the histological grade of VAIN and to investigate any correlation between clinical and colposcopic features and high-grade VAIN.

2. Materials and Methods

All women affected by VAIN and who were attending the Preventive Gynecologic Unit of the European Institute of Oncology, Milan, Italy, from January 2000 to June 2022, were retrieved from hospital file archives and selected for a retrospective analysis.

The local Institutional Review Board approved the study protocol (IEO protocol UID 3821, date of approval: 27 October 2022) and written formal consent for the use of data for scientific purposes was signed by each subject.

Patients were included if the following criteria were met: (a) age at diagnosis of 25 years or older; (b) colposcopic-guided vaginal biopsies because of an abnormal pap smear or a previous history of any HPV-related lower genital tract diseases; (c) histologic confirmation of any grade of VAIN, including VAIN3 with stromal microinvasion; (c) available data about colposcopic findings. Patients were excluded in the case of (a) denied informed consent; (b) negative histology; or (c) diagnosis of invasive vaginal carcinoma.

Data regarding sociodemographic, clinical, laboratory and pathological characteristics of patients were recorded in a dedicated database.

Colposcopies were performed by staining with a 5% acetic solution and a 3% Lugol's solution (Schiller test), by expert colposcopists working at the Preventive Gynecologic Unit of the European Institute of Oncology. Abnormal colposcopic findings were described as grade 1 if minor (thin acetowhite epithelium, fine punctuation, fine mosaic) or grade 2 if major (dense acetowhite epithelium, coarse punctuation, coarse mosaic), according to the 2011 Colposcopic Terminology of the International Federation for Cervical Pathology and Colposcopy (IFCPC) [21,22]. All records of colposcopies performed before the introduction of the 2011 IFCPC Colposcopic Terminology were revised accordingly. Location of the lesion (vaginal vault, upper, middle and/or lower thirds), and uni/multifocality, vascular and papillary (defined as an acetowhite exophytic lesion not to be misdiagnosed as condyloma) patterns were reported separately.

Single or multiple colposcopic-guided biopsies were taken from suspicious vaginal lesions with the worst colposcopic characteristics. Dedicated gynecological pathologists working at the Pathology Division of our Institute performed all pathologic diagnoses. In the case of multifocal lesions and different grades of VAIN, the worst pathologic diagnosis and the related colposcopic pattern was considered for our analysis.

When possible, the Cobas 4800 HPV test (Cobas; Roche Diagnostics), an HR-HPV DNA assay with concurrent partial genotyping, was performed on liquid-based cervical (LBC) specimens at the time of colposcopy. The Cobas test is a Real-Time PCR-based assay able to detect HR-HPV genotypes 16 and 18 in separate channels, as well as a group of 12 other HR-HPV types (31, 33, 35, 39, 45, 51, 52, 56, 58, 59, 66 and 68) in another channel. It is a fully automated test and includes an internal control (B-globin) as a marker of sample adequacy.

Statistical Analysis

Categorical patients' characteristics at diagnosis were summarized by counts and percent, age by mean and standard deviation and cross-tabulated by VAIN grade. Between VAIN grade groups, comparisons were done by using Fisher's exact test for categorical variables and the F-test for age (one-way analysis of variance). Lesion type and vascularity were significantly associated with colposcopic grade and then entered two separated multivariate logistic regression analyses in order to estimate their association with VAIN grade as risk factors. Results are presented as Odds Ratios (OR) with 95% Confidence Intervals (CI). All tests were two-tailed and considered significant at the 5% level. All analyses were done using SAS 9.4 (Cary, NC, USA).

3. Results

After applying inclusion and exclusion criteria, 255 women affected by VAIN and attending the Preventive Gynecologic Unit of the European Institute of Oncology, Milan, Italy, from January 2000 to June 2022, were selected for our retrospective analysis.

VAIN 1, 2 and 3 were diagnosed in 52, 55 and 148 women, respectively.

The main clinical characteristics of patients are summarized by VAIN grade at diagnosis in Table 1.

The mean age of women at first diagnosis was 52.4 ± 12.8 years, with no significant difference among patients diagnosed with different histological grade of VAIN. About a third of cases was a current or former smoker (34.1%, $p = 0.01$) and more than half of patients reported previous pregnancies (55.4%, $p = 0.02$). Both variables were significantly associated with the diagnosis of VAIN, even according to histological grade.

Previous hysterectomy for CIN2+ was reported by 38.0% of women affected by VAIN, especially VAIN3 (45.3%, $p = 0.02$). Prior cervical cancer occurred in 49 patients undergoing hysterectomy (3 squamocellular carcinoma and 46 adenocarcinoma, $p = 0.16$), diagnosed as FIGO stage IA, IB and IIA-B in 29.4, 52.9 and 17.7% of cases ($p = 0.17$), respectively.

There was a significant correlation ($p < 0.001$) between cytology and histological grade of VAIN: 59.1% of VAIN1 were preceded by ASCUS-LSIL, whereas 73.1% of VAIN3 by ASCH-HSIL.

No other clinical variables, including immunosuppression, hormonal therapy, prior diagnosis of cervical or other cancers, previous or concomitant CIN, HPV-related VIN (vulvar intraepithelial neoplasia) or AIN (anal intraepithelial neoplasia), were significantly associated with VAIN and histological grade.

Table 1. Patients' characteristics summary statistics [a] by VAIN grade at diagnosis.

Characteristic	Category	All Patients n = 255	VAIN 1 n = 52	VAIN 2 n = 55	VAIN 3 n = 148	p-Value
Age (years) at first diagnosis		52.4 (12.8)	51.4 (12.2)	50.1 (13.4)	53.7 (12.7)	0.18
Current/former smoker		86 (34.1)	18 (34.6)	27 (50.9)	41 (27.9)	0.01
Parity		129 (55.4)	21 (42.9)	21 (46.7)	87 (62.6)	0.02
Immunosuppression		29 (11.5)	5 (9.6)	5 (9.1)	19 (13.0)	0.77
Hormonal therapy		40 (15.7)	8 (15.4)	7 (12.7)	25 (16.9)	0.82
Previous hysterectomy	CIN2+	97 (38.0)	13 (25.0)	17 (30.9)	67 (45.3)	
	Other	14 (5.5)	3 (5.8)	6 (10.9)	5 (3.4)	
	No hysterectomy	144 (56.5)	36 (69.2)	32 (58.2)	76 (51.4)	0.02
Previous cervical cancer	Yes	56 (22.1)	12 (23.5)	6 (10.9)	38 (25.9)	
	No/Other tumors [b]	197 (77.9)	39 (76.5)	49 (89.1)	109 (74.2)	0.06
Previous CIN	No/CIN1	150 (59.3)	33 (63.5)	31 (56.4)	86 (58.9)	
	CIN2-3	103 (40.7)	19 (44.7)	24 (43.6)	60 (41.1)	0.75
Concomitant CIN	No/CIN1	224 (87.8)	48 (92.3)	47 (85.5)	129 (87.2)	
	CIN2-3	31 (12.2)	4 (7.7)	8 (14.6)	19 (12.8)	0.52
Previous VIN	No	232 (91.7)	47 (92.2)	51 (92.7)	134 (91.2)	
	VIN3	21 (8.3)	4 (7.8)	4 (7.3)	13 (8.8)	1.00
Concomitant VIN	No	233 (91.4)	48 (92.3)	51 (92.7)	134 (90.5)	
	VIN1	4 (1.6)	2 (3.9)	0	2 (1.4)	
	VIN2	1 (0.4)	0	1 (1.8)	0	
	VIN3	17 (6.7)	2 (3.9)	3 (5.5)	12 (8.1)	0.34
Previous AIN	No	247 (97.6)	49 (96.1)	53 (96.4)	145 (98.6)	
	AIN2	1 (0.4)	0	1 (1.8)	0	
	AIN3	5 (2.0)	2 (3.9)	1 (1.8)	2 (1.4)	0.28
Concomitant AIN	No	253 (99.6)	51 (98.1)	54 (100)	148 (100)	
	AIN1	1 (0.4)	1 (1.9)	0	0	0.20
HR-HPV	HR+ with 16 and/or 18	71 (44.4)	11 (30.6)	14 (36.8)	46 (53.5)	
	HR+ without 16 and 18	63 (39.4)	14 (36.8)	20 (52.6)	26 (30.2)	
	Negative	26 (16.3)	8 (22.2)	4 (10.5)	14 (16.3)	0.05
Cytology	Negative	7 (3.1)	2 (4.1)	2 (4.0)	3 (2.3)	
	ASCUS-LSIL	67 (29.3)	29 (59.2)	15 (30.0)	23 (17.7)	
	ASCH-HSIL	145 (63.3)	17 (34.7)	33 (66.0)	95 (73.1)	
	SCC	10 (4.4)	1 (2.0)	0	9 (6.9)	<0.001

[a] n (column %) for categorical variable, Mean (SD) for Age; SD = Standard deviation; [b] including 153 women with no history of any cancer and 44 women with a previous history of other non-HPV-related tumors (i.e., breast cancer, Hodgkin's lymphoma, colorectal cancer, endometrial cancer); VAIN = Vaginal Intraepithelial Neoplasia; CIN = Cervical Intraepithelial Neoplasia; VIN = Vulvar Intraepithelial Neoplasia; AIN = Anal Intraepithelial Neoplasia; HR-HPV = High-risk Human Papillomavirus; ASCUS = Atypical Squamous Cells of Undetermined Significance; LSIL = Low Squamous Intraepithelial Lesion; ASCH = Atypical Squamous Cells cannot exclude HSIL; HSIL = High Squamous Intraepithelial Lesion; SCC = Squamous Cell Carcinoma.

Interestingly, the HPV test was positive for HR-HPV with 16 and/or 18 and other HR-HPV not 16–18 in 44.4% and 39.4% of patients, respectively. Most women affected by VAIN3 were positive for HR-HPV with 16 and/or 18 (53.5%), however borderline significant ($p = 0.05$), probably due to the large number of missing data regarding the Cobas result in our population ($n = 95$).

Colposcopic findings in relation to the histological grade of VAIN are detailed in Table 2, including 10 VAIN3 with stromal microinvasion in the VAIN3 category.

Table 2. Patients' colposcopic features summary statistics [a] by VAIN grade at diagnosis.

Characteristic	Category	VAIN Grade				
		All Patients $n = 255$	VAIN 1 $n = 52$	VAIN 2 $n = 55$	VAIN 3 [b] $n = 148$	p-Value
Grade	G1	134 (53.4)	45 (88.2)	41 (74.6)	48 (33.1)	
	G2	117 (46.6)	6 (11.8)	14 (25.4)	97 (66.9)	<0.001
Lesion type	Flat	145 (59.2)	41 (80.4)	38 (70.4)	66 (47.1)	
	Papillary	100 (40.8)	10 (19.6)	16 (29.6)	74 (52.9)	<0.001
Multifocality	Unifocal	141 (56.6)	34 (65.4)	29 (53.7)	78 (54.6)	
	Multifocal	108 (43.4)	18 (34.6)	25 (46.3)	65 (45.4)	0.36
Vascular pattern	No	196 (80.3)	51 (98.1)	51 (92.7)	94 (68.6)	
	Yes	48 (19.7)	1 (1.9)	4 (7.3)	43 (31.4)	<0.001
Vaginal localization	Vault	98 (38.7)	15 (28.9)	21 (38.2)	62 (42.5)	
	Upper third	114 (45.1)	24 (46.2)	24 (43.6)	66 (45.2)	
	Middle third	26 (10.3)	10 (19.2)	8 (14.6)	8 (5.5)	
	Lower third	15 (5.9)	3 (5.8)	2 (3.6)	10 (6.9)	0.09

[a] n (column %); [b] Including $n = 10$ VAIN3 with stromal microinvasion; VAIN = Vaginal Intraepithelial Neoplasia; G = Grade.

Most VAIN1 (88.2%) were characterized by colposcopic grade G1, and most VAIN3 (66.9%) were characterized by colposcopic grade G2 ($p < 0.001$) (Figure 1). A flat lesion was detected in 80.4% of VAIN1, whereas a papillary lesion was in 52.9% of VAIN3 ($p < 0.001$) (Figure 2). A vascular pattern was present in only 19.7% of VAIN, but there was a significant linear correlation according to histological grade ($p < 0.001$). Indeed, about one-third of VAIN3 (31.4%) showed a vascular pattern (Figure 3).

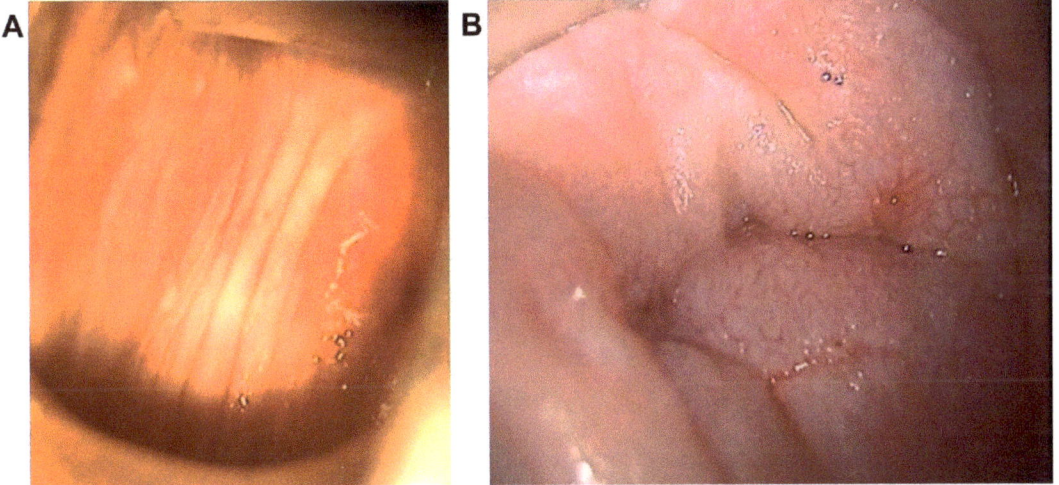

Figure 1. Colposcopic grade according to the 2011 IFCPC Colposcopic Terminology. (**A**): Grade 1 or minor, as shown by the colposcopic pattern (thin acetowhite epithelium) of a patient diagnosed with VAIN1, located at the upper third of the right vaginal wall. (**B**): Grade 2 or major, as shown by the colposcopic pattern (coarse mosaic) of a patient diagnosed with VAIN3, located at the vaginal vault, after previous hysterectomy for CIN3.

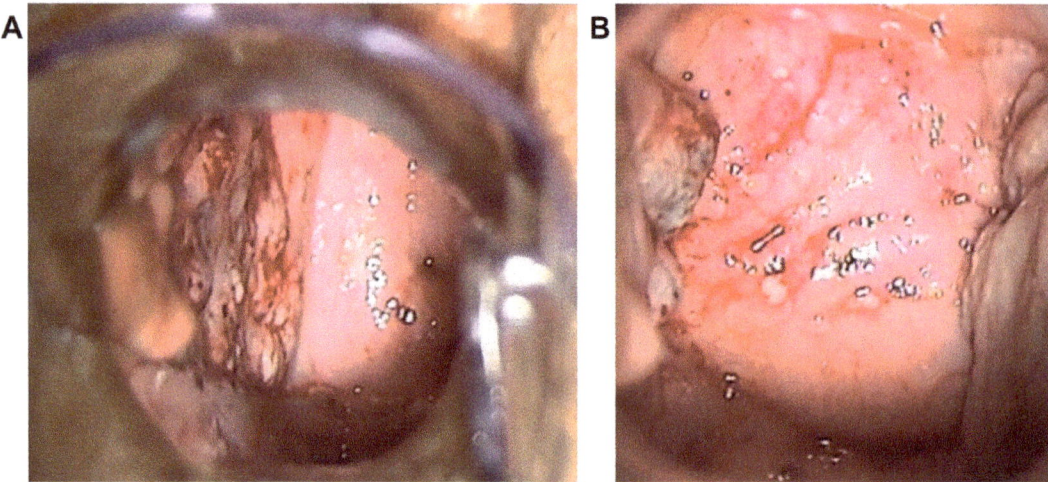

Figure 2. Papillary pattern. Multiple papillary lesions with both regular and irregular surface, located at the whole right vaginal wall in a patient diagnosed with VAIN3 at a colposcopic overview (**A**) and at a magnified colposcopic vision (**B**).

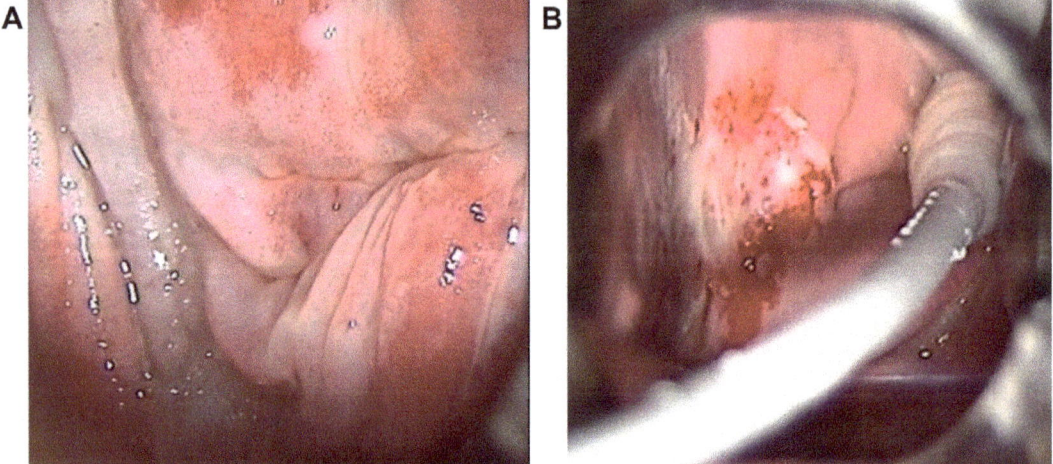

Figure 3. Vascular pattern. Colposcopic findings showing: dense acetowhite epithelium with coarse punctuation at the posterolateral right vaginal fornices and upper-third walls in a young woman (35 years) affected by VAIN3 (**A**); and dense acetowhite epithelium with fragile vessels at the upper-middle third of the right vaginal wall in a post-menopausal woman (62 years) affected by VAIN2 (**B**).

No significant association was found for multifocal lesions ($p = 0.36$) and vaginal localization ($p = 0.09$) by VAIN grade at diagnosis.

When considered as a separate category, VAIN3 with stromal microinvasion was significantly associated with colposcopic grade G2 (100%), papillary lesions (90.0%) and vascular pattern (44.4%) with a p-value <0.001 for all variables, as shown in Table 3 (Figure 4).

Table 3. Patients' colposcopic features summary statistics [a] by VAIN grade at diagnosis, considering microinvasive VAIN3 as a separate category.

Characteristic	Category	VAIN					
		All Patients $n = 255$	VAIN 1 $n = 52$	VAIN 2 $n = 55$	VAIN 3 $n = 138$	VAIN 3 Microinvasive $n = 10$	p-Value
Grade	G1	134 (53.4)	45 (88.2)	41 (74.6)	48 (35.6)	0	
	G2	117 (46.6)	6 (11.8)	14 (25.4)	87 (64.4)	10 (100)	<0.001
Lesion type	Flat	145 (59.2)	41 (80.4)	38 (70.4)	66 (50.4)	0	
	Papillary	100 (40.8)	10 (19.6)	16 (29.6)	65 (49.6)	9 (90.0)	<0.001
Multifocality	Unifocal	141 (56.6)	34 (65.4)	29 (53.7)	76 (56.7)	2 (22.2)	
	Multifocal	108 (43.4)	18 (34.6)	25 (46.3)	58 (43.3)	7 (77.8)	0.11
Vascularity	No	196 (80.3)	51 (98.1)	51 (92.7)	89 (69.5)	5 (55.6)	
	Yes	48 (19.7)	1 (1.9)	4 (7.3)	39 (30.5)	4 (44.4)	<0.001
Vaginal localization	Vault	98 (38.7)	15 (28.9)	21 (38.2)	58 (42.7)	4 (40.0)	
	Upper third	114 (45.1)	24 (46.2)	24 (43.6)	61 (44.9)	5 (50.0)	
	Middle third	26 (10.3)	10 (19.2)	8 (14.6)	8 (5.9)	0	
	Lower third	15 (5.9)	3 (5.8)	2 (3.6)	9 (6.6)	1 (10.0)	0.23

[a] n (column %); VAIN = Vaginal Intraepithelial Neoplasia; G = Grade.

However, a sensitivity analysis showed that these colposcopic variables were still statistically significantly correlated with VAIN grade even after excluding all cases with microinvasive VAIN3 (Table S1).

Old medical reports of women firstly diagnosed with VAIN farther away from current times had some missing clinical and colposcopic data. The distribution of missing data by VAIN grade at diagnosis was evaluated as a possible selection bias for different variables (Table S2). Only the distributions of missing data for parity ($n = 22$, $p = 0.03$) and vascular pattern ($n = 11$, $p = 0.02$) were significant. In particular, all missing data regarding vascular pattern were in VAIN3 category. However, the arbitrary imputation of the missing data to the presence of the vascular pattern did not change the significance of the association with the histological grade of VAIN (data not shown).

Since lesion type and vascularity were significantly associated with colposcopic grade (Table S3), two separated multivariate logistic regression analyses were performed in order to estimate their association with high-grade VAIN as risk factors.

As shown in Table 4, at multivariate analysis, colposcopic grade G2 was significantly associated with a greater risk of developing both VAIN 2 (OR = 4.77, 95%CI: 1.40–16.2, $p = 0.01$) and VAIN3 (OR = 20.4, 95%CI: 6.67–61.4, $p < 0.001$).

When excluding the colposcopic grade from the multivariate logistic regression (Table 5), only papillary lesion represented a predictive factor for VAIN2 (OR = 2.90, 95%CI: 1.07–7.89, $p = 0.03$), whereas a previous hysterectomy for CIN2+ (OR = 2.37, 95%CI: 1.02–5.36, $p = 0.04$), papillary lesion (OR = 4.33, 95%CI: 1.79–10.5, $p = 0.001$) and vascular pattern (OR = 14.4, 95%CI: 1.86–112, $p = 0.01$) significantly led to a higher risk of VAIN3.

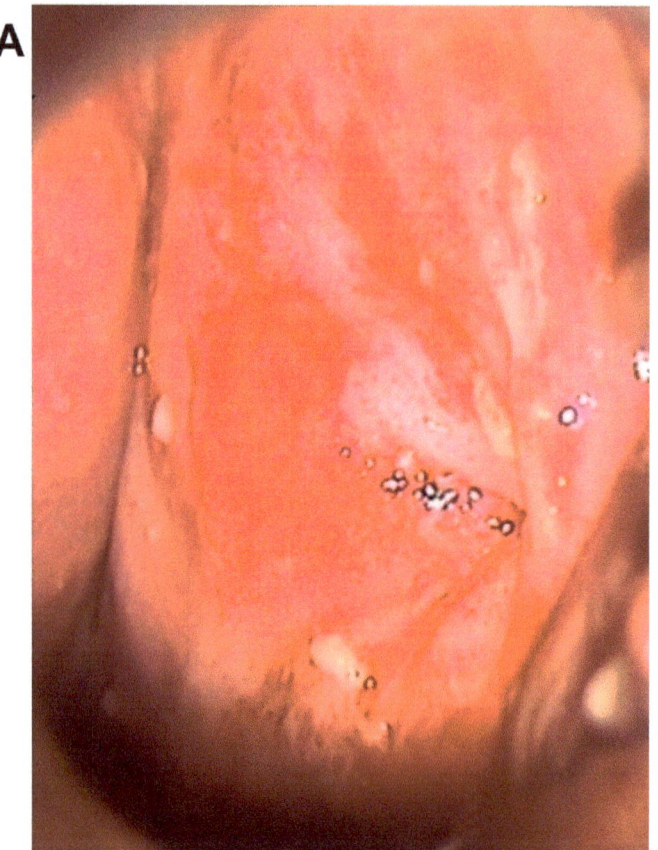
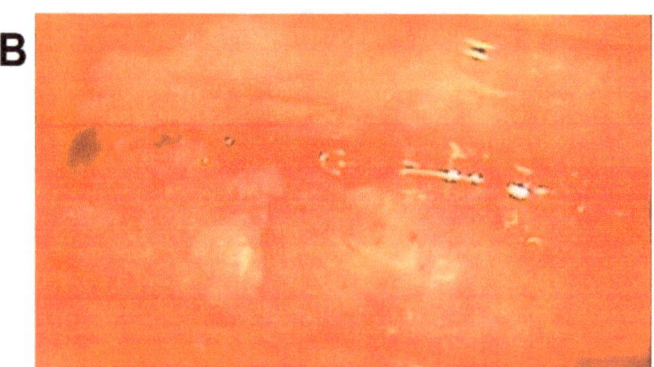

Figure 4. Colposcopic patterns associated with microinvasive VAIN3. Abnormal colposcopic findings of grade 2, vascular patterns and papillary lesions with regular (**A**) and/or irregular (**B**) surface in two women affected by VAIN3 with stromal microinvasion, both located at the vaginal vault, after previous hysterectomy for cervical cancer.

Table 4. Multivariate analysis of variance of risk factors for VAIN excluding lesion type and vascularity.

VAIN Grade	Factor	Level	OR (95% CI)	p-Value
VAIN2 vs. VAIN1	Smoking	No	Ref	
		Yes	1.53 (0.62,3.78)	0.36
	Previous hysterectomy	No hysterectomy	Ref	
		CIN2+	1.20 (0.43,3.38)	0.73
		Other	1.11 (0.19,6.50)	0.91
	Colposcopic Grade	G1	Ref	
		G2	4.77 (1.40,16.2)	0.01
VAIN3 [a] vs. VAIN1	Smoking	No	Ref	
		Yes	0.61 (0.25,1.47)	0.27
	Previous hysterectomy	No hysterectomy	Ref	
		CIN2+	2.15 (0.89,5.24)	0.09
		Other	1.46 (0.28,7.64)	0.66
	Colposcopic Grade	G1	Ref	
		G2	20.4 (6.67,61.4)	<0.001

[a] Including n = 10 VAIN3 with stromal microinvasion; VAIN = Vaginal Intraepithelial Neoplasia; OR = Odds Ratio; CI = Confidence Interval; CIN = Cervical Intraepithelial Neoplasia; G = Grade.

Table 5. Multivariate analysis of variance of risk factors for VAIN excluding colposcopic grade.

VAIN Grade	Factor	Level	OR (95% CI)	p-Value
VAIN2 vs. VAIN1	Smoking	No	Ref	
		Yes	1.49 (0.60,3.67)	0.40
	Previous hysterectomy	No hysterectomy	Ref	
		CIN2+	1.27 (0.45,3.56)	0.65
		Other	0.91 (0.15,5.69)	0.92
	Lesion type	Flat	Ref	
		Papillary	2.90 (1.07,7.89)	0.03
	Vascularity	No	Ref	
		Yes	2.81 (0.25,31.5)	0.40
VAIN3 [a] vs. VAIN1	Smoking	No	Ref	
		Yes	0.79 (0.35,1.78)	0.57
	Previous hysterectomy	No hysterectomy	Ref	
		CIN2+	2.37 (1.02,5.36)	0.04
		Other	1.04 (0.20,5.36)	0.96
	Lesion type	Flat	Ref	
		Papillary	4.33 (1.79,10.5)	0.001
	Vascularity	No	Ref	
		Yes	14.4 (1.86,112)	0.01

[a] Including n = 10 VAIN3 with stromal microinvasion; VAIN = Vaginal Intraepithelial Neoplasia; OR = Odds Ratio; CI = Confidence Interval; CIN = Cervical Intraepithelial Neoplasia.

4. Discussion

Our findings confirmed that smoking, parity, previous hysterectomy for CIN2+ and abnormal cytology should be considered as potential risk factors for VAIN, and a significant association is maintained by histologic grade. In addition, abnormal colposcopic findings, including grade G2, papillary and vascular patterns, are predictive of the development of high-grade VAIN, even at multivariate analysis.

According to our results, current or former smoking was significantly associated with the risk of VAIN, as already well-known in previous literature [23–25]. Sherman et al. also showed that smoking is significantly associated with the occurrence of high-grade VAIN in women infected by HR-HPV [6], as a possible consequence of a biological interaction between smoke and the viral protein of HR-HPV genotypes. Due to the large number of missing data regarding HR-HPV status, it was not possible to investigate the same correlation in our study population.

In our analysis, parity was related with a significantly increased risk of developing VAIN and, in particular, high-grade VAIN, as opposed to previous findings [26]. However, it was not possible to exclude a selection bias due to the significant distribution of missing data for parity by VAIN grade at diagnosis.

It is well-established that women with a previous history of CIN or cervical cancer, who underwent hysterectomy, remain at a higher life-time risk of VAIN and should be carefully screened for HPV-related vaginal and vulvar disease throughout their lives [26,27]. Our study confirmed that prior hysterectomy for CIN2+ should be considered as a risk factor for high-grade VAIN. Indeed, VAIN after hysterectomy usually arises near the vaginal cuff [7], since HPV infection is often multifocal and may affect other sites of the female lower genital tract. Moreover, the grade of VAIN may be affected by the severity of previous cervical disease [26] and women with a history of CIN2+ should be extensively counselled regarding the future risk of VAIN before hysterectomy. Previous hysterectomy for HPV-related cervical lesions has also been recognized as a risk factor for progression to vaginal cancer [28].

Unlike other authors [22], we did not find any correlation between age at diagnosis and the histological grade of VAIN. However, Zhou et al. also reported a poor rank correlation [22], whereas Boonlikit et al. did not show any significant distribution of patients' age among different VAIN grade groups [17]. The mean age of our patients was 52.4 ± 12.8 years. Therefore, we did not investigate whether the post-menopausal status correlated with an increased risk of VAIN because of a thinner vaginal epithelium that results in more susceptibility to changes in the vaginal microbiome and HPV infections [26].

Even immunosuppression was not associated with the development of VAIN in our cohort, as opposed to previous studies [29], probably due to the small proportion of immunosuppressed patients (11.5%).

Most diagnoses of VAIN were preceded by an abnormal pap smear result, thus supporting the assumption that cytology, in combination with a HR-HPV test, is an effective tool for early diagnosis of VAIN, even after hysterectomy, since its sensitivity is not inferior to that for CIN2+ detection [5]. We did not investigate whether cytology positivity was higher in patients with a previous hysterectomy, as recently shown by Zhang et al. in a large retrospective series of VAIN. However, the combined use of cytology and HPV testing could curb this issue, since no statistically significant difference in co-testing positivity was identified in women with or without a history of previous hysterectomy [30]. HR-HPV status was known only in 160 out of 255 enrolled patients. Most of the missing data were found in women with a first diagnosis of VAIN in the early 2000s, when HPV testing was neither applied for primary screening nor routinely performed as a triage test after abnormal cytology. In our cohort with an available Cobas result, 83.8% of cases were affected by HR-HPV infection, with or without HPV 16 and 18, as reported by previous literature [26]. Most of the women affected by VAIN3 were positive for HR-HPV with 16 and/or 18 (53.5%). As already explained, this association was only borderline significant, due to the large number of missing Cobas results, but is in agreement with previous data [31]. HPV 16, 52, 56 and 58 have been identified as the most prevalent genotypes in high-grade VAIN [30], while many LR and HR genotypes have been linked to the development of low-grade VAIN. HPV type distribution is even more heterogeneous in case of coexisting cervical lesions, although a recent study by Zhang et al. showed that different HPV genotypes are independent causative agents of coexisting CIN and VAIN [32]. Furthermore, specific HPV genotypes, particularly HPV 16, have been related to a greater risk of VAIN persistence, progression and recurrence [28]. Therefore, HPV genotyping could be a useful tool for risk-stratification of patients affected by VAIN.

Regarding the diagnostic accuracy of colposcopy in relation to the histological grade of VAIN, our study confirmed that colposcopic grade G2 and vascularity were significantly associated with VAIN3, including VAIN3 with stromal microinvasion. These associations have been widely demonstrated by other authors [17,19,20], that already observed specific abnormal colposcopic findings, such as grade 2 and vascular punctuation, more commonly in women diagnosed with VAIN3 rather than with VAIN2 or VAIN1. Interestingly, our study included a larger proportion of women diagnosed with VAIN3, when compared to previous studies, and also considered microinvasive VAIN3 as a separate category [17,19]. Moreover, in our cohort we found colposcopic grade 2 in 46.6% of women, that is a prevalence roughly double that previously reported by Sopracordevole et al. (22.7%) [19].

The correlation between vascularity and high-grade VAIN has been already explained by Boonlikit et al., as a consequence of the lack of vascular structure in very mature squamous vaginal epithelium. Thus, vascular patterns appear later, as distinct from the cervical dysplastic process, in which vascular punctuation appears early due to the immature squamous metaplasia of the transformation zone [17].

Conversely, our results showed a significant association between papillary lesions and VAIN3, and in particular, microinvasive VAIN3. This is totally different from the evidence of other authors who detected micropapillary patterns more frequently in women affected by low-grade VAIN [19,20,22]. The exact meaning of this colposcopic feature is still unclear and lacking. According to our experience, if the papillary pattern is caused by a persistent HPV infection, as already suggested [19,20,22], it should be considered as the expression of dysplastic progression towards high-grade VAIN. Another possible explanation of this relevant difference could derive from the absence of this specific feature in the 2011 IFCPC colposcopic terminology [21]. In fact, a recent study found poor concordance between the diagnosis based on the 2011 IFCPC colposcopic classification and vaginal histology for the high-grade VAIN category (only 35.71%), with a substantial false negative rate (42.86%), thus suggesting that the IFCPC nomenclature should be improved and better standardized for vaginal lesions [22].

Notably, we did not find any significant difference among VAIN grade groups regarding lesions number, as against that sustained by Zhou et al. [20]. Even vaginal localization was not significantly associated with the histological grade of VAIN. Nevertheless, the prevalence of VAIN in the vaginal vault (38.7%) and in the upper third of vaginal walls (45.1%) was much higher than in the lower two thirds (16.2%), in agreement with previously reported frequencies [3,22,33,34].

To the best of our knowledge, this is the first study to investigate and portray colposcopic characteristics of not only low- and high-grade VAIN, but also VAIN3 with stromal microinvasion, that should always be correctly identified before choosing a therapeutic approach.

The main strengths of the study are related to the higher proportion of high-grade VAIN in our population and the data homogeneity, because all colposcopies were performed at a referral oncologic center, only by trained colposcopists, with particular expertise in the diagnosis and treatment of vaginal lesions. On the contrary, limits of the study include selection bias related to the single center retrospective design of the study and the amount of missing data in old medical reports.

A better defined and standardized application of the 2011 ICFPC colposcopic terminology for vaginal lesions could be useful for correct diagnosis and management of VAIN. Indeed, identifying risk factors and colposcopic patterns predictive for high-grade VAIN would help the colposcopist to sample the area most likely to contain VAIN3 or stromal invasion, especially in large and multifocal lesions, which could simultaneously hold different grades of VAIN.

Appropriate diagnosis of VAIN3, with or without stromal microinvasion, is mandatory to choose the optimal management, which still remains challenging and controversial for high-grade VAIN. Several therapeutic regimens, including conservative surveillance, ablative procedures and surgical excisions, have been proposed over time, due to a high recurrence rate of VAIN2-3 despite the type of treatment [4,35–38]. Hence, proper and accurate diagnosis could allow for more personalized risk-based management, based on risk factors, colposcopic patterns and the histologic grade of VAIN.

5. Conclusions

The risk of high-grade VAIN should not be underestimated in women with a history of current or former smoking and previous hysterectomy for CIN2+, which also represents a risk factor for recurrence and progression to vaginal cancer. Colposcopic findings, including grade 2, papillary and vascular patterns, are predictive factors for VAIN3 with or without stromal microinvasion. Accurate colposcopic and histologic diagnosis is crucial for the optimal management of vaginal pre-cancers and cancers. In addition, HPV genotyping could be a helpful tool for risk stratification and prompt identification of women with VAIN3 at higher risk of persistence, progression and recurrence.

Supplementary Materials: The following supporting information can be downloaded at: https://www.mdpi.com/article/10.3390/diagnostics13020176/s1, Table S1: Patients' colposcopic features summary statisticsa by VAIN grade at diagnosis; Table S2: Missing data distribution by VAIN grade at diagnosis; Table S3: Colposcopic Grade association with Lesion type and Vascularity.

Author Contributions: Conceptualization, A.D.I., M.E.G., N.S. and E.P.P.; Methodology, A.D.I., D.R., M.E.G. and B.G.; Software, A.D.I., D.R. and B.G.; Validation, A.D.I. and D.R.; Formal Analysis, D.R. and S.B.; Investigation, A.D.I., M.E.G., N.S., F.B., S.M., A.M.V.U. and E.P.P.; Resources, A.D.I., M.E.G. and I.P.; Data Curation, A.D.I., D.R. and S.B.; Writing—Original Draft Preparation, A.D.I. and D.R.; Writing—Review and Editing, A.D.I., M.E.G., N.S., S.M., A.M.V.U., I.P., D.F. and E.P.P.; Visualization, A.D.I., D.R., N.S. and E.P.P.; Supervision, F.B. and D.F.; Project Administration, A.D.I. All authors have read and agreed to the published version of the manuscript.

Funding: This research received no external funding.

Institutional Review Board Statement: The study was conducted according to the guidelines of the Declaration of Helsinki, and approved by the Institutional Review Board of the European Institute of Oncology, Milan, Italy (IEO protocol number UID 3821, date of approval: 27 October 2022).

Informed Consent Statement: Informed consent was obtained from all subjects involved in the study.

Data Availability Statement: The data presented in this study are available on request from the corresponding author. The data are not publicly available due to patients' privacy restrictions. The data are safely stored in a private database of the European Institute of Oncology, Milan, Italy.

Acknowledgments: This work was partially supported by the Italian Ministry of Health with Ricerca Corrente and 5x1000 funds.

Conflicts of Interest: The authors declare no conflict of interest. None of the authors received financial support or funding for this work.

References

1. Sillman, F.H.; Fruchter, R.G.; Chen, Y.S.; Camilien, L.; Sedlis, A.; McTigue, E. Vaginal intraepithelial neoplasia: Risk factors for per-sistence, recurrence, and invasion and its management. *Am. J. Obstet. Gynecol.* **1997**, *176*, 93–99. [CrossRef] [PubMed]
2. Dodge, J.A.; Eltabbakh, G.H.; Mount, S.L.; Walker, R.; Morgan, A. Clinical Features and Risk of Recurrence among Patients with Vaginal Intraepithelial Neoplasia. *Gynecol. Oncol.* **2001**, *83*, 363–369. [CrossRef] [PubMed]
3. Gurumurthy, M.; Cruickshank, M.E. Management of Vaginal Intraepithelial Neoplasia. *J. Low. Genit. Tract Dis.* **2012**, *16*, 306–312. [CrossRef] [PubMed]
4. Hodeib, M.; Cohen, J.G.; Mehta, S.; Rimel, B.; Walsh, C.S.; Li, A.J.; Karlan, B.Y.; Cass, I. Recurrence and risk of progression to lower genital tract malignancy in women with high grade VAIN. *Gynecol. Oncol.* **2016**, *141*, 507–510. [CrossRef]
5. Cong, Q.; Song, Y.; Wang, Q.; Zhang, H.; Gao, S.; Sui, L. A retrospective study of cytology, high-risk HPV and colposcopy results of vaginal intraepithelial neoplasia patients. *Biomed. Res. Int.* **2018**, *8*, 5894801. [CrossRef]
6. Sherman, J.F.; Mount, S.L.; Evans, M.F.; Skelly, J.; Simmons-Arnold, L.; Eltabbakh, G.H. Smoking increases the risk of high-grade vaginal intraepithelial neoplasia in women with oncogenic human papillomavirus. *Gynecol. Oncol.* **2008**, *110*, 396–401. [CrossRef]
7. Schockaert, S.; Poppe, W.; Arbyn, M.; Verguts, T.; Verguts, J. Incidence of vaginal intraepithelial neoplasia after hysterectomy for cervical intraepithelial neoplasia: A retrospective study. *Am. J. Obstet. Gynecol.* **2008**, *199*, 113.e1–113.e5. [CrossRef]
8. Liao, J.B.; Jean, S.; Wilkinson-Ryan, I.; Ford, A.E.; Tanyi, J.L.; Hagemann, A.R.; Lin, L.L.; McGrath, C.M.; Rubin, S.C. Vaginal intraepithelial neoplasia (VAIN) after radiation therapy for gynecologic malignancies: A clinically recalcitrant entity. *Gynecol. Oncol.* **2011**, *120*, 108–112. [CrossRef]
9. Zhou, F.-Y.; Zhou, Q.; Zhu, Z.-Y.; Hua, K.-Q.; Chen, L.-M.; Ding, J.-X. Types and viral load of human papillomavirus, and vaginal microbiota in vaginal intraepithelial neoplasia: A cross-sectional study. *Ann. Transl. Med.* **2020**, *8*, 1408. [CrossRef]

10. Kurman, R.J. *WHO Classification of Tumours of Female Reproductive Organs*; International Agency for Research on Cancer: Lyon, France, 2014.
11. Darragh, T.M.; Colgan, T.J.; Thomas Cox, J.; Heller, D.S.; Henry, M.R.; Luff, R.D.; McCalmont, T.; Nayar, R.; Palefsky, J.M.; Stoler, M.H.; et al. The Lower Anogenital Squamous Terminology Standardization project for HPV-associated lesions: Background and consensus recommendations from the College of American Pathologists and the American Society for Colposcopy and Cervical Pathology. *Int. J. Gynecol. Pathol.* **2013**, *32*, 76–115. [CrossRef]
12. Reich, O.; Regauer, S.; Marth, C.; Schmidt, D.; Horn, L.-C.; Dannecker, C.; Menton, M.; Beckmann, M. Precancerous Lesions of the Cervix, Vulva and Vagina According to the 2014 WHO Classification of Tumors of the Female Genital Tract. *Geburtshilfe Und Frauenheilkd.* **2015**, *75*, 1018–1020. [CrossRef] [PubMed]
13. Sopracordevole, F.; Barbero, M.; Clemente, N.; Fallani, M.G.; Cattani, P.; Agarossi, A.; De Piero, G.; Parin, A.; Frega, A.; Boselli, F.; et al. High-grade vaginal intraepithelial neoplasia and risk of progression to vaginal cancer: A multicentre study of the Italian Society of Colposcopy and Cervico-Vaginal Pathology (SICPCV). *Eur. Rev. Med. Pharmacol. Sci.* **2016**, *20*, 818–824. [PubMed]
14. Sopracordevole, F.; De Piero, G.; Clemente, N.; Buttignol, M.; Mancioli, F.; Di Giuseppe, J.; Canzonieri, V.; Giorda, G.; Ciavattini, A. Vaginal intraepithelial neoplasia: Histopathological upgrading of lesions and evidence of occult vaginal cancer. *J. Low. Genit. Tract. Dis.* **2016**, *20*, 70–74. [CrossRef] [PubMed]
15. Gunderson, C.C.; Nugent, E.K.; Elfrink, S.H.; Gold, M.A.; Moore, K.N. A contemporary analysis of epidemiology and management of vaginal intraepithelial neoplasia. *Am. J. Obstet. Gynecol.* **2013**, *208*, 410.e1–410.e6. [CrossRef]
16. Gillet, E.; Meys, J.F.; Verstraelen, H.; Bosire, C.; De Sutter, P.; Temmerman, M.; Broeck, D.V. Bacterial vaginosis is associated with uterine cervical human papillomavirus infection: A meta-analysis. *BMC Infect. Dis.* **2011**, *11*, 10. [CrossRef]
17. Boonlikit, S.; Noinual, N. Vaginal intraepithelial neoplasia: A retrospective analysis of clinical features and colpohistology. *J. Obstet. Gynaecol. Res.* **2010**, *36*, 94–100. [CrossRef]
18. Indraccolo, U.; Baldoni, A. A Simplified Classification for Describing Colposcopic Vaginal Patterns. *J. Low. Genit. Tract Dis.* **2012**, *16*, 75–79. [CrossRef]
19. Sopracordevole, F.; Barbero, M.; Clemente, N.; Fallani, M.G.; Cattani, P.; Agarossi, A.; De Piero, G.; Parin, A.; Frega, A.; Boselli, F.; et al. Colposcopic patterns of vaginal intraepithelial neoplasia: A study from the Italian Society of Colposcopy and Cervico-Vaginal Pathology. *Eur. J. Cancer Prev.* **2018**, *27*, 152–157. [CrossRef]
20. Sopracordevole, F.; Clemente, N.; Barbero, M.; Agarossi, A.; Cattani, P.; Garutti, P.; Fallani, M.G.; Pieralli, A.; Boselli, F.; Frega, A.; et al. Colpo-scopic patterns of vaginal intraepithelial neoplasia: A focus on low-grade lesions. *Eur. Rev. Med. Pharmacol. Sci.* **2017**, *21*, 2823–2828.
21. Bornstein, J.; Bentley, J.; Bösze, P.; Girardi, F.; Haefner, H.; Menton, M.; Perrotta, M.; Prendiville, W.; Russell, P.; Sideri, M.; et al. 2011 Colposcopic Terminology of the International Federation for Cervical Pathology and Colposcopy. *Obstet. Gynecol.* **2012**, *120*, 166–172. [CrossRef]
22. Zhou, Q.; Zhang, F.; Sui, L.; Zhang, H.; Lin, L.; Li, Y. Application of 2011 International Federation for Cervical Pathology and Colposcopy Terminology on the Detection of Vaginal Intraepithelial Neoplasia. *Cancer Manag. Res.* **2020**, *12*, 5987–5995. [CrossRef] [PubMed]
23. Daling, J.R.; Madeleine, M.M.; Schwartz, S.M.; Shera, K.A.; Carter, J.J.; McKnight, B.; Porter, P.L.; Galloway, D.A.; McDougall, J.K.; Tamimi, H. A population-based study of squamous cell vaginal cancer: HPV and cofactors. *Gynecol. Oncol.* **2002**, *84*, 263–270. [CrossRef] [PubMed]
24. Tolstrup, J.; Munk, C.; Thomsen, B.L.; Svare, E.; Brule, A.J.V.D.; Grønbæk, M.K.; Meijer, C.; Kjær, S.K. The role of smoking and alcohol intake in the development of high-grade squamous intraepithelial lesions among high-risk HPV-positive women. *Acta Obstet. Gynecol. Scand.* **2006**, *85*, 1114–1119. [CrossRef] [PubMed]
25. Madsen, B.S.; Jensen, H.L.; Brule, A.J.V.D.; Wohlfahrt, J.; Frisch, M. Risk factors for invasive squamous cell carcinoma of the vulva and vagina—Population-based case–control study in Denmark. *Int. J. Cancer* **2008**, *122*, 2827–2834. [CrossRef] [PubMed]
26. Li, H.; Guo, Y.-L.; Zhang, J.-X.; Qiao, J.; Geng, L. Risk factors for the development of vaginal intraepithelial neoplasia. *Chin. Med. J.* **2012**, *125*, 1219–1223.
27. Cao, D.; Wu, D.; Xu, Y. Vaginal intraepithelial neoplasia in patients after total hysterectomy. *Curr. Probl. Cancer* **2020**, *45*, 100687. [CrossRef]
28. Ao, M.; Zheng, D.; Wang, J.; Gu, X.; Xi, M. Risk factors analysis of persistence, progression and recurrence in vaginal intraepithelial neoplasia. *Gynecol. Oncol.* **2021**, *162*, 584–589. [CrossRef]
29. Bradbury, M.; Xercavins, N.; García-Jiménez, A.; Pérez-Benavente, A.; Franco-Camps, S.; Cabrera, S.; Sánchez-Iglesias, J.L.; De La Torre, J.; Díaz-Feijoo, B.; Gil-Moreno, A.; et al. Vaginal Intraepithelial Neoplasia: Clinical Presentation, Management, and Outcomes in Relation to HIV Infection Status. *J. Low. Genit. Tract Dis.* **2019**, *23*, 7–12. [CrossRef]
30. Zhang, L.; Wang, Q.; Zhang, H.; Xie, Y.; Sui, L.; Cong, Q. Screening History in Vaginal Precancer and Cancer: A Retrospective Study of 2131 Cases in China. *Cancer Manag. Res.* **2021**, *13*, 8855–8863. [CrossRef]
31. Insinga, R.P.; Liaw, K.-L.; Johnson, L.G.; Madeleine, M.M. A systematic review of the prevalence and attribution of human papil-lomavirus types among cervical, vaginal, and vulvar precancers and cancers in the United States. *Cancer. Epidemiol. Bi-omarkers. Prev.* **2008**, *17*, 1611–1622. [CrossRef]

32. Zhang, S.; Saito, M.; Okayama, K.; Okodo, M.; Kurose, N.; Sakamoto, J.; Sasagawa, T. HPV Genotyping by Molecular Mapping of Tissue Samples in Vaginal Intraepithelial Neoplasia (VaIN) and Vaginal Squamous Cell Carcinoma (VaSCC). *Cancers* **2021**, *13*, 3260. [CrossRef] [PubMed]
33. Jentschke, M.; Hoffmeister, V.; Soergel, P.; Hillemanns, P. Clinical presentation, treatment and outcome of vaginal intraepithelial neoplasia. *Arch. Gynecol. Obstet.* **2015**, *293*, 415–419. [CrossRef] [PubMed]
34. Lamos, C.; Mihaljevic, C.; Aulmann, S.; Bruckner, T.; Domschke, C.; Wallwiener, M.; Paringer, C.; Fluhr, H.; Schott, S.; Dinkic, C.; et al. Detection of Human Papillomavirus Infection in Patients with Vaginal Intraepithelial Neoplasia. *PLoS ONE* **2016**, *11*, e0167386. [CrossRef] [PubMed]
35. Frega, A.; Sopracordevole, F.; Assorgi, C.; Lombardi, D.; DESanctis, V.; Catalano, A.; Matteucci, E.; Milazzo, G.N.; Ricciardi, E.; Moscarini, M. Vaginal intraepithelial neoplasia: A therapeutical dilemma. *Anticancer. Res.* **2013**, *33*, 29–38. [PubMed]
36. Ratnavelu, N.; Patel, A.; Fisher, A.D.; Galaal, K.; Cross, P.; Naik, R. High-grade vaginal intraepithelial neoplasia: Can we be selective about who we treat? *BJOG* **2013**, *120*, 887–893. [CrossRef]
37. Kim, M.-K.; Lee, I.H.; Lee, K.H. Clinical outcomes and risk of recurrence among patients with vaginal intraepithelial neoplasia: A comprehensive analysis of 576 cases. *J. Gynecol. Oncol.* **2018**, *29*, e6. [CrossRef]
38. Yu, D.; Qu, P.; Liu, M. Clinical presentation, treatment, and outcomes associated with vaginal intraepithelial neoplasia: A ret-rospective study of 118 patients. *J. Obstet. Gynaecol. Res.* **2021**, *47*, 1624–1630. [CrossRef]

Disclaimer/Publisher's Note: The statements, opinions and data contained in all publications are solely those of the individual author(s) and contributor(s) and not of MDPI and/or the editor(s). MDPI and/or the editor(s) disclaim responsibility for any injury to people or property resulting from any ideas, methods, instructions or products referred to in the content.

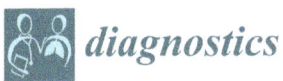

Article

Tips and Tricks for Early Diagnosis of Cervico-Vaginal Involvement from Extramammary Paget's Disease of the Vulva: A Referral Center Experience

Anna Daniela Iacobone [1,2,*], Maria Elena Guerrieri [1], Eleonora Petra Preti [1], Noemi Spolti [1], Gianluigi Radici [1], Giulia Peveri [3,4], Vincenzo Bagnardi [5], Giulio Tosti [6], Angelo Maggioni [7], Fabio Bottari [2,8], Chiara Scacchi [9] and Mariacristina Ghioni [10]

1 Preventive Gynecology Unit, European Institute of Oncology IRCCS, 20141 Milan, Italy
2 Department of Biomedical Sciences, University of Sassari, 07100 Sassari, Italy
3 Department of Clinical Sciences and Community Health, University of Milan, 20122 Milan, Italy
4 Department of Medical Epidemiology and Biostatistics, Karolinska Institutet, 17177 Stockholm, Sweden
5 Department of Statistics and Quantitative Methods, University of Milan-Bicocca, 20126 Milan, Italy
6 Dermato-Oncology Unit, European Institute of Oncology IRCCS, 20141 Milan, Italy
7 Department of Gynecology, European Institute of Oncology IRCCS, 20141 Milan, Italy
8 Division of Laboratory Medicine, European Institute of Oncology IRCCS, 20141 Milan, Italy
9 Division of Diagnostic Cytology, European Institute of Oncology IRCCS, 20141 Milan, Italy
10 Division of Pathology, European Institute of Oncology IRCCS, 20141 Milan, Italy
* Correspondence: annadaniela.iacobone@ieo.it

Abstract: Cervico-vaginal (CV) localization of extra-mammary Paget's disease (EMPD) of the vulva is extremely rare. In order to investigate the incidence risk and the pathognomonic clinical and pathological features of this condition, a retrospective analysis was conducted including 94 women treated for vulvar EMPD at the European Institute of Oncology, Milan, Italy, from October 1997 to May 2020. Overall nine patients developed CV involvement from EMPD, with a cumulative incidence of 2.5% (95% CI: 0.5–8.0%) at 5 years, 6.5% (95% CI: 1.9–15.1%) at 10 years and 14.0% (95% CI: 4.8–27.8%) at 15 years, respectively. All cases except one were firstly detected by abnormal glandular cytology. None reported vaginal bleeding or other suspicious symptoms. The colposcopic findings were heterogeneous and could sometimes be misdiagnosed. Cervical and/or vaginal biopsies were always performed for histopathological diagnosis by identification of Paget cells in the epithelium or stroma. Most patients developed invasive EMPD (5/9) of the cervix and/or vagina and underwent hysterectomy with partial or total colpectomy. CV involvement from EMPD should not be underestimated in women with a long-standing history of vulvar Paget's disease. Liquid-based cytology with immunocytochemistry represents a valuable tool for early diagnosis and should be routinely performed during the required lifelong follow-up.

Keywords: vulvar extramammary Paget's disease (EMPD); cervico-vaginal involvement; atypical glandular cytology; colposcopic-guided biopsy; Paget cells

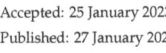

Citation: Iacobone, A.D.; Guerrieri, M.E.; Preti, E.P.; Spolti, N.; Radici, G.; Peveri, G.; Bagnardi, V.; Tosti, G.; Maggioni, A.; Bottari, F.; et al. Tips and Tricks for Early Diagnosis of Cervico-Vaginal Involvement from Extramammary Paget's Disease of the Vulva: A Referral Center Experience. *Diagnostics* **2023**, *13*, 464. https://doi.org/10.3390/diagnostics13030464

Academic Editor: Edward J. Pavlik

Received: 20 October 2022
Revised: 24 January 2023
Accepted: 25 January 2023
Published: 27 January 2023

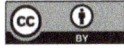

Copyright: © 2023 by the authors. Licensee MDPI, Basel, Switzerland. This article is an open access article distributed under the terms and conditions of the Creative Commons Attribution (CC BY) license (https:// creativecommons.org/licenses/by/ 4.0/).

1. Introduction

Extramammary Paget's disease (EMPD) of the vulva is a rare vulvar neoplasia with an unclear pathophysiology that usually occurs in the apocrine gland-rich skin of postmenopausal Caucasian women [1]. Vulvar EMPD predominantly manifests as an intraepithelial tumor (primary EMPD) but can also appear with stromal invasion or in association with an underlying lower genital tract or distant adenocarcinoma (secondary EMPD) [2].

The clinical presentation is various and includes erythematous, scaly or eczematous plaque on the vulva and perineum with occasional erosions or ulcerations, hypopigmentation and nodules. Itching and burning pain are the most common symptoms. Due to the overlap of signs and symptoms with other vulvar diseases, the diagnosis is confirmed by histological assessment on punch or excision biopsy. It is also well known that EMPD often appears as multifocal and/or with the histological extent of the disease far beyond the visible macroscopic lesion [3]. Moreover, despite surgical excision, local recurrence has been reported in up to 73% of cases and negative resection margins cannot ensure relapse-free survival [4]. On the contrary, Matsuo et al. recently showed that positive surgical margins are significantly associated with an increased risk of local but not distant recurrence [5]. Nevertheless, alternative therapeutic regimens have been advocated over time, including laser excision and ablation, topical therapy with imiquimod, photodynamic therapy and radiotherapy, since multiple surgical instances for recurrences lead to the destruction of vulvar anatomy with psychosocial consequences.

The cervical and vaginal localization of EMPD has only been described in the case reports as an extremely rare extension of recurrent vulvar EMPD and was firstly described in 1988 by Costello et al. [6].

While investigations based on age and anatomical site to distinguish between primary and secondary EMPD are well established, little is known about how to early diagnose cervico-vaginal (CV) localization of EMPD.

The objective of the present study was to investigate the incidence risk of CV involvement from EMPD of the vulva in women referred to a tertiary cancer center and to identify the pathognomonic clinical and pathological features of this rare evolution of vulvar EMPD.

2. Materials and Methods

All women affected by EMPD of the vulva and attending the Preventive Gynecologic Unit of the European Institute of Oncology, Milan, Italy, from October 1997 to May 2020, were retrieved from hospital file archives and enrolled in a retrospective analysis.

The local Institutional Review Board approved the study protocol (IEO protocol number UID 2408, date of approval: 22 June 2020) and written informed consent for the use of data for scientific purposes was obtained from all subjects prior to treatment.

Patients were included if the following criteria were met: (a) age at diagnosis of 18 years or older; (b) histologic confirmation of vulvar EMPD; (c) available data regarding follow-up. Patients were excluded in the case of different histology of vulvar neoplasia.

The data regarding clinical and pathological characteristics of the patients were recorded in a dedicated database.

The histological characteristics of first diagnosis, vulvar recurrence and cervical and/or vaginal localization were retrieved from surgical and pathological reports. All histological diagnoses were conducted by dedicated gynecological pathologists working at the Pathology Division of our Institute. Vulvar EMPD was classified according to the classification of Wilkinson and Brown as either primary, if Paget cells were of cutaneous origin, or secondary, in the case of vulvar skin involvement derived from an internal noncutaneous malignancy. The primary vulvar EMPD was further classified as exclusively intraepithelial (Type 1a), associated with stromal invasion (Type 1b) and as a manifestation of a primary vulvar adenocarcinoma (Type 1c). Secondary vulvar EMPD could be associated with anal or rectal adenocarcinoma (Type 2a), urothelial carcinoma (Type 2b) and distant tumors, including hepatocellular and breast carcinomas (Type 2c) [7].

Follow-up was routinely scheduled at the dedicated Vulvar Pathology Clinic of our Institute.

Apart from primary HPV screening, a pap smear was routinely performed once a year, also in women older than 65 years. In the case of abnormal cytology, women underwent colposcopy with cervical and/or vaginal guided biopsies. When atypical glandular cells were detected, endocervical curettage, endometrial biopsy and transvaginal ultrasound were always performed to rule out the origin of abnormal cells from endocervix, endometrium, ovary or Fallopian tube. If not available, HPV testing was conducted to exclude HPV-related disease.

A dedicated database was prospectively filled at each follow-up visit.

Therapeutic approaches, including surgery and alternative treatments such as topical therapy with imiquimod, photodynamic therapy and radiotherapy, as well as the type and timing of any persistence or recurrence, invasive disease and cervico-vaginal (CV) localization of EMPD were registered.

To improve the accuracy of the survival data, telephone interviews and consultation of civil registries were allowed in the case of patients lost to follow-up.

Statistical Analysis

Patients' history, characteristics at diagnosis, therapeutic pathway and follow-up occurrences were summarized as the count and percentage for the categorical variables, as a mean and range for the continuous variables, and as the median and range for the skewed variables. The cumulative incidence function (CIF) of the CV localization was computed considering death as a competing event. The overall survival was estimated by the Kaplan–Meier (KM) method, and a survival curve was represented. Statistical analyses were performed using SAS statistical software version 9.4 (SAS Institute Inc., Cary, NC, USA).

3. Results

After applying the inclusion and exclusion criteria, 94 women affected by vulvar EMPD and treated at the European Institute of Oncology, from October 1997 to May 2020, were selected for our retrospective analysis.

The mean age of patients at the time of first diagnosis was 63.3 years (range: 31–88) and the median follow-up time was 7 years + 10 months (range: 2 months–30 years + 7 months).

The main clinical and pathological characteristics of the enrolled women at first diagnosis and during follow-up are shown in Table 1.

Most of the patients (81%) were affected by intraepithelial EMPD (Type 1a) at first diagnosis. Invasive EMPD occurred in only 36% of cases, including 17 patients diagnosed at first occurrence and 17 during follow-up. The histology of the invasive EMPD patients is listed in Table 1.

Persistence or recurrence was very common, taking place in 86% of cases and, thus, often requiring multiple surgical instances (median: 2; range: 0–11). The histology of persistence/recurrence of EMPD is detailed in Table 1. Alternative treatments were applied, especially in the case of relapse, including local therapy with imiquimod (63%), photodynamic therapy (5%) and radiotherapy (12%).

After excluding one patient with an unknown death date, the 5 year overall survival was 90.5% (95% CI: 81.8–95.1%), as shown in Figure 1.

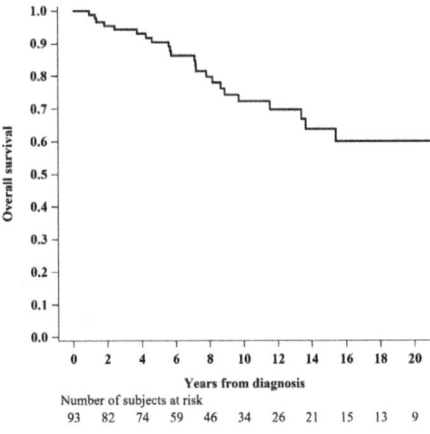

Figure 1. Overall survival of women affected by vulvar EMPD (N = 93).

Table 1. Clinical and pathological characteristics of women affected by vulvar EMPD at first diagnosis and during follow-up (N = 94).

Variable	N (%)
Histology at diagnosis	
1a	76 (81)
1b	10 (11)
1c	7 (7)
N+	1
2a	1 (1)
Previous or concurrent cancer	
No	67 (71)
Breast	14 (15)
Endometrial	2 (2)
Bladder–Urethral	3 (3)
Colorectal	1 (1)
Vulvar squamous	4 (4)
Other	3 (3)
Surgery	
No	2 (2)
Yes	92 (98)
Imiquimod	
No	32 (34)
Yes	59 (63)
Missing	3 (3)
Photodynamic therapy	
No	87 (93)
Yes	5 (5)
Missing	2 (2)
Radiotherapy	
No	81 (86)
Yes	11 (12)
Missing	2 (2)
Persistence or recurrence	
No	12 (13)
Yes	81 (86)
Unknown	1 (1)
Histology at persistence or recurrence	
1a	47 (58)
1b	9 (11)
1c	3 (4)
N+	1
2a	3 (4)
Invasive mammary PD	1 (1)
N+	1
Unknown histology	18 (22)
Invasive EMPD	
No	60 (64)
Yes	34 (36)
Time of diagnosis of invasive EMPD	
At diagnosis of EMPD	17 (50)
During the follow-up	17 (50)
Histology of invasive EMPD	
1b	19 (56)
1c	11 (32)
N+	1
2a invasive	2 (6)
N+	2
Invasive mammary PD	1 (3)
N+	1

Table 1. Cont.

Variable	N (%)
Invasive PD of the urethra	1 (3)
Abnormal pap smear	
No	82 (87)
Yes	11 (12)
Unknown	1 (1)
Cervico-vaginal localization	
No	84 (89)
Yes	9 (10)
Unknown	1 (1)

Overall, nine women developed CV localization of EMPD, with a cumulative incidence of 2.5% (95% CI: 0.5–8.0%) at 5 years, 6.5% (95% CI: 1.9–15.1%) at 10 years and 14.0% (95% CI: 4.8–27.8%) at 15 years, respectively (Figure 2).

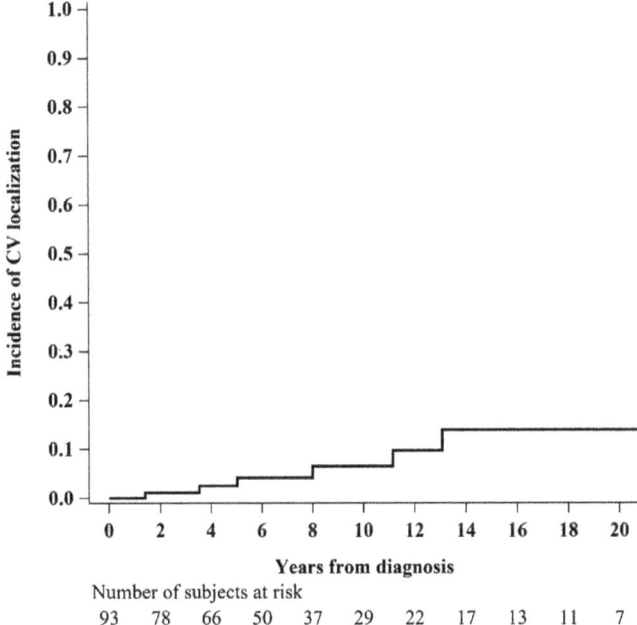

Figure 2. Cumulative incidence function of cervico-vaginal (CV) localization of vulvar EMPD, considering death as a competing event (N = 93).

The main characteristics of women who developed CV involvement from vulvar EMPD are reported in Table 2, including histology at diagnosis and at vulvar recurrence and the timing and type of CV localization. The majority of women (6/9) showed an intraepithelial vulvar EMPD (Type 1a) at first diagnosis, but three of them developed an invasive disease (Type 1b) at recurrence. The CV localizations occurred after a median time of 133 months (range: 16–334) from the first diagnosis of vulvar EMPD. All cases except one were firstly detected by abnormal pap smear and histologically confirmed by cervical and vaginal colposcopic-guided biopsies.

Table 2. Principal characteristics of women with cervico-vaginal (CV) localization of vulvar EMPD (N = 9).

Subject ID	Age at Diagnosis (Years)	Histology of Vulvar EMPD at First Diagnosis	Histology of Vulvar EMPD at Recurrence	Time to Abnormal Cytology (Months)	Time to Diagnosis of CV Localization (Months)	Site of CV Localization	Histology of CV Localization
1	52	1a	1a	155	157	Cervical and vaginal	Intraepithelial EMPD *
2	42	1a	1a	251	260	Cervical and vaginal N+	Invasive EMPD
3	67	1a	1b	94	95	Vaginal	Invasive EMPD
4	59	1a	1a	132	133	Cervical and vaginal	Invasive urothelial carcinoma
5	62	1a	1b	251	255	Cervical and vaginal	Intraepithelial EMPD
6	86	1a	1b	NA	60	Vaginal	Invasive EMPD
7	46	1b	1b	333	334	Cervical and vaginal	Invasive EMPD
8	70	1c	1c	15	16	Cervical and vaginal	Invasive EMPD
9	74	2a	Invasive mucinous intestinal-type adenocarcinoma	30	42	Cervical N+	Invasive mucinous intestinal-type adenocarcinoma

* Developed invasive EMPD of the urethra after CV localization.

Most patients (5/9) developed invasive EMPD of the cervix and/or vagina. In the case of invasive or unusual disease, magnetic resonance imaging (MRI) of the lower abdomen and total body positron emission tomography (PET) were performed to rule out pelvic node or distant metastases. Interestingly, one woman with vulvar EMPD Type 1a at the onset developed invasive cervico-vaginal involvement with node metastasis after 251 months from the initial diagnosis. CV intraepithelial EMPD occurred in only two patients, among which one later developed invasive EMPD of the urethra. Two CV localizations manifested with other associated diseases: invasive urothelial carcinoma and invasive mucinous intestinal-type adenocarcinoma with node metastasis.

Most of the women underwent hysterectomy with partial or total colpectomy based on the site of extravulvar EMPD localization. The patient with node metastases was treated with chemotherapy in association with anti-HER2 (human epidermal growth factor 2)-targeted monoclonal antibodies. Instead, the patient diagnosed with cervical invasive mucinous intestinal-type adenocarcinoma refused any treatment because of comorbidities and died nine months after the diagnosis. Radiotherapy was offered to the woman who developed an unresectable and advanced form of invasive EMPD of the urethra.

3.1. Clinical Features

None of the women reported suspicious symptoms, such as vaginal bleeding or discharge. Almost all cases were detected by abnormal glandular cytology. An HPV DNA test resulted negative in all patients. Endometrial biopsy and transvaginal ultrasound ruled out the origin of abnormal glandular cells from endometrium, ovary and Fallopian tube in all cases.

3.2. Cytology

Liquid-based cervical cytology revealed the presence of atypical or frankly malignant glandular cells in eight out of nine cases affected by CV localization of vulvar EMPD. The Paget cells were round to columnar with an increased nuclear/cytoplasmic (N/C) ratio and vacuolated cytoplasm. Since HER2 is frequently expressed in genital and anal EMPD (15–60% of cases) [8], a cell block was set-up with residual cellularity and HER2 expression explored by immunocytochemistry in four cases in order to support the diagnosis (Figure 3).

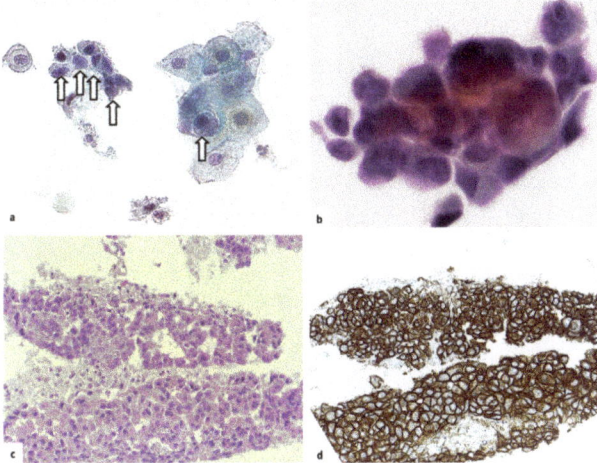

Figure 3. Cervical cytology of EMPD: (**a**,**b**) liquid-based cytology; (**c**,**d**) cell block. Note the (arrow) Paget cells as round or columnar cells with an increased N/C ratio (**a**, 20×), arranged in small clusters (**b**, 40×) on liquid-based cytology and highlighted on the cell block (**c**, 20×) by HER2 expression (**d**, 20×).

3.3. Colposcopy

Colposcopy with endocervical curettage and guided ectocervical and/or vaginal biopsies was performed in all patients diagnosed with atypical glandular cells on pap smear in order to assess the nature of the atypical cells, the extent of the disease and make the best therapeutic decision.

The colposcopic findings were heterogeneous in our CV localizations of EMPD and could sometimes be misdiagnosed as high-grade intraepithelial squamous lesions. After acetic acid wash, major abnormal colposcopic findings were revealed in all patients. However, some cases showed dense acetowhite epithelium with a sharp border, whereas other cases appeared as micropapillary lesions with ridge sign or large papillae with irregular surface and fragile vessels. Coarse punctuation was common in almost all cases of CV EMPD. The location of lesions could be inside or outside the transformation zone of the cervix and in the vaginal fornices or walls. Most of the lesions were multifocal and with a wide extension (Figure 4).

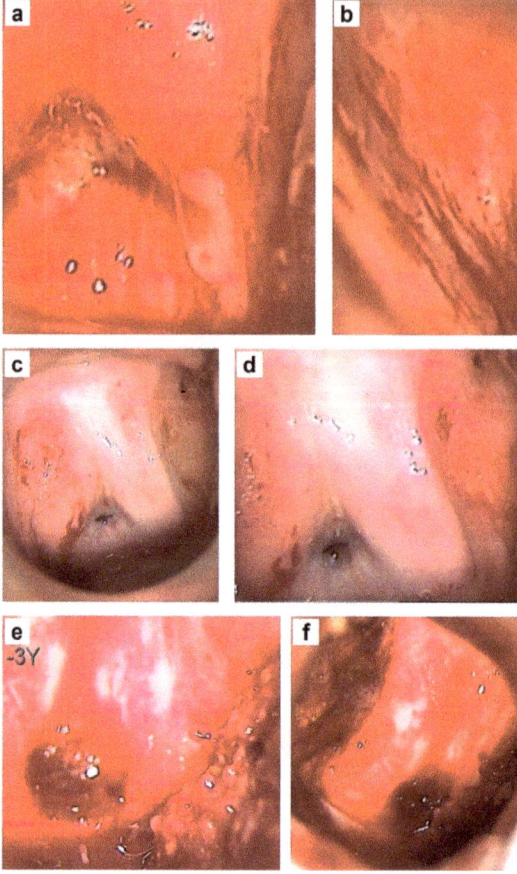

Figure 4. Heterogeneous colposcopic findings in women diagnosed with CV involvement from vulvar EMPD: (**a,b**) Dense acetowhite epithelium with sharp borders and coarse punctuation: inside the transformation zone of the cervix and in the left vaginal fornix (**a**); in the middle third of the left vaginal wall (**b**). (**c,d**) Micropapillary lesions with ridge sign and coarse punctuation: outside the transformation zone of the cervix (**c**); in the upper third of the left vaginal wall (**d**). (**e,f**) Large papillae with an irregular surface and fragile vessels: in the left vaginal wall (**e**); in the right and left vaginal walls with a wide extension (**f**).

3.4. Histopathological Diagnosis

As in vulvar EMPD, the diagnostic clue in CV localization is the presence of Paget cells in the epithelium or stroma. Paget cells are large cells with abundant pale cytoplasm, large vesicular nuclei and prominent nucleoli, arranged as single cells or cell clusters throughout the epithelium and/or in the stroma (Figure 5). The diagnosis is not so difficult in cases with a long history of vulvar EMPD, but it could represent a challenge in some instances. Among the differential diagnoses, it is mandatory to consider intraepithelial or invasive squamous cells carcinoma and malignant melanoma in the first instance and to take into account the involvement by an internal regional cancer (colon or urinary bladder, mainly). A diagnostic immunohistochemical panel is recommended for excluding EMPD mimics [3], comprising cytokeratin (CK)7, CK20, p63, SOX10 and carcinoembryonic antigen (CEA). EMPD is typical CK7-positive, CK20-positive or negative, p63-negative, SOX10-negative and CEA-positive unlike squamous cell carcinoma which is p63-positive and malignant melanoma which is SOX10-positive. To rule out the possibility of spread from an internal tumor, CDX-2 (negative in EMPD and positive in colon cancer) and uroplakin-III (negative in EMPD and positive in urothelial carcinoma) are helpful.

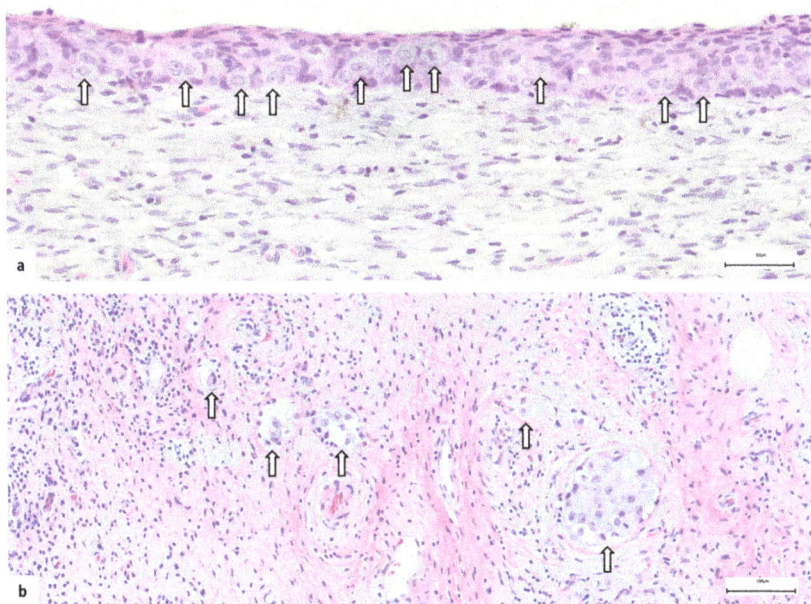

Figure 5. Cervical EMPD: (**a**) intraepithelial and (**b**) invasive. Note the (arrow) Paget cells, with clear cytoplasm and prominent nucleoli, arranged as single cells or little clusters in the ectocervical epithelium (**a**) and as gland-like structures in the cervical stroma (**b**).

4. Discussion

CV involvement from EMPD occurred in 9.6% (9/94) of women affected by vulvar EMPD and attending the Preventive Gynecologic Unit of the European Institute of Oncology, Milan, Italy, from October 1997 to May 2020.

This rare condition has already been reported by a few case reports in previous years [9–13]. Only Gu at al. reported a higher prevalence (15.6%) of patients with vulvar EMPD who developed CV localization during the course of their disease. However, a potential bias in their results is the limited number (only 19) of women who were retrospectively analyzed and among whom three were diagnosed with CV EMPD after an abnormal pap smear [14]. This could obviously lead to an overestimation of this rare evolution of vulvar Paget's disease.

Nevertheless, cervix and/or vagina could be involved more than usually expected, as a direct contiguous extension from the vulva. Indeed, it is already well known that vulvar EMPD could histologically extend beyond the visible lesion, even if primary and intraepithelial [10,11].

In addition, CV EMPD can be incidentally diagnosed on exfoliative cytology smears, though not differentiating between intraepithelial and invasive disease, as widely reported previously in the literature [15,16]. Therefore, a Papanicolaou smear should be routinely performed even in the cases of benign appearance of the cervix and vagina [10].

However, when atypical glandular cells are detected on a pap smear, endocervix, endometrium, ovary and Fallopian tube should be always investigated as a potential source, since related malignancies are more common than Paget's disease [17].

A clinical history of EMPD in women with abnormal glandular cytology could be helpful for pathological diagnosis and is often crucial for a differential diagnosis. Indeed, immunocytochemistry is not usually necessary but represents an additional valuable tool to distinguish Paget cells from high-grade squamous lesions on liquid-based cytology specimens of suspicious glandular lesions in women with known EMPD of the vulva [18].

Although only described by rare case reports [6,10,14], Papanicolaou smear still plays a fundamental role for the early detection of Paget cells in the cervix and/or vagina. This assumption is very noteworthy in our recent time when HPV testing alone has been advocated as the best cost-effective strategy for cervical cancer screening [19,20]. All of our cases of CV EMPD had a negative HPV DNA test result and would not be identified by HPV primary screening. Moreover, in most cases, CV EMPD occurred in women older than 65 years of age when routine screening was usually discontinued. Hence, according to our experience, there is a strong clinical rationale to routinely perform pap smear in older patients with a history of vulvar Paget's disease.

Colposcopic findings when Paget cells are detected in the pap smear have been reported as normal or minor abnormal in the past literature [10]. In our retrospective analysis, colposcopic findings were major abnormal in all patients with CV localizations of EMPD, but widely heterogeneous and could sometimes be misdiagnosed as high-grade intraepithelial squamous lesions. Thus, colposcopic-guided biopsies are mandatory for full assessment in order to confirm histopathological diagnosis of EMPD after an abnormal glandular cytology, as already suggested by other authors [9,21].

Interestingly, according to our experience, the cumulative incidence of CV localization of vulvar EMPD increases with an increasing survival time: 2.5% at 5 years, 6.5% at 10 years and 14.0% at 15 years. The risk of CV EMPD should always be considered in women with longstanding, extensive and recurrent vulvar disease. Long-term follow-up with routine liquid-based cervical cytology is highly recommended.

To the best of our knowledge, the present study is the largest case series of women diagnosed with CV involvement from EMPD of the vulva. Furthermore, this is the first paper that retrospectively analyzes and describes all pathognomonic clinical and pathological features of this condition in order to identify which steps might be useful for early diagnosis by clinicians.

Early diagnosis of this disease manifestation is a key step in choosing the correct therapeutic management. Surgical approach is always the first choice in the case of CV localization of EMPD in the absence of lymph node metastasis. The role of chemotherapy and radiotherapy for this disease is not well defined unlike vulvar squamous cell carcinoma and should be reserved only for unresectable advanced disease and/or with lymph node metastases [22,23]. However, combined chemotherapy and anti-HER2-targeted therapy represents a promising strategy in patients with advanced or recurrent EMPD of the vulva [24].

The limits of this study include selection bias related to the single-center retrospective analysis and the small sample of events, which did not allow for a logistic regression analysis to investigate risk factors for the development and occurrence of CV EMPD.

5. Conclusions

CV involvement from EMPD is a rare condition but should not be underestimated in women with a long-standing history of vulvar Paget's disease. It can be promptly detected by cytology, which is a valuable and reliable tool for early diagnosis and should be routinely performed during the required lifelong follow-up.

Author Contributions: Conceptualization, A.D.I., M.E.G., E.P.P. and N.S.; Methodology, A.D.I., M.E.G., C.S. and M.G.; Software, A.D.I., M.E.G. and G.P.; Validation, A.D.I. and V.B.; Formal Analysis, G.P. and V.B.; Investigation, A.D.I., M.E.G., E.P.P., N.S. and G.R.; Resources, A.D.I., E.P.P., N.S., G.T. and A.M.; Data Curation, A.D.I., M.E.G. and G.P.; Writing—Original Draft Preparation, A.D.I. and M.G.; Writing—Review and Editing, A.D.I., M.E.G., G.R., G.T. and F.B.; Visualization, A.D.I., C.S. and M.G.; Supervision, F.B. and A.M.; Project Administration, A.D.I. All authors have read and agreed to the published version of the manuscript.

Funding: This research received no external funding.

Institutional Review Board Statement: The study was conducted according to the guidelines of the Declaration of Helsinki and approved by the Institutional Review Board of the European Institute of Oncology, Milan, Italy (IEO protocol number: UID 2408; date of approval: 22 June 2020).

Informed Consent Statement: Informed consent was obtained from all subjects involved in the study.

Data Availability Statement: The data presented in this study are available upon request from the corresponding author. The data are not publicly available due to the patients' privacy restrictions. The data are safely stored in a private database of the European Institute of Oncology, Milan, Italy.

Acknowledgments: This work was partially supported by the Italian Ministry of Health with Ricerca Corrente and 5×1000 funds.

Conflicts of Interest: The authors declare no conflict of interest. None of the authors received financial support or funding for this work.

References

1. Morris, C.R.; Hurst, E.A. Extramammary Paget disease: A review of the literature—Part I: History, epidemiology, pathogenesis, presentation, histopathology, and diagnostic work-up. *Dermatol. Surg.* **2020**, *46*, 151–158. [CrossRef]
2. Zhang, G.; Zhou, S.; Zhong, W.; Hong, L.; Wang, Y.; Lu, S.; Pan, J.; Huang, Y.; Su, M.; Crawford, R.; et al. Whole-exome sequencing reveals frequent mutations in chromatin remodeling genes in mammary and extramammary Paget's diseases. *J. Investig. Dermatol.* **2019**, *139*, 789–795. [CrossRef] [PubMed]
3. Kibbi, N.; Owen, J.L.; Worley, B.; Wang, J.X.; Harikumar, V.; Downing, M.B.; Aasi, S.Z.; Aung, P.P.; Barker, C.A.; Bolotin, D.; et al. Evidence-Based Clinical Practice Guidelines for Extramammary Paget Disease. *JAMA Oncol.* **2022**, *8*, 618–628. [CrossRef] [PubMed]
4. Preti, M.; Micheletti, L.; Borella, F.; Cosma, S.; Marrazzu, A.; Gallio, N.; Privitera, S.; Tancredi, A.; Bevilacqua, F.; Benedetto, C. Vulvar Paget's disease and stromal invasion: Clinico-pathological features and survival outcomes. *Surg. Oncol.* **2021**, *38*, 101581. [CrossRef] [PubMed]
5. Matsuo, K.; Nishio, S.; Matsuzaki, S.; Iwase, H.; Kagami, S.; Soeda, S.; Usui, H.; Nishikawa, R.; Mikami, M.; Enomoto, T. Surgical margin status and recurrence pattern in invasive vulvar Paget's disease: A Japanese Gynecologic Oncology Group study. *Gynecol. Oncol.* **2021**, *160*, 748–754. [CrossRef]
6. Costello, T.J.; Wang, H.H.; Schnitt, S.J.; Ritter, R.; Antonioli, D.A. Paget's disease with extensive involvement of the female genital tract initially detected by cervical cytosmear. *Arch. Pathol. Lab. Med.* **1988**, *112*, 941–944.
7. Wilkinson, E.J.; Brown, H.M. Vulvar Paget disease of urothelial origin: A report of three cases and a proposed classification of vulvar Paget disease. *Hum. Pathol.* **2002**, *33*, 549–554. [CrossRef]
8. Tokuchi, K.; Maeda, T.; Kitamura, S.; Yanagi, T.; Ujiie, H. HER2-Targeted Antibody-Drug Conjugates Display Potent Antitumor Activities in Preclinical Extramammary Paget's Disease Models: In Vivo and Immunohistochemical Analyses. *Cancers* **2022**, *14*, 3519. [CrossRef]
9. Lloyd, J.; Evans, D.J.; Flanagan, A.M. Extension of extramammary Paget disease of the vulva to the cervix. *J. Clin. Pathol.* **1999**, *52*, 538–540. [CrossRef]

10. Westacott, L.; Cominos, D.; Williams, S.; Knight, B.; Waterfield, R. Primary cutaneous vulvar extramammary Paget's disease involving the endocervix and detected by Pap smear. *Pathology* **2013**, *45*, 426–428. [CrossRef]
11. Hardy, L.E.; Baxter, L.; Wan, K.; Ayres, C. Invasive cervical adenocarcinoma arising from extension of recurrent vulval Paget's disease. *BMJ Case Rep.* **2020**, *13*, e232424. [CrossRef] [PubMed]
12. Geisler, J.P.; Gates, R.W.; Shirrell, W.; Parker, S.M.; Maloney, C.D.; Wiemann, M.C.; Geisler, H.E. Extramammary Paget's disease with diffuse involvement of the lower female genito-urinary system. *Int. J. Gynecol. Cancer* **1997**, *7*, 84–87. [CrossRef]
13. Chen, Q.; Qiu, Y.; Xu, L.; Tang, X.; Yang, K.; Wang, W. Cytological diagnosis of patients with extramammary Paget's disease of the vagina. *Int. J. Clin. Exp. Pathol.* **2018**, *11*, 3765–3769. [PubMed]
14. Gu, M.; Ghafari, S.; Lin, F. Pap smears of patients with extramammary Paget's disease of the vulva. *Diagn. Cytopathol.* **2005**, *32*, 353–357. [CrossRef] [PubMed]
15. Castellano Megías, V.M.; Ibarrola de Andrés, C.; Martínez Parra, D.; Lara Lara, I.; Pérez Palacios, C.; Conde Zurita, J.M. Cytology of extramammary Paget's disease of the vulva. A case report. *Acta Cytol.* **2002**, *46*, 1153–1157. [CrossRef]
16. Klapsinou, E.; Terzakis, E.; Arnogiannaki, N.; Daskalopoulou, D. Paget's disease of the vulva detected in vulvar and vaginal brushing smears. *Acta Cytol.* **2010**, *54*, 898–902.
17. Perkins, R.B.; Guido, R.S.; Castle, P.E.; Chelmow, D.; Einstein, M.H.; Garcia, F.; Huh, W.K.; Kim, J.J.; Moscicki, A.-B.; Nayar, R.; et al. 2019 ASCCP Risk-Based Management Consensus Guidelines Committee. 2019 ASCCP Risk-Based Management Consensus Guidelines for Abnormal Cervical Cancer Screening Tests and Cancer Precursors. *J. Low. Genit. Tract. Dis.* **2020**, *24*, 102–131. [CrossRef] [PubMed]
18. Gilliland, K.; Knapik, J.; Wilkinson, E.J. Cytology of vulvar/vaginal Paget disease: Report of a case and review of the literature. *J. Low. Genit. Tract. Dis.* **2013**, *17*, e26–e30. [CrossRef]
19. Kyrgiou, M.; Arbyn, M.; Bergeron, C.; Bosch, F.X.; Dillner, J.; Jit, M.; Kim, J.; Poljak, M.; Nieminen, P.; Sasieni, P.; et al. Cervical screening: ESGO-EFC position paper of the European Society of Gynaecologic Oncology (ESGO) and the European Federation of Colposcopy (EFC). *Br. J. Cancer* **2020**, *123*, 510–517. [CrossRef]
20. Jeronimo, J.; Castle, P.E.; Temin, S.; Denny, L.; Gupta, V.; Kim, J.J.; Luciani, S.; Murokora, D.; Ngoma, T.; Qiao, Y.; et al. Secondary Prevention of Cervical Cancer: ASCO Resource-Stratified Clinical Practice Guideline. *J. Glob. Oncol.* **2016**, *3*, 635–657. [CrossRef]
21. Davis, G.; Anderson, L.; Pather, S. Extramammary paget's disease mimicking localized malignancy on cervical cytology. *Diagn. Cytopathol.* **2016**, *44*, 931–934. [CrossRef]
22. Tomao, F.; Di Tucci, C.; Marchetti, C.; Perniola, G.; Bellati, F.; Panici, P.B. Role of chemotherapy in the management of vulvar carcinoma. *Crit. Rev. Oncol. Hematol.* **2012**, *82*, 25–39. [CrossRef] [PubMed]
23. Ni, L.; Sinha, S.; Rara, M.; Phuong, C.; Chen, L.-M.; Hsu, I.-C.J.; Yoshida, E.J. The role of adjuvant radiation therapy in older patients with node-positive vulvar cancer: A national cancer database analysis. *Gynecol Oncol.* **2022**, *167*, 189–195. [CrossRef] [PubMed]
24. Talia, K.L.; Banet, N.; Buza, N. The role of HER2 as a therapeutic biomarker in gynaecological malignancy: Potential for use beyond uterine serous carcinoma. *Pathology* **2023**, *55*, 8–18. [CrossRef] [PubMed]

Disclaimer/Publisher's Note: The statements, opinions and data contained in all publications are solely those of the individual author(s) and contributor(s) and not of MDPI and/or the editor(s). MDPI and/or the editor(s) disclaim responsibility for any injury to people or property resulting from any ideas, methods, instructions or products referred to in the content.

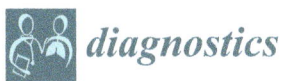

Article

Mapping HPV 16 Sub-Lineages in Anal Cancer and Implications for Disease Outcomes

Daniel Guerendiain [1,2,*], Laila Sara Arroyo Mühr [3], Raluca Grigorescu [4], Matthew T. G. Holden [2] and Kate Cuschieri [1]

1. Scottish HPV Reference Laboratory, Royal Infirmary of Edinburgh, 51 Little France Crescent, Edinburgh EH16 4SA, UK
2. School of Medicine, University of St Andrews, St Andrews KY16 9TF, UK
3. International HPV Reference Center, Department of Laboratory Medicine, Karolinska Institutet, 141 86 Stockholm, Sweden
4. Department of Pathology, Royal Infirmary of Edinburgh, 51 Little France Crescent, Edinburgh EH16 4SA, UK
* Correspondence: dgr7@st-andrews.ac.uk or daniel.guerendiain@nhslothian.scot.nhs.uk

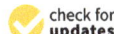

Citation: Guerendiain, D.; Mühr, L.S.A.; Grigorescu, R.; Holden, M.T.G.; Cuschieri, K. Mapping HPV 16 Sub-Lineages in Anal Cancer and Implications for Disease Outcomes. *Diagnostics* 2022, 12, 3222. https://doi.org/10.3390/diagnostics12123222

Academic Editors: Fabio Bottari and Anna Daniela Iacobone

Received: 31 October 2022
Accepted: 9 December 2022
Published: 19 December 2022

Publisher's Note: MDPI stays neutral with regard to jurisdictional claims in published maps and institutional affiliations.

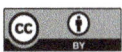

Copyright: © 2022 by the authors. Licensee MDPI, Basel, Switzerland. This article is an open access article distributed under the terms and conditions of the Creative Commons Attribution (CC BY) license (https://creativecommons.org/licenses/by/4.0/).

Abstract: The incidence of anal cancer is rising worldwide. As identified in cervical cancer management, an improvement in the early detection and management of anal pre-cancer is essential. In other cancers associated with human papillomavirus (HPV), HPV 16 sub-lineages have been shown to be associated with disease status and prognosis. However, in anal cancer, they have been under-explored. A total of 119 HPV 16-positive anal cancer lesions diagnosed between 2009 and 2018 in Scotland and 134 HPV 16-positive residual rectal swabs from asymptomatic men collected in 2016/7 were whole genome sequenced. The association of HPV 16 sub-lineages with underlying disease status (cancer vs. asymptomatic) and overall survival in anal cancer samples was assessed (comparing A1 vs non-A1 sub-lineages). A1 was the dominant sub-lineage present in the anal cancer (76.5%) and the asymptomatic (76.1%) cohorts. A2 was the second most dominant sub-lineage in both groups (16.8% and 17.2%, respectively). We did not observe significant associations of sub-lineage with demographics, clinical variables or survival (A1 vs. non-A1 sub-lineages (HR 0.83, 0.28–2.46 $p = 0.743$)). HPV 16 sub-lineages do to not appear to cluster with disease vs asymptomatic carriage or be independently associated with outcomes in anal cancer patients. Further international studies on anal HPV sub-lineage mapping will help to determine whether this is a consistent observation.

Keywords: human papillomavirus; HPV 16 sub-lineages; anal cancer

1. Introduction

Anal cancer is one of the six cancers shown to have a human papillomavirus (HPV) aetiology [1]. Most HPV-positive anal cancers are caused by HPV type 16 (HPV 16), and in a recent population-based assessment in Scotland, in cases diagnosed between 2009–2018, HPV 16 was detected in 93.3% of the HPV positive cases [2], higher than the amount of HPV 16 attributable to cervical cancer [3].

Additionally, as with other HPV-driven cancers, anal cancer incidence is increasing worldwide, including in the USA and Europe [4–7].

HPVs are formally classified as "types" based on the nucleotide sequence of the open reading frame (ORF) coding for the major capsid protein: L1 [8]. HPV types differ by more than 10% of their primary sequence compared to their most closely related type [8]. Phenotypic differences in HPV types with respect to disease risk and tissue tropism are well-established, and this knowledge has informed the development of effective vaccines and HPV-based cervical screening assays. However, below the level of HPV type exist lineages (with 2–10% variation) and sub-lineages (0.5% to 2% variation) [9], and the implications of this level of variation on clinical outcomes of infection is less established.

For HPV 16, four lineages have been identified (lineages A, B, C and D), as well as 16 sub-lineages: A, including A1–A3 (previously named European) and A4 (Asian) sub-lineages; B, including B1 (African-1, Afr1a) and B2 (African-1, Afr1b), B3 and B4 sub-lineages; C1 (African-2, Afr2a), C2, C3 and C4; and D, including D1 (North American, NA1), D2 (Asian-American, AA2), D3 (Asian-American, AA1) and D4 sub-lineages [9].

Although some investigators have assessed the global distribution of sub-lineages, the majority have focused on cervical cancers rather than other HPV-driven cancers. In 2013, Cornet et al. looked at the HPV lineages in cervical cancers and showed that European sub-lineages (A1–A3) were the most common in all regions of the world, except in sub-Saharan Africa and East Asia, whereas the African sub-lineages dominated in the northern sub-Saharan region of Africa, and the Asian variant in East Asia [10]. Nicolás-Párraga et al. (2016) found similar results, with A1–3 present in 95.65% of the cases in Europe, 78.26% in Central/South America (D in 21.73%) and 80% in Asia (12% A4 and 7.69% D) [11].

In terms of HPV 16 sub-lineages present in the anus, data is relatively sparce. Volpini et al. (2017) investigated the HPV 16 variants in anal samples collated in Brazil, finding that 70.8% were classified as A1–3 sub-lineages and 29.2% as "other" [12]. A recent systematic review, performed by Ferreira et al. (2021) of genetic variants of HPV-16 in men, found HPV 16 lineages vary according to anatomical and geographical regions, but they found that European samples had a high prevalence (86.59%) of HPV 16 lineage A [13].

In the context of cervical disease, evidence suggests that sub-lineages and variants may be independently associated with poor clinical outcomes. Mirabello et al. (2015) [14] revealed a higher risk of disease associated with B/C/D lineages as a group compared to the A lineage. Clifford et al. (2019). also found an increased cervical cancer risk for A3, A4 and D-(sub-) lineages vs the A1 sub-lineage. A more recent study by Lang Kuhs et al. (2022) looked into the genetic variation of HPV 16 and its association with clinical outcomes in HPV 16-positive oropharyngeal cancer patients. They investigated different high-risk single nucleotide polymorphisms (SNPs) and found that those with one or more high-risk SNPs had a median survival time of 3.96 years compared to 18.67 years for those with no high-risk SNPs. Most of these SNPs were common to the D2 sub-lineage, which have also been associated with higher risk of cancer in the cervix [14]. However equivalent studies on anal cancer are rare.

We recently identified that the viral load of HPV16 in anal cancer may be informative for prognosis [2]. Now, due to the information published on the association of HPV 16 sub-lineages and cancer risk yet the comparative absence of data in the anal context, we aimed to better understand the pattern and dominance of HPV 16 sub-lineages in a population-based cohort of anal cancer and to determine whether significant associations with sub-lineage and demographic or clinical variables existed). Data obtained from the cancer cohort was contextualized and compared to variant profile in anal samples obtained from an asymptomatic population.

2. Material and Methods

2.1. Sample Collection

A total of 150 HPV 16-positive anal cancers and 182 DNA extracts from residual rectal swabs obtained from asymptomatic men were selected for HPV 16 sub-lineage identification through whole genome sequencing (WGS).

2.1.1. Anal Cancer Cohort, Collection and Annotation

For the present work, we used the same anal cancer (n = 150) sample set as described in detail in Guerendiain et al. (2022) [2]. Briefly, nucleic acid extract associated with archived formalin-fixed, paraffin-embedded tissue was genotyped using the Seegene Anyplex II 28 (Seoul, Korea), followed by storage at −80 °C. Anal cancer biopsy samples were taken between 2009 and 2018 as part of the management of patients with anal disease from 3 of the 14 territorial health boards in Scotland (NHS Lothian, NHS Borders and NHS Fife).

HPV typing was performed at the Scottish HPV Reference Laboratory, Edinburgh, UK. One 10 μm section per sample was obtained and incubated in Seegene Universal Lysis Buffer (LB) at 65 °C overnight. DNA extraction was performed using the Microlab Nimbus IVD (Hamilton, Reno, USA) with the StarMAg Universal cartridge Kit (Seegene), following manufacturers' instructions. Mastermix was prepared with the Nimbus and PCR on the CFX Real-Time PCR instrument (Biorad, CA, USA).

As described in Guerendiain et al. (2022), clinico-demographic information was obtained in January 2020, specifically the patient's age, sex, stage of cancer (using the American Joint Committee on Cancer (AJCC) TNM system) [15], response to treatment, date of diagnosis and vital (dead/alive) status. Age and stage of cancer were considered at the time of diagnosis. Vital status information and date of death data was censored in July 2020.

Cases categorized according to the various clinical and demographic variables are summarized in Table 1. Age was stratified in 4 different groups: <50, 50–59, 60–69 and ≥0. Response to treatment was organized in 3 groups: yes, no or unknown, following the ESMO guidelines for anal cancer [16]. Cancer stage was aggregated in 5 groups: I, II, III, IV and unknown, following the AJCC system effective January 2018 [15].

Table 1. Anal cancer cohort: clinical characteristics and demographics with valid NGS analysis.

Variable	Level	$n = 119$	%
Sex	Female	90	75.6
	Male	29	24.4
Age	<50	15	12.6
	50–59	32	26.9
	60–69	39	32.8
	70 and over	33	27.7
Stage	I	18	15.1
	II	48	40.3
	III	36	30.2
	IV	16	13.4
	Unknown	1	0.8
Response to treatment	Yes	95	79.8
	No	17	14.3
	Unknown	7	5.9
Vital status	Alive	87	73.1
	Deceased	30	25.2
	Unknown	2	1.7

2.1.2. Residual Rectal Swabs from Asymptomatic Men

To contextualize the sequences observed in the anal cancers, a disease-free control group of anonymized residual rectal swabs obtained from asymptomatic men attending sexual health clinics were collated for downstream WGS. These samples had previously been genotyped as a consequence of immunization surveillance in Scotland [17]. DNA was extracted from the residual rectal swabs by Qiagen MDx (Hilden, Germany) or Seegene Universal Extraction System, obtaining an eluate volume of 100 μL. HPV genotyping was performed using the Seegene Anyplex II and the Optiplex HPV Genotyping Kit (Heildelberg, Germany), detecting 28 and 24 different HPV types, respectively.

A total of 182 anonymized DNA extracts from residual rectal swabs were collated. Samples had originally been collected in the years 2016–2017 and were included if positive for HPV 16.

2.2. Governance

Use of samples for the present project was approved by the Southeast of Scotland National Research for Scotland Bioresource (NRS) (application reference SR 1283 and SR1364). A favorable ethical opinion to conduct the research was provided by University of St Andrews Teaching and Research Ethics Committee, reference MD 14482.

2.3. PCR Target-Enrichment for Deep Sequencing of HPV 16

HPV 16 whole genome material was amplified using 47 overlapping amplicons described in Cullen et al. [18] and optimized by Arroyo et al. [19] Briefly, primer sets were divided into five different reactions to decrease self-dimer and cross-primer dimer formation. PCRs were performed using Qiagen Multiplex PCR Master Mix (Qiagen, Hilden, Germany) and 0.2 µM of each primer, according to manufacturers' instructions. PCR amplification products were pooled together according to sample name prior to library preparation.

2.4. Library Preparation

Libraries were prepared using the Illumina DNA prep kit (San Diego, CA, USA) following the manufacturer's instructions, using 450 ng of DNA in 35 µL as input. Sequencing was performed using the Illumina MiSeq instrument and the Illumina MiSeq reagent kit v2 500 cycles (2 × 250 bp). Libraries were normalized to 4 nM in combination with 12.5 pM of PhiX (Illumina).

2.5. Quality Control and Quality Analysis

HPV 16-positive (SiHa) and HPV-negative (water) controls were added at the DNA extraction step and carried through the PCR, library preparation and data analysis stages. Individual amplification products were assessed using a Bioanalyzer (Santa Clara, CA, USA). Quality control for library preparation included both controlling the library size using an Agilent Tapestation (Santa Clara, CA, USA) and determining the DNA concentration using the Qubit dsDNA High-Sensitivity Assay Kit (ThermoFisher, Waltham, MA, USA).

As a further quality control for analysis of the sequence data generated, a subset of 25 fastq files were sent to the International HPV Reference Laboratory in Karolinska, Sweden for independent bioinformatic analysis and sub-lineage identification.

2.6. Bioinformatic Analysis

Reads obtained from Illumina were de-multiplexed and converted to fastq files. All fastq files were quality and adaptor trimmed using Trimmomatic (v0.39) [20]. Only high-quality paired reads (-phred 33 -leading 3 -trailing 3- slidingWindow: 4:15) with 150 bp were used for further analysis. FASTQC tools were further used to assess whether any adaptors remained [21]. High-quality reads were then mapped to the HPV 16 reference genome from the Papillomavirus Episteme (PaVE) [22] using bwa (v0.7.17) [23], to create a sam file. Due to the circular HPV genome, the reference genome was modified by adding the 258 nucleotides from the beginning to the end of the genome sequence to not lose coverage of amplicons 46 and 47. SAMtools (v1.14) [24] was then used to convert files from sam to bam and to curate files for the variant calling. BCFtools (v1.14), mpileup and consensus tools were used for the variant calling and for the generation of a consensus sequence [25], using default parameters. Positions not covered were annotated as Ns.

New consensus files were aligned using MAFFT (v7.490) with default parameters [26]. A manual edit was performed when required. Maximum likelihood trees were inferred using RaxML (v2.0.8) [27] with the GTR substitution model (ML + transfer bootstrap expectation + consensus, 1 run, 100 reps). Visualization of the trees generated by RaxML was performed using Figtree (v1.4.4). Each sample was assigned with a sub-lineage corresponding to the nearest neighbor.

Sub-lineages references were obtained from the PAVE for each of the HPV 16 sub-lineages: A1 (K02718.1), A2 (AF536179.1), A3 (HQ644236.1), A4 (AF534061.1), B1 (AF536180.1), B2 (HQ644298.1), B3 (HQ644298.1), B4 (KU053914.1), C1 (AF472509.1), C2 (HQ644244.1),

C3 (KU053920.1), C4 (KU053925.1), D1 (HQ644257.1), D2 (AY686579.1), D3 (AF402678.1) and D4 (AF402678.1) A sub-lineage assignment was performed for all specimens excluding those with <100× median depth or low genome coverage (<80% genome coverage).

2.7. Assessment of Variants According to Clinic-Demographic Characteristics and Survival Analysis

To assess the relationship between HPV sub-lineages and different factors (two or more independent variables), a univariate logistic regression analysis was performed between HPV 16 sub-lineages (HPV 16 A1-positive vs. HPV 16 non-A1-positive), age at diagnosis, collection year and health board of diagnosis. Adjustment was performed for age group (<50, 50–59, 60–69 and 70 or over), sex, response to treatment, stage of cancer and vital status (dead or alive). Comparison was performed between A1 vs. non-A1 sub-lineages due to the small number of samples identified from the different sub-lineages. The non-A1 group includes the following sub-lineages: A2, A3, A4, B1, B2, B3, B4, C1, C2, C3, C4, D1, D2, D3 and D4.

Odds ratios (OR) were calculated to quantify the strength of the association between HPV 16 sub-lineages and the demographic and clinical data. All the statistics were obtained using R-studio macOS, (version 1.2.1335) [28]. The distribution of sub-lineages in anal cancers vs. the asymptomatic population was assessed with sequences from the two groups displayed in a phylogenetic tree.

Overall survival by HPV 16 sub-lineages (HPV 16 A1-positive vs. HPV 16 non-A1-positive) was analyzed using the Kaplan-Meier method. The univariate and multivariate hazard ratios of HPV 16 sub-lineages (HPV 16 A1-positive vs. HPV 16 non-A1-positive) for all-cause death were derived using the cox proportional hazard model. A univariate and multivariate model was derived; age (<50, 50–59, 60–69, 70+), sex, stage (I, II, III, IV) and response to treatment (no, yes) were adjusted for. All the statistical analyses were performed using R-studio (version 1.2.1335) [29]. Differences in prevalence of the HPV 16 sub-lineages between the anal cancer cohort and asymptomatic control cohort are presented descriptively.

3. Results

A total of 182 asymptomatic/control samples and 150 anal cancer samples were subjected to WGS. In the anal cancer cohort, 119/150 (79.3%) samples passed the quality parameters, and in the asymptomatic men cohort, 134/182 (73.6%) were valid. This left a total of 253 samples for inclusion for detailed sequencing/phylogenetic analysis. Twenty-five of these sequences were also analyzed by the International HPV Reference Center as a further quality control for analysis. Results showed 100% agreement.

3.1. Distribution of HPV 16 Sub-Lineages in Anal Cancers

Of the 119 cancer cases with sufficient read depth (>100× median depth and >80% genome), the HPV 16 sub-lineage A1 was identified in 91 anal cancer samples (76.5%), followed by A2, which was identified in 20/119 (16.8%) of samples. A4 was detected in 5/119 samples (4.2%). Two samples were classified as B1 (1.7%), one as A3 (0.8%) and one as D1 (0.8%). Further detail of HPV 16 sub-lineages in anal cancers is described in detail in Table 2 and Figure 1.

Table 2. HPV 16 sub-lineages identified in the anal cancer and asymptomatic cohorts.

	Anal Cancer		Asymptomatic Group	
Sub-Lineage	N	% (N = 119)	N	% (N = 134)
HPV 16 A1	91	76.5%	102	76.1%
HPV 16 A2	20	16.8%	23	17.2%
HPV 16 A3	1	0.8%	0	0%
HPV 16 A4	5	4.2%	0	0%

Table 2. *Cont.*

Sub-Lineage	Anal Cancer		Asymptomatic Group	
	N	% (N = 119)	N	% (N = 134)
HPV 16 B1	2	1.7%	2	1.5%
HPV 16 B2	0	0.0%	1	0.7%
HPV 16 B3	0	0.0%	0	0%
HPV 16 B4	0	0.0%	0	0%
HPV 16 C1	0	0.0%	2	1.5%
HPV 16 C2	0	0.0%	0	0%
HPV 16 C3	0	0.0%	0	0%
HPV 16 C4	0	0.0%	0	0%
HPV 16 D1	1	0.8%	4	3.0%
HPV 16 D2	0	0.0%	0	0%
HPV 16 D3	0	0.0%	0	0%
HPV 16 D4	0	0.0%	0	0%
Total	119		134	

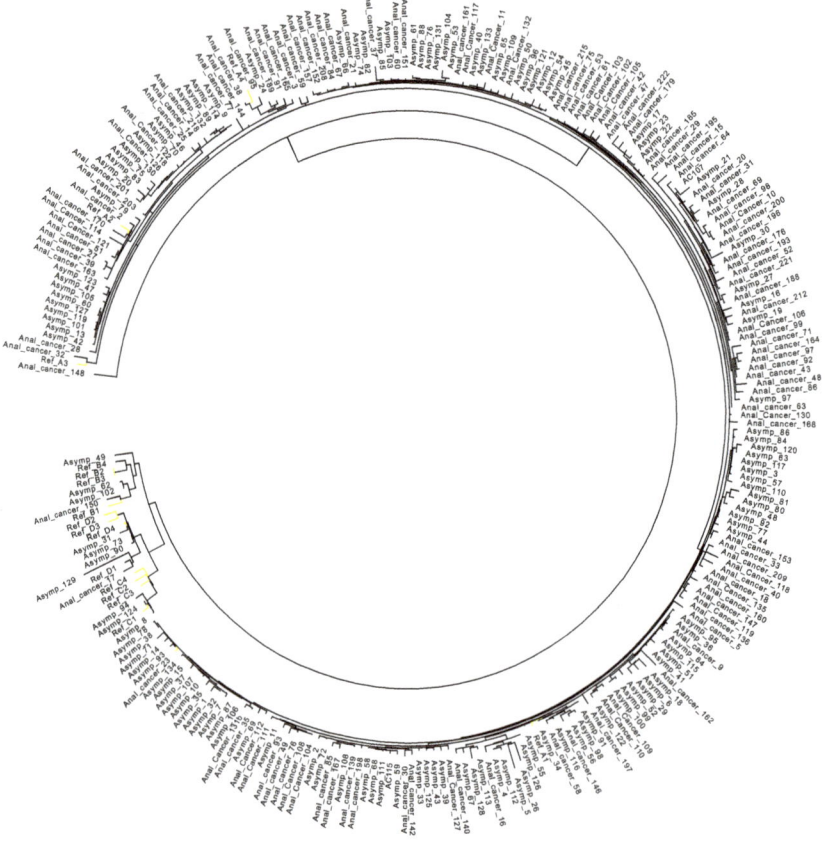

Figure 1. Phylogenetic tree representing the HPV 16 sub-lineages present in the anal sample and control groups.

3.2. HPV 16 Sub-Lineages in the Control Cohort

Of the 134 control samples, most samples were classified (76.1%) as A1, followed by A2, identified in 23/134 (17.2%) of samples. D1 sub-lineage was identified in 4/134 samples (3.0%), and C1 and B1 were identified in two cases each (1.5%). B2 was present in 1/134 (0.7%). Table 2 describes the number of cases identified for each sub-lineage, and Figure 1 contains the phylogenetic tree obtained from the control cohort.

3.3. Differences in Prevalence of HPV 16 Sub-Lineages between Anal Cancer and Control Cohort

No major differences in the proportion of A1 and A2 sub-lineages were observed between the case vs. control cohorts, being 76.4% vs. 76.0% and 16.2% vs. 17.0%, respectively. Whereas the case cohort revealed the presence of the A4 sub-lineage in 4.2% of anal cancers, this sub-lineage was not present in the control cohort. Conversely, the C lineage was present in 1.5% of control specimens and was not detected in cancer cases. Finally, there was a slight increase in the D1 sub-lineage observed in the control vs. case cohort (3.0% vs. 0.8%).

3.4. Association of HPV 16 Sub-Lineages with Demographic and Clinical Variables

From the 119 anal cancers, four samples did not contain vital status information and were not included in the analysis. Due to the dominance of the A1 sub-lineage, the logistic analysis and odds ratio analysis were performed based on the presence or absence of the HPV 16 sub-lineage A1.

No significant differences in A1 positivity with sex, age, response to treatment, stage or vital status were observed. This observation was consistent for the adjusted analysis (Table 3).

Table 3. Influence of A1 sub-lineage presence stratified by demographic and clinical variables. The comparator for the odds ratio (univariate and adjusted) is A1 absence.

Variable	Level	Unadjusted OR (95% CIs)	p Value	Adjusted OR (95% CIs)	p Value
Sex	Male	1		1	
	Female	1.12 (0.39–2.92)	0.827	1.09 (0.37–3.00)	0.87
Age	<50	1		1	
	50–59	1.20 (0.27–4.80)	0.8	1.11 (0.24–4.56)	0.89
	60–69	1.50 (0.34–5.93)	0.57	1.82 (0.40–7.67)	0.416
	70 and over	1.37 (0.30–5.67)	0.666	1.63 (0.34–7.41)	0.529
Response to treatment	No	1		1	
	Yes	1.02 (0.26–3.26)	0.968	1.18 (0.34–7.41)	0.528
Stage	I	1		1	
	II	1.36 (0.37–4.62)	0.625	1.28 (0.33–4.51)	0.706
	III	1.60 (0.40–6.11)	0.486	1.56 (0.38–6.06)	0.522
	IV	1.80 (0.36–10.40)	0.478	3.03 (0.42–29.47)	0.289
Vital Status	Alive	1		1	
	Deceased	1.01 (0.39–2.85)	0.983	0.92 (0.25–3.81)	0.907

3.5. HPV 16 Sub-Lineages and Overall Survival

For the Kaplan-Meier estimator, overall survival was calculated by classifying HPV 16 sub-lineages into A1 presence or absence. No differences in overall survival were found between both sub-lineage groups (p = 0.57), Figure 2.

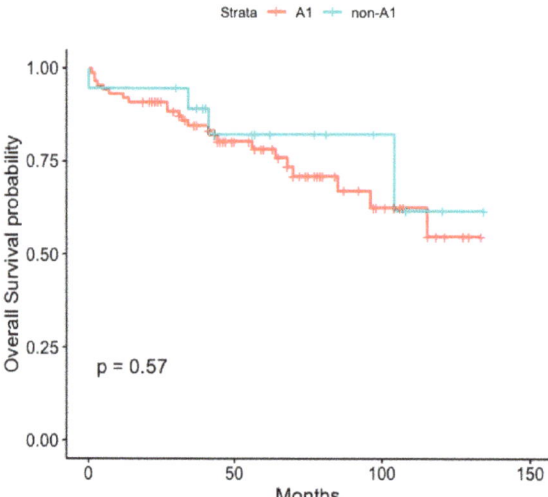

Figure 2. Kaplan-Meier survival curve stratified by HPV 16 sub-lineages (A1 vs. Non-A1). Survival time expressed in months from the diagnosis date. Data censored on 31 July 2020.

Table 4 shows overall survival stratified by the clinical and demographic variables (age group, sex, cancer stage and response to treatment), with HPV 16 sub-lineages categorized into the two groups (A1 vs. non-A1) with A1 as the reference. Non-A1 (vs. A1) was not associated with improved overall survival in the univariate analysis, with a hazard ratio (HR) of 0.87 (0.37–2, $p = 0.751$). Variables associated with worse overall survival in the univariate model were stage IV vs. stage I with HR of 15.7 (3.38–72.8), $p < 0.001$ and response to treatment vs. no response to treatment with HR of 0.11 (0.05–0.25) $p < 0.001$. After adjustment for age, gender, stage and response to treatment, non-A1 sub-lineages did not significantly influence the overall survival compared to A1, with a HR 0.83 (0.28–2.46, $p = 0.743$).

Table 4. Hazard ratio of HPV 16 sub-lineages (univariate and multivariate) derived from Cox regression ($N = 115$) in anal cancer samples collected between 2009 to 2018 in the southeast of Scotland.

Variable	Level	Unadjusted HR (95% Cis)	p Value	Adjusted HR (95% Cis)	p Value
HPV 16 sub-lineage	A1 ($n = 88$)	1		1	
	Non-A1 ($n = 27$)	0.87 (0.37–2)	0.751	0.83 (0.28–2.46)	0.743
Sex	Male	1		1	
	Female	1.2 (0.48–2.9)	0.71	0.88 (0.32–2.39)	0.795
Age	<50	1		1	
	50–59	1.10 (0.33–3.70)	0.877	0.83 (0.21–3.26)	0.788
	60–69	0.85 (0.26–2.8)	0.795	2.67 (0.607–11.72)	0.194
	70 and over	1.54 (0.48–5.0)	0.466	5.56 (1.082–28.58)	0.04
Stage	I	1		1	
	II	1.7 (0.37–8.1)	0.49	2.34 (0.47–11.74)	0.302
	III	2.4 (0.50–11.6)	0.274	2.26 (0.42–12.27)	0.344
	IV	15.7 (3.38–72.8)	<0.001	15.95 (2.45–10.3.82)	0.004
Response to treatment	No	1		1	
	Yes	0.11 (0.05–0.25)	<0.001	0.12 (0.03–0.39)	<0.001

If only A1 and A2 samples were considered, no significant differences in HR were found when using A1 as the reference (HR 0.74, 0.25–2.1, p = 0.575).

3.6. Integration

Although it was not the main aim of the study, the absence of part of the HPV 16 genome was identified in 13/119 (10.92%) of the anal cancer samples. This absence indicates the potential integration of the HPV16 in the human genome. The E2 gene was the most frequently missing region, followed by E4, E5 and L2 E1 and L1 (see Table 5 for details). Notably, all cases retained E6 and E7 oncogenes. Due to the small number of cases in which integration was detected, no further analysis was performed. No integration was detected in the asymptomatic cohort.

Table 5. HPV integration identified in the anal cancer cohort.

HPV Genes Integration in the Anal Cancer Samples (n = 13)	N
L1 only	1
E1 only	1
E1, E2, E4	1
E2, E5, part E2	1
E2, E4, E5, L2, L1	3
E1, E2, E4, E5 and part L2	2
E1, E2, E4, E5, L2 and part L1	3
E1, E2, E4, E5, L2 and L1 complete	1

4. Discussion

Previously, we described that 93.3% of HPV-positive anal cancer cases diagnosed in Scotland between 2019 and 2018 were caused by HPV 16. In this study, we have identified that 76% of cases belonged to the A1 sub-lineage, followed by A2 (16%).

In the control group of asymptomatic men, a similar prevalence of A1 and A2 was observed. Differences identified were the presence of A4 in the anal cancers (4.7%), which was absent in the control group; presence of the C lineage only detected in the control group; and the presence of the sub-lineage D1 in the control group (3%), which had a lower prevalence of 0.81% in the cancers. This higher prevalence of sub-lineages A1 and A2 is consistent with previously published studies in European cohorts. Gonçalves et al. (2022) found a higher prevalence of the A lineage in the anal canal of asymptomatic men, mainly A1 [29], and Nicolás-Párraga et al. (2016) found that A1–3 sub-lineages were identified in 96.1% of the European cases [30]. Beyond Europe, Volpini et al. (2017) investigated the HPV 16 variants in cervical and anal samples collated in Brazil and determined that proportionally less of the anal cancer samples (70.8%) were classified as A1–3 sub-lineages [12].

The data collated in the study add to the limited information on the pattern and implications of HPV sub-lineages in the anus. Though we did not see significant associations with demographic and underlying disease status, these observations need to be confirmed or refuted by future studies with larger sample sizes.

To our knowledge, no other studies have investigated the association of HPV 16 sub-lineages in anal cancer and overall survival. We did not observe that A1 vs. non -A1 sub-lineages influenced overall survival in the univariate and adjusted analysis. Interestingly, a recent study was reported by Lang Kuhs et al. (2022) in which the authors looked into the genetic variation of HPV 16 and its association with clinical outcomes in HPV 16-positive oropharyngeal cancer patients [31]. They investigated different high-risk single nucleotide polymorphisms (SNPs) and found that those with one or more high-risk SNPs had significantly shorter median survival times. Most of these SNPs were common to the D2 sub-lineage, which has also been associated with a higher risk of cancer in the cervix [14]. Due to the absence of D2 cases in the present study, we were not able to explore this in the present work; however, the identification of these high-risk SNPs may be very helpful for patient and treatment management.

Although we identified potential integration of the HPV16 genome (calculated through the loss of the sequence), due to the small number, we did not perform any further analysis, including in relation to implications for survival. Given the relative lack of information on the extent and implications of integration in anal cancer, we would assert that this is an area that would benefit from further study.

We acknowledge this study has limitations; the asymptomatic population were all men, whereas the cancer population had a majority of female (75.63%) samples compared to males (24.37%); this was due to pragmatic reasons relating to available material. However, data did not show differences in the distribution of HPV 16 sub-lineages between women and men in the anal cancer group. Additionally, as discussed earlier, we believe the observations made in the present work would benefit from validation in a larger sample of cases and controls and would hope this study serves as a primer for such. Though the number of cases of cancers was not trivial (n = 253), particularly given that the Scottish European age-standardized rate (EASR) (per 100,000 person-years at risk) was 2.6 in 2017, we appreciate that detecting rarer sub-lineages with precision can take large sample sizes.

In the UK, there is no screening program for anal cancer. However, since 2017, there has been an opportunistic vaccination program for MSM, and in 2019, the national HPV vaccination became gender neutral. In term of vaccines, a study from Godi et al. (2019) reported that HPV 16 lineage variants B, C and D exhibited slightly (<two-fold) reduced sensitivity to nonavalent vaccine sera compared to lineage A [32].

Therefore, the high prevalence of lineage A in the samples included in this study could be interpreted as positive for vaccine efficacy, particularly given that gender-neutral vaccination is now a part of core policy in the UK and several other countries.

This study has demonstrated the technical feasibility of detecting HPV 16 sub-lineages in anal cancer samples and residual material from rectal swabs. Though some differences in the presence of non-A sub-lineages were detectable between the cancer and asymptomatic population, the consistency, magnitude and implications of these would benefit from further study. The domination of lineage A is consistent with existing European data and suggests that sub-lineage identification in itself may not be informative for prognostication.

Author Contributions: D.G. was involved in the planning of experiments, delivered the end-to-end whole genome sequencing process and performed data analysis, including the analysis of next-generation sequencing data. D.G. also drafted the manuscript. L.S.A.M. assisted with the planning of laboratory experiments, supporting with quality checking/analysis of data, including sequencing data, and performing critical appraisal of the manuscript. R.G. performed original data retrieval on the clinical cohort, including the collation of clinical-demographic variables, and supported critical appraisal of the manuscript. M.T.G.H. was the lead academic supervisor for the project and was involved in advising on experimental methodology and technology, providing support for data analysis and performing critical appraisal of the manuscript. K.C. was the principal clinical investigator for the project and supported with interaction with the bio-resource and pathology team for sample collation, advising on experimental and analytical methodology, providing support for data analysis and assisting in the drafting and critical appraisal of the manuscript. All authors have read and agreed to the published version of the manuscript.

Funding: This research received no external funding.

Institutional Review Board Statement: Use of samples for the present project was approved by the Southeast of Scotland National Research for Scotland Bioresource (NRS) (application reference SR 1283 (24 September 2019) and SR1364 (22 January 2020)). Favorable ethical opinion to conduct the research was provided by University of St Andrews Teaching and Research Ethics Committee, reference MD 14482 (5 July 2019).

Informed Consent Statement: Not applicable.

Data Availability Statement: Request for data in anonymized form can be made available upon reasonable request to the senior author and following due process of governance and the Scottish Data Protection Regulations. GenBank submission IDs 2637056 and 2638666.

Conflicts of Interest: D.G.: Received gratis consumables from Seegene to support the HPV genotyping of the anal cancer samples. K.C.: K.C.'s institution has received research funding or gratis consumables to support research from the following commercial entities in the last 3 years: Cepheid, Euroimmun, GeneFirst, SelfScreen, Hiantis, Seegene, Roche, Abbott and Hologic. All other authors have nothing to declare.

Abbreviations

Human papillomavirus (HPV), hazard ratio (HR), European age-standardized rate (EASR), human immunodefiency virus (HIV), deoxyribonucleic acid (DNA), overall survival (OS), National Health Service (NHS), whole genome sequencing (WGS).

References

1. De Sanjosé, S.; Serrano, B.; Tous, S.; Alejo, M.; Lloveras, B.; Quirós, B.; Clavero, O.; Vidal, A.; Ferrándiz-Pulido, C.; Pavón, M.; et al. Burden of Human Papillomavirus (HPV)-Related Cancers Attributable to HPVs 6/11/16/18/31/33/45/52 and 58. *JNCI Cancer Spectr.* **2018**, *2*, pky045. [CrossRef] [PubMed]
2. Guerendiain, D.; Grigorescu, R.; Kirk, A.; Stevenson, A.; Holden, M.T.G.; Pan, J.; Kavanagh, K.; Graham, S.V.; Cuschieri, K. HPV status and HPV16 viral load in anal cancer and its association with clinical outcome. *Cancer Med.* **2022**, *11*, 4193–4203. [CrossRef] [PubMed]
3. Cuschieri, K.; Brewster, D.; Williams, A.R.W.; Millan, D.; Murray, G.; Nicoll, S.; Imrie, J.; Hardie, A.; Graham, C.; Cubie, H.A. Distribution of HPV types associated with cervical cancers in Scotland and implications for the impact of HPV vaccines. *Br. J. Cancer* **2010**, *102*, 930–932. [CrossRef]
4. Islami, F.; Ferlay, J.; Lortet-Tieulent, J.; Bray, F.; Jemal, A. International trends in anal cancer incidence rates. *Int. J. Epidemiol.* **2017**, *46*, 924–938. [CrossRef] [PubMed]
5. Robinson, D.; Coupland, V.; Moller, H. An analysis of temporal and generational trends in the incidence of anal and other HPV-related cancers in Southeast England. *Br. J. Cancer* **2009**, *100*, 527–531. [CrossRef] [PubMed]
6. Anal Cancer Incidence Statistics | Cancer Research, UK. Available online: https://www.cancerresearchuk.org/health-professional/cancer-statistics/statistics-by-cancer-type/anal-cancer/incidence#heading-Two (accessed on 11 September 2021).
7. Anal Cancer—Cancer Stat Facts. Available online: https://seer.cancer.gov/statfacts/html/anus.html (accessed on 11 September 2021).
8. De Villiers, E.-M.; Fauquet, C.; Broker, T.R.; Bernard, H.-U.; zur Hausen, H. Classification of papillomaviruses. *Virology* **2004**, *324*, 17–27. [CrossRef]
9. Burk, R.D.; Harari, A.; Chen, Z. Human papillomavirus genome variants. *Virology* **2013**, *445*, 232–243. [CrossRef]
10. Cornet, I.; Gheit, T.; Iannacone, M.R.; Vignat, J.; Sylla, B.S.; Del Mistro, A.; Franceschi, S.; Tommasino, M.; Clifford, G.M.; on behalf of the IARC HPV Variant Study Group. HPV16 genetic variation and the development of cervical cancer worldwide. *Br. J. Cancer* **2012**, *108*, 240–244. [CrossRef]
11. Clifford, G.M.; Tenet, V.; Georges, D.; Alemany, L.; Pavón, M.A.; Chen, Z.; Yeager, M.; Cullen, M.; Boland, J.F.; Bass, S.; et al. Human papillomavirus 16 sub-lineage dispersal and cervical cancer risk worldwide: Whole viral genome sequences from 7116 HPV16-positive women. *Papillomavirus Res.* **2019**, *7*, 67–74. [CrossRef]
12. Volpini, L.P.B.; Boldrini, N.A.T.; de Freitas, L.B.; Miranda, A.E.; Spano, L.C. The high prevalence of HPV and HPV16 European variants in cervical and anal samples of HIV-seropositive women with normal Pap test results. *PLoS ONE* **2017**, *12*, e0176422. [CrossRef]
13. Ferreira, M.T.; Gonçalves, M.G.; López, R.V.M.; Sichero, L. Genetic variants of HPV-16 and their geographical and anatomical distribution in men: A systematic review with meta-analysis. *Virology* **2021**, *558*, 134–144. [CrossRef] [PubMed]
14. Mirabello, L.; Yeager, M.; Cullen, M.; Boland, J.F.; Chen, Z.; Wentzensen, N.; Zhang, X.; Yu, K.; Yang, Q.; Mitchell, J.; et al. HPV16 Sublineage Associations with Histology-Specific Cancer Risk Using HPV Whole-Genome Sequences in 3200 Women. *J. Natl. Cancer Inst.* **2016**, *108*, djw100. [CrossRef] [PubMed]
15. American Joint Committee on Cancer. *AJCC Cancer Staging Manual*, 8th ed.; Springer: Berlin/Heidelberg, Germany, 2017; p. 275. Available online: www.cancerstaging.orgajcc@facs.org (accessed on 11 September 2021).
16. Glynne-Jones, R.; Nilsson, P.; Aschele, C.; Goh, V.; Peiffert, D.; Cervantes, A.; Arnold, D. Anal cancer: ESMO-ESSO-ESTRO Clinical Practice Guidelines for diagnosis, treatment and follow-up. *Ann. Oncol.* **2014**, *25*, iii10–iii20. [CrossRef] [PubMed]
17. Cameron, R.L.; Cuschieri, K.; Pollock, K.G.J. Baseline HPV prevalence in rectal swabs from men attending a sexual health clinic in Scotland: Assessing the potential impact of a selective HPV vaccination programme for men who have sex with men. *Sex. Transm. Infect.* **2019**, *96*, 55–57. [CrossRef] [PubMed]

18. Cullen, M.; Boland, J.F.; Schiffman, M.; Zhang, X.; Wentzensen, N.; Yang, Q.; Chen, Z.; Yu, K.; Mitchell, J.; Roberson, D.; et al. Deep sequencing of HPV16 genomes: A new high-throughput tool for exploring the carcinogenicity and natural history of HPV16 infection. *Papillomavirus Res.* **2015**, *1*, 3–11. [CrossRef] [PubMed]
19. Arroyo-Mühr, L.S.; Lagheden, C.; Hultin, E.; Eklund, C.; Adami, H.-O.; Dillner, J.; Sundström, K. Human papillomavirus type 16 genomic variation in women with subsequent in situ or invasive cervical cancer: Prospective population-based study. *Br. J. Cancer* **2018**, *119*, 1163–1168. [CrossRef] [PubMed]
20. Bolger, A.M.; Lohse, M.; Usadel, B. Trimmomatic: A flexible trimmer for Illumina sequence data. *Bioinformatics* **2014**, *30*, 2114–2120. [CrossRef] [PubMed]
21. Babraham Bioinformatics—FastQC: A Quality Control Tool for High Throughput Sequence Data. 2010. Available online: https://www.bioinformatics.babraham.ac.uk/projects/fastqc/ (accessed on 18 April 2022).
22. PaVE. Available online: https://pave.niaid.nih.gov/explore/reference_genomes/human_genomes (accessed on 31 October 2022).
23. Li, H.; Durbin, R. Fast and accurate short read alignment with Burrows—Wheeler transform. *Bioinformatics* **2009**, *25*, 1754–1760. [CrossRef]
24. Li, H.; Handsaker, B.; Wysoker, A.; Fennell, T.; Ruan, J.; Homer, N.; Marth, G.; Abecasis, G.; Durbin, R. 1000 Genome Project Data Processing Subgroup. The Sequence Alignment/Map format and SAMtools. *Bioinformatics* **2009**, *25*, 2078–2079. [CrossRef]
25. Li, H. A statistical framework for SNP calling, mutation discovery, association mapping and population genetical parameter estimation from sequencing data. *Bioinformatics* **2011**, *27*, 2987–2993. [CrossRef]
26. Kazutaka, K.; Misakwa, K.; Kei-ichi, K.; Miyata, T. MAFFT: A novel method for rapid multiple sequence alignment based on fast Fourier transform. *Nucleic Acids Res.* **2002**, *30*, 3059–3066. [CrossRef]
27. Stamatakis, A. RAxML version 8: A tool for phylogenetic analysis and post-analysis of large phylogenies. *Bioinformatics* **2014**, *30*, 1312–1313. [CrossRef] [PubMed]
28. Team, R. Rstudio: Integrated Development for r. Rstudio, pbc, Boston, MA. 2020. Available online: http://www.Rstudio.Com (accessed on 3 March 2022).
29. Gonçalves, M.G.; Ferreira, M.T.; López, R.V.M.; Ferreira, S.; Sirak, B.; Baggio, M.L.; Lazcano-Ponce, E.; Nyitray, A.G.; Giuliano, A.R.; Villa, L.L.; et al. Prevalence and persistence of HPV-16 molecular variants in the anal canal of men: The HIM study. *J. Clin. Virol.* **2022**, *149*, 105128. [CrossRef] [PubMed]
30. Nicolás-Párraga, S.; Gandini, C.; Pimenoff, V.N.; Alemany, L.; Sanjosé, S.; Bosch, F.X.; Bravo, I.G.; the RIS HPV TT and HPV VVAP Study Groups. HPV16 variants distribution in invasive cancers of the cervix, vulva, vagina, penis, and anus. *Cancer Med.* **2016**, *5*, 2909–2919. [CrossRef] [PubMed]
31. Kuhs, K.L.; Faden, D.; Chen, L.; Smith, D.; Pinheiro, M.; Wood, C.; Davis, S.; Yeager, M.; Boland, J.; Cullen, M.; et al. Genetic variation within the human papillomavirus type 16 genome is associated with oropharyngeal cancer prognosis. *Ann. Oncol.* **2022**, *33*, 638–648. [CrossRef] [PubMed]
32. Godi, A.; Kemp, T.J.; Pinto, L.A.; Beddows, S. Sensitivity of Human Papillomavirus (HPV) Lineage and Sublineage Variant Pseudoviruses to Neutralization by Nonavalent Vaccine Antibodies. *J. Infect. Dis.* **2019**, *220*, 1940–1945. [CrossRef] [PubMed]

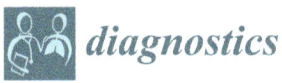

Systematic Review

Prevalence of Human Papilloma Virus Infection in Bladder Cancer: A Systematic Review

Narcisa Muresu [1,†], Biagio Di Lorenzo [2,†], Laura Saderi [2,†], Illari Sechi [1], Arcadia Del Rio [3], Andrea Piana [1,*] and Giovanni Sotgiu [2]

1. Department of Medicine, Surgery and Pharmacy, University of Sassari, 07100 Sassari, Italy; narcisamuresu@outlook.com (N.M.); illasechi@uniss.it (I.S.)
2. Clinical Epidemiology and Medical Statistics Unit, Department of Medical, Surgical and Experimental Medicine, University of Sassari, 07100 Sassari, Italy; dilorbiagio@gmail.com (B.D.L.); lsaderi@uniss.it (L.S.); gsotgiu@uniss.it (G.S.)
3. Department of Biomedical Science, University of Sassari, 07100 Sassari, Italy; delrio.arcadia2@gmail.com
* Correspondence: piana@uniss.it
† These authors contributed equally to this work.

Abstract: The etiology of bladder cancer is known to be associated with behavioral and environmental factors. Moreover, several studies suggested a potential role of HPV infection in the pathogenesis with controversial results. A systematic review was conducted to assess the role of HPV. A total of 46 articles that reported the prevalence of HPV infection in squamous (SCC), urothelial (UC), and transitional cell carcinomas (TCC) were selected. A pooled prevalence of 19% was found, with a significant difference in SCC that was mainly driven by HPV-16. Moreover, infection prevalence in case-control studies showed a higher risk of bladder cancer in HPV-positive cases (OR: 7.84; p-value < 0.00001). The results may suggest an etiologic role of HPV in bladder cancer. HPV vaccine administration in both sexes could be key to prevent the infection caused by high-risk genotypes.

Keywords: human papillomavirus; HPV; bladder cancer; HPV detection; urothelial carcinoma; transitional cell carcinoma

1. Introduction

Bladder cancer (BCa) is the 10th most prevalent cancer globally, with >572,000 and >212,000 incident cases and deaths [1]. The highest rates of BCa are registered in Southern and Western Europe and North America, with a higher incidence in men [2]. Several risk factors were found; most of them are related to personal behavior (i.e., diet and smoking), socioeconomic status (i.e., the accessibility to health services and delay in diagnosis), and environmental and occupational exposure to chemical substances or infectious diseases [3]. Moreover, epidemiological studies revealed a higher risk in men and a worse prognosis in black males [4]. BCa histological subtypes can vary: urothelial BCa, previously classified as transitional cell carcinoma (TCC) and the predominant histological type, accounts for ~90% and is mainly related to chemical exposure, whereas squamous cell carcinoma (SCC, 5%) is associated with chronic inflammation and persistent infections (Schistosoma spp. in Africa) [5]. Adenocarcinoma (2%), sarcoma, and small cell carcinoma are less incident forms [6].

While the role played by human papillomavirus (HPV) in the development of cervical, anogenital, and oropharyngeal cancers was proven [7–9], the causative relationship between HPV and BCa still remains controversial, with a high variable prevalence attributed to the study design, the enrolled population, and the HPV detection methods [10]. Understanding the role of HPV in BCa could have relevant diagnostic, therapeutic, and preventive implications. The current systematic review is aimed to assess the prevalence of HPV infection in BCa, focusing on patients' clinical and epidemiological characteristics.

2. Materials and Methods

2.1. Search Strategy

A systematic literature review aimed at retrieving papers focused on the prevalence of HPV infection in BCa was carried out from its inception to 31st December 2021. The literature search was performed using PubMed and Scopus, selecting the key words "Human Papillomavirus", "HPV", or "Papillomavirus" and "bladder cancer" or "bladder carcinoma", combined in different strings. No restrictions related to age of patients, setting, or time of the study were chosen.

Lists of references of all selected articles were screened to find other eligible studies not included in the above-mentioned databases.

2.2. Study Selection and Inclusion Criteria

Case-control, cross-sectional, and cohort studies reporting HPV infection prevalence were selected.

The following inclusion criteria were considered:
(1) Studies dealing with patients with primary BCa;
(2) Studies describing molecular and non-molecular HPV detection methods on fresh or FFPE (Formalin Fixed Paraffin Embedded) bladder biopsies;
(3) Studies focused on the following medical conditions: SCC, urothelial carcinoma (UC), and transitional cell carcinoma (TCC);

Articles were excluded for the following reasons:
(1) Review articles, abstracts, letters, commentaries, correspondences, case-reports, and case-series enrolling <10 subjects;
(2) Use of languages other than English;
(3) Secondary malignancies located in the bladder.

Article selection and data extraction were performed by two Authors and double-checked (M.N. and D.B.), while discrepancies of opinions or disagreement were resolved by a third investigator (S.G.).

2.3. Data Extraction

Qualitative and quantitative variables were collected in an ad hoc electronic form.

The following variables were collected: first author's last name; title of the article; year and country/countries of the study; period of the study; epidemiological study design; sample size; sex and age; type of samples; HPV detection methods; histological subtypes; tumor grading; HPV prevalence.

No ethical approval was needed given the anonymized and aggregated nature of the data.

2.4. Study Quality Assessment

Inter-rater agreement was ~100% for the phases of study selection and data extraction, and the few inconsistencies were resolved by consensus and with the support of a third investigator (G.S.).

Guidelines of the Preferred Reporting Items for Systematic Reviews and Meta-Analysis (PRISMA) were followed to guide the process of the systematic review [11].

The Newcastle–Ottawa Scale [12] was used to assess the quality of the included case-control studies by evaluating selection, comparability, and exposure criteria, through four, two, and three items, respectively. The Joanna Briggs Institute Critical Appraisal tools (JBI), applied for analytical cross-sectional studies where the control group is missing, consists of eight items aimed at evaluating the risk of bias: high, moderate, or low risk of bias was assigned when positive answers were $\leq$49%, between 50% and 75%, or >75%, respectively [13] (Table S1a,b).

2.5. Statistical Analysis

Qualitative and quantitative variables were summarized with absolute and relative (percentage) frequencies and means/medians [standard deviation (SD), interquartile range (IQR)] respectively.

Forest plots were used to show pooled risk differences of the selected outcomes and interval (95% confidence interval, CI) estimates, as well as the weight of the sample size of the recruited studies. The I2 indicator (low, medium, and high heterogeneity expressed as <25%, ≥25%–<50%, ≥50%, respectively) showed the association between true variability and overall variation.

Fixed and random-effects models were chosen depending on the estimated between-study heterogeneity. A two-tailed *p*-value less than 0.05 was deemed statistically significant. The statistical software Stata version 17 (StataCorp, College Station, TX, USA) and StatsDirect version 3.1.12 (StatsDirect Ltd., Willar, UK).

3. Results

3.1. Study Selection

A total of 637 articles were identified through electronic database searches; 162 (26.2%) were excluded for being duplicates, and then, a total of 475 studies were screened by titles and abstracts. Fifty-six (11.8%) full texts were evaluated, and ten (17.9%) were excluded for the following reasons: tissue samples did not include bladder tissues (n = 5), full text was not available (n = 2), case-report (n = 1), review (n = 1), and dataset described in another study (n = 1). A total of 46 (46/56; 82.1%) manuscripts were included in the review (Table 1; Figure 1).

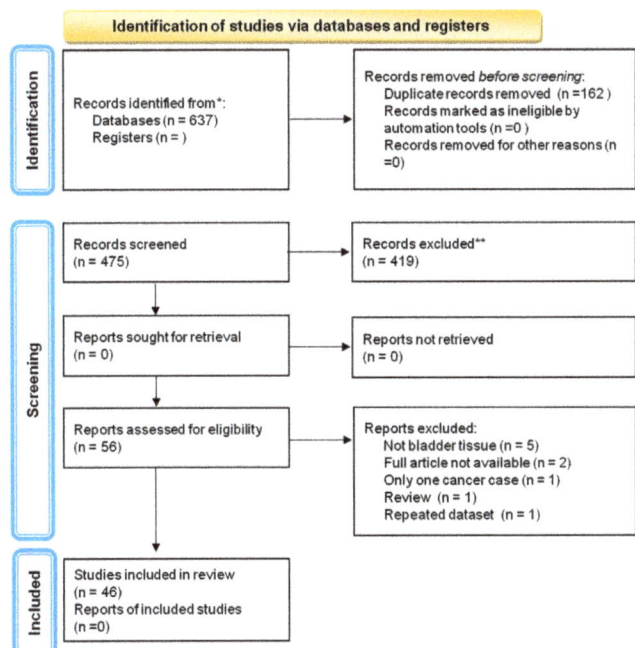

Figure 1. PRISMA 2020 flow diagram for new systematic reviews, which included searches of databases and registers only.

Table 1. Characteristics of the included studies (n = 46).

Ref.	First Author	Year	Title	Type of Study	Multicentre/Single Centre	Country/Ies	Study Period
[14]	Abdollahzadeh P, et al.	2017	Association Between Human Papillomavirus and Transitional Cell Carcinoma of the Bladder	Case/control study	Single	Iran	2008–2011
[15]	Aggarwal S, et al.	2009	Koilocytosis: correlations with high-risk HPV and its comparison on tissue sections and cytology, urothelial carcinoma	Retrospective observational study	Single	India	-
[16]	Alexander RE, et al.	2012	p16 expression is not associated with human papillomavirus in urinary bladder squamous cell carcinoma	Retrospective observational study	Single	USA	1992–2011
[17]	Alexander RE, et al.	2013	Human papillomavirus is not an etiologic agent of urothelial inverted papillomas	Retrospective observational study	Multi	USA Spain Italy France	1985–2005
[18]	Alexander RE, et al.	2014	The expression patterns of p53 and p16 and an analysis of a possible role of HPV in primary adenocarcinoma of the urinary bladder	Retrospective observational study	Multi	USA Spain Italy France	-
[19]	Badawi H, et al.	2008	Role of human papillomavirus types 16, 18, and 52 in recurrent cystitis and urinary bladder cancer among Egyptian patients	Case/control study	Single	Egypt	2001–2006
[20]	Barghi MR, et al.	2005	Correlation between human papillomavirus infection and bladder transitional cell carcinoma	Case/control study	Single	Iran	1999–2002
[21]	Ben Selma W, et al.	2010	Investigation of human papillomavirus in bladder cancer in a series of Tunisian patients	Observational study	Single	Tunisia	2003–2004
[22]	Berrada N, et al.	2013	Human papillomavirus detection in Moroccan patients with bladder cancer	Prospective study	Single	Morocco	-
[23]	Chan KW, et al.	1997	Prevalence of six types of human papillomavirus in inverted papilloma and papillary transitional cell carcinoma of the bladder: an evaluation by polymerase chain reaction	Retrospective observational study	Single	China	1987–1994

Table 1. *Cont.*

Ref.	First Author	Year	Title	Type of Study	Multicentre/Single Centre	Country/Ies	Study Period
[24]	Chapman-Fredricks JR, et al.	2013	High-risk human papillomavirus DNA detected in primary squamous cell carcinoma of urinary bladder	Retrospective observational study	Single	USA	-
[25]	Collins K, et al.	2020	Prevalence of high-risk human papillomavirus in primary squamous cell carcinoma of urinary bladder	Retrospective observational study	Single	Texas	2009–2019
[26]	Cooper K, et al.	1997	Human papillomavirus and schistosomiasis associated bladder cancer	Retrospective observational study	Single	South Africa	-
[27]	De Gaetani C, et al.	1999	Detection of human papillomavirus DNA in urinary bladder carcinoma by in situ hybridisation	Retrospective observational study	Single	Italy	1995–1997
[28]	Fioriti D, et al.	2003	Urothelial bladder carcinoma and viral infections: different association with human polyomaviruses and papillomaviruses	Comparative study	Single	Italy	-
[29]	Gazzaniga P, et al.	1998	Prevalence of papillomavirus, Epstein-Barr virus, cytomegalovirus, and herpes simplex virus type 2 in urinary bladder cancer	Retrospective observational study	Single	Italy	-
[30]	Golovina DA, et al.	2016	Loss of Cell Differentiation in HPV-Associated Bladder Cancer	Retrospective observational study	Single	Russia	-
[31]	Gopalkrishna V, et al.	1995	Detection of human papillomavirus DNA sequences in cancer of the urinary bladder by in situ hybridisation and polymerase chain reaction	Retrospective observational study	Single	India	-
[32]	Gould VE, et al.	2010	Human papillomavirus and p16 expression in inverted papillomas of the urinary bladder	Case/control study	Single	USA	-
[33]	Helal Tel A, et al.	2006	Human papilloma virus and p53 expression in bladder cancer in Egypt: relationship to schistosomiasis and clinicopathologic factors	Observational study	Single	Egypt	-
[34]	Javanmard B, et al.	2019	Human Papilloma Virus DNA in Tumor Tissue and Urine in Different Stage of Bladder Cancer	Retrospective observational study	Single	Iran	2014–2016
[35]	Kamel D, et al.	1995	Human papillomavirus DNA and abnormal p53 expression in carcinoma of the urinary bladder	Retrospective observational study	Single	Finland	1987–1992

Table 1. *Cont.*

Ref.	First Author	Year	Title	Type of Study	Multicentre/Single Centre	Country/ies	Study Period
[36]	Kim KH, et al.	1995	Analysis of p53 tumor suppressor gene mutations and human papillomavirus infection in human bladder cancers	Retrospective observational study	Single	Korea	-
[37]	Kim SH, et al.	2014	Detection of human papillomavirus infection and p16 immunohistochemistry expression in bladder cancer with squamous differentiation	Case/control study	Single	Korea	2001–2011
[38]	LaRue H, et al.	1995	Human papillomavirus in transitional cell carcinoma of the urinary bladder	Retrospective observational study	Single	Canada	-
[39]	Llewellyn MA, et al.	2018	Defining the frequency of human papillomavirus and polyomavirus infection in urothelial bladder tumours	Retrospective observational study	Single	UK	2005–2011
[40]	Lopez-Beltran A, et al.	1996a	Human papillomavirus DNA as a factor determining the survival of bladder cancer patients	Retrospective observational study	Single	Spain	-
[41]	López-Beltrán A, et al.	1996b	Human papillomavirus infection and transitional cell carcinoma of the bladder: Immunohistochemistry and in situ hybridization	Observational study	Single	Spain	-
[42]	Mete UK, et al.	2018	Human Papillomavirus in Urothelial Carcinoma of Bladder: An Indian study	Case/control study	Single	India	-
[43]	Moghadam SO, et al.	2020	Association of human papilloma virus (HPV) infection with oncological outcomes in urothelial bladder cancer	Prospective study	Single	Iran	-
[44]	Musangile FY, et al.	2021	Detection of HPV infection in urothelial carcinoma using RNAscope: Clinicopathological characterization	Retrospective observational study	Single	Japan	2013–2019
[45]	Pichler R, et al.	2015	Low prevalence of HPV detection and genotyping in non-muscle invasive bladder cancer using single-step PCR followed by reverse line blot	Prospective study	Single	Austria	-
[46]	Samarska IV, et al.	2019	Condyloma Acuminatum of Urinary Bladder: Relation to Squamous Cell Carcinoma	Observational study	Single	*	-

Table 1. Cont.

Ref.	First Author	Year	Title	Type of Study	Multicentre/Single Centre	Country/Ies	Study Period
[47]	Sarier M, et al.	2019	Is There any Association between Urothelial Carcinoma of the Bladder and Human Papillomavirus? A Case-Control Study	Case/control study	Single	Turkey	Jan–Dec 2018
[48]	Schmid SC, et al.	2015	Human papilloma virus is not detectable in samples of urothelial bladder cancer in a central European population: a prospective translational study	Prospective study	Single	Germany	-
[49]	Shaker OG, et al.	2013	Is there a correlation between HPV and urinary bladder carcinoma?	Case/control study	Single	Egypt	-
[50]	Shigehara K, et al.	2011	Etiologic role of human papillomavirus infection in bladder carcinoma	Case/control study	Single	Japan	1997–2009
[51]	Shigehara K, et al.	2013	Etiological correlation of human papillomavirus infection in the development of female bladder tumor	Prospective study	Single	Japan	1996–2010
[52]	Simoneau M, et al.	1999	Low frequency of human papillomavirus infection in initial papillary bladder tumors	Retrospective observational study	Single	Canada	1990–1992
[53]	Steinestel J, et al.	2013	Overexpression of p16INK4a in Urothelial Carcinoma In Situ Is a Marker for MAPK-Mediated Epithelial-Mesenchymal Transition but Is Not Related to Human Papillomavirus Infection	Case/control study	Single	Germany	2001–2011
[54]	Tekin MI, et al.	1999	Human papillomavirus associated with bladder carcinoma? Analysis by polymerase chain reaction	Case/control study	Single	Turkey	-
[55]	Tenti P, et al.	1996	p53 overexpression and human papillomavirus infection in transitional cell carcinoma of the urinary bladder: correlation with histological parameters	Retrospective observational study	Single	Italy	-
[56]	Westenend PJ, et al.	2001	Human papillomaviruses 6/11, 16/18 and 31/33/51 are not associated with squamous cell carcinoma of the urinary bladder	Retrospective observational study	Single	Netherlands	-

Table 1. *Cont.*

Ref.	First Author	Year	Title	Type of Study	Multicentre/Single Centre	Country/Ies	Study Period
[57]	Yan Y, et al.	2021	Human Papillomavirus Prevalence and Integration Status in Tissue Samples of Bladder Cancer in the Chinese Population	Retrospective observational study	Single	China	2015–2019
[58]	Yavuzer D, et al.	2011	Role of human papillomavirus in the development of urothelial carcinoma	Retrospective observational study	Single	Turkey	-
[59]	Youshya S, et al.	2005	Does human papillomavirus play a role in the development of bladder transitional cell carcinoma? A comparison of PCR and immunohistochemical analysis	Retrospective observational study	Single	England	-

* not specified.

3.2. Quality Assessment

Twelve (34.3%) cross-sectional studies were deemed at moderate risk of bias, whereas 23 (65.7%) were classified as low-risk (Table 2). Nine (81.8%) cross-sectional studies were deemed to be medium-quality, whereas two (18.2%) were high-quality (Table 3).

Table 2. JBI risk of bias assessment table. Eight items per study were evaluated and the risk of bias was calculated on the number of positive answers. y = yes, n = no, u = unclear. Moderate = where positive answers were between 50% and 75%; low = where positive answers were above 75%.

Ref.	First Author	Were the Criteria for Inclusion in the Sample Clearly Defined?	Were the Study Subjects and the Setting Described in Detail?	Was the Exposure Measured in a Valid and Reliable Way?	Were Objective, Standard Criteria Used for Measurement of the Condition?	Were Confounding Factors Identified?	Were Strategies to Deal with Confounding Factors Stated?	Were the Outcomes Measured in a Valid and Reliable Way?	Was Appropriate Statistical Analysis Used?	% YES	Risk
[15]	Aggarwal S; 2009	y	y	y	y	y	n	y	u	75	Low
[16]	Alexander RE; 2012	y	y	y	y	y	n	y	n	75	Low
[17]	Alexander RE; 2013	y	y	y	y	y	n	y	n	75	Low
[18]	Alexander RE; 2014	y	y	y	y	y	n	y	n	75	Low
[21]	Ben Selma W; 2010	y	y	y	y	y	n	y	n	75	Low
[22]	Berrada N; 2013	y	y	y	y	y	y	y	n	88	Low
[23]	Chan KW; 1997	y	y	y	y	n	n	y	y	75	Low
[24]	Chapman-Fredricks JR; 2013	y	y	y	y	y	y	y	n	88	Low
[25]	Collins K; 2020	y	y	y	y	y	y	y	y	100	Low
[26]	Cooper K; 1997	y	n	y	y	y	n	y	n	63	Moderate
[27]	De Gaetani C; 1999	y	n	y	y	y	n	y	y	75	Low
[28]	Fioriti D; 2003	y	n	y	n	y	n	y	n	50	Moderate
[29]	Gazzaniga P; 1998	y	n	y	y	y	y	y	n	75	Low
[30]	Golovina DA; 2016	y	y	y	y	y	y	y	y	100	Low
[31]	Gopalkrishna V; 1995	y	n	y	n	y	y	y	n	63	Moderate
[33]	Helal Tel A; 2006	y	y	y	n	y	y	y	y	88	Low
[34]	Javanmard B; 2019	y	n	y	n	y	n	y	y	63	Moderate
[35]	Kamel D; 1995	y	n	y	y	n	n	y	n	50	Moderate
[36]	Kim KH; 1995	y	n	y	y	n	n	y	n	50	Moderate
[38]	LaRue H; 1995	y	y	y	y	n	n	n	n	50	Moderate
[39]	Llewellyn MA; 2018	y	y	y	y	n	y	y	y	63	Moderate
[40]	Lopez-Beltran A; 1996a	y	y	y	y	y	y	y	y	100	Low
[41]	López-Beltrán A; 1996b	y	y	y	y	y	y	y	n	88	Low
[43]	Moghadam SO; 2020	y	y	y	y	y	y	y	y	100	Low
[44]	Musangile FY; 2021	y	y	y	y	y	n	y	y	88	Low
[45]	Pichler R; 2015	y	y	y	y	y	y	y	y	100	Low
[46]	Samarska IV; 2019	y	y	y	n	y	y	y	n	75	Low
[48]	Schmid SC; 2015	y	y	y	y	y	n	y	n	75	Low
[51]	Shigehara K; 2013	y	n	y	y	y	y	y	y	88	Low
[52]	Simoneau M; 1999	y	n	y	y	n	n	y	n	50	Moderate
[55]	Tenti P; 1996	y	y	y	y	n	y	y	n	75	Low
[56]	Westenend PJ; 2001	y	n	y	y	y	n	y	n	63	Moderate
[57]	Yan Y; 2021	y	n	y	y	y	y	y	y	88	Low
[58]	Yavuzer D; 2011	y	y	y	y	n	n	y	n	63	Moderate
[59]	Youshya S; 2005	y	n	y	y	y	n	y	n	63	Moderate

Table 3. NOS quality assessment table. Each study was awarded one star per item within the selection and exposure categories. A maximum of two stars could be awarded for comparability. The score is the sum of the awarded stars and ranges from zero to nine.

		Selection				Comparability		Exposure			Score
Ref.	First Author	Is the Case Definition Adequate?	Representativeness of the Cases	Selection of Controls	Definition of Controls	Based on the Design or Analysis	Ascertainment of Exposure	Same Method of Ascertainment for Cases and Controls	Non-Response Rate		
[14]	Abdollahzadeh P; 2017	*	*	*	*	*		*	*		5/9
[19]	Badawi H; 2008	*	*	*	*	*	*	*	*		7/9
[20]	Barghi MR; 2005	*	*	*	*	*	*	*	*		6/9
[32]	Gould VE; 2010	*	*	*	*	*	*	*	*		6/9
[37]	Kim SH; 2014	*	*	*	*	*	*	*	*		6/9
[42]	Mete UK; 2018	*	*	*	*	*		*	*		5/9
[47]	Sarier M; 2019	*	*	*	*	*		*	*		5/9
[49]	Shaker OG; 2013	*	*	*	*	*		*	*		5/9
[50]	Shigehara K; 2011	*	*	*	*	*		*	*		5/9
[53]	Steinestel J; 2013	*	*	*	*	*		*	*		5/9
[54]	Tekin MI; 1999	*	*	*	*		*	*			5/9

"*": Each study was awarded one star per item. The score is the sum of the awarded stars, ranged from 0 to 9 (high-quality, >7 stars; medium-quality, 4–6 stars; poor-quality, <4 stars).

3.3. Study Characteristics

Studies were published during the period 1995 [31,35,36,38]–2021 [44,57]. Patients were enrolled between 1985 [17] and 2019 [57]. The epidemiological study types were observational retrospective (26, 56.5%) [15–18,23–27,29–31,34–36,38–40,44,46,52,55–59], case-control (11, 23.9%) [14,19,20,32,37,42,47,49,50,53,54], prospective (8, 17.4%) [21,22,33,41,43,45,48,51], and comparative (1, 2.2%) [28]. Most of them were single-center (44/46, 95.7%) [14–16,19–59], and only two (4.3%) were multi-center [17,18]. Single-center studies were performed in Europe (18, 40.9%) [27–30,35,39–41,45–48,53–56,58,59], Asia (14, 31.8%) [14,15,20,23,31,34,36,37,42–44,50,51,57], America (6, 13.6%) [16,24,25,32,38,52], and Africa (6, 13.6%) [19,21,22,26,33,49].

3.4. Characteristics of the Study Samples

The sample size ranged from 10 [31] to 689 [39] patients, for a total of 3975 subjects. Information on gender was reported by 36 (73.5%) studies [14–17,19–22,24–34,37,40–48,50,51,53,55–58], including 555 and 1969 females and males, respectively. The mean/median age ranged from 47 [26] to 74.8 [44] years (Table S2).

The majority of the samples were FFPE (2706/3518; 76.9%) [14–18,20–26,30–38,40–46,48–51, 53,55,56,58,59], and only 812 (23.1%) were fresh tissue specimens [19,28,29,42,47,48,50,54,57,59]. Information on the type of specimen was not available for three (3/46; 6.5%) studies [27,39,52].

Histological classification was available for 42/46 (91.3%): TCC were the most prevalent (1445/2792; 51.8%) type, followed by UC (1098/2792; 39.3%) and SCC (249/2792; 8.9%) (Table S3).

Sixteen (34.8%) studies [14,21,27,30,35,38,40,41,45,48,50–52,54,55], for a total of 1428 samples, reported the grading, following the recommendations of the American Joint Committee on Cancer [AJCC Cancer Staging Manual. 7th ed. New York, NY: Springer; 2010.]. A total of 580 (40.6%), 513 (35.9%), and 335 (23.5%) tumors were classified as moderate (G2), poor (G3), and well (G1) differentiated, respectively. 1049 specimens [15,20,22,33,34, 36,37,42,43,45,47,49,51,57,58] were classified according to the guidelines of the European Association of Urology [60], with 541 (51.6%) low- and 508 (48.4%) high- grade lesions (Table S3).

The most frequent HPV detection method was molecular (38/46; 82.6%) [15,19–24,26, 28–48,50–55,57–59], whereas a non-molecular technique (i.e., immunohistochemistry–IHC and/or in situ hybridization–ISH) was employed in 34 (73.9%) studies [14,16–18,23–25,27,31–33,35,37,41,43,44,46,49–51,55,56,59] (Table S4)

3.5. Outcomes

Pooled HPV prevalence was 19% (95% CI: 13%-26%; I2: 96.4%) (Figure 2) ranging from 0% [17,21,26,41,47,52,55,57,58] to 83% [48]. 619/3682 (16.8%) BCa samples were positive (Table 4).

No risk differences were found between females and males [pooled risk difference (95% CI): 0.0046 (−0.0545; 0.0636); p-value: 0.87999; I2: 13.5%] (Figure S1). No statistically significant risk differences were found when prevalences related to patients in stage $\leq$T1 and $\geq$T2 stage were compared [pooled risk difference (95% CI) = −0.0659 (−0.173; 0.0411); p-value: 0.22746; I2: 45.2%], as well as in patients with G1 and G2/G3 tumors, [pooled risk difference (95% CI): −0.0451 (−0.1447; 0.0546); p-value: 0.37542; I2: 75.9%] (Figures S2 and S3).

Pooled prevalence stratified by histological subtypes was 36.5% (95% CI: 15.9–60.1%; I2: 88.2%), 32.5% (95% CI: 23.8–41.8%; I2: 90.7%), and 18.5% (95% CI: 3.8–40.9%; I2: 97.3%) for SCC, TCC, and UC, respectively (Figure 3), with a statistically significant difference between the prevalence in SCC vs. TCC (p-value: 0.0002) and vs. UC (p-value < 0.0001).

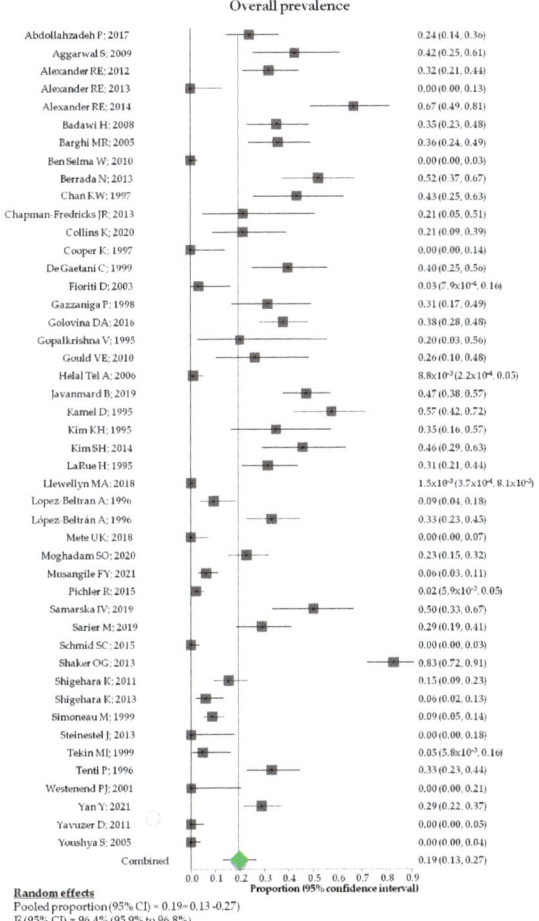

Figure 2. Forest plot of HPV pooled prevalence in bladder cancer. Adapted from [14–59].

Table 4. Overall HPV prevalence among the selected studies. If different prevalence values were outlined in the studies, the value from the standard detection technique (or the highest in case of comparison between standard methods) was reported in the table below.

Ref.	First Author	Overall HPV Prevalence	Ref.	First Author	Overall HPV Prevalence
[14]	Abdollahzadeh P; 2017	16/67 (23.9)	[37]	Kim SH; 2014	16/35 (45.7)
[15]	Aggarwal S; 2009	14/33 (42.4)	[38]	LaRue H; 1995	22/70 (31.4)
[16]	Alexander RE; 2012	22/69 (31.9)	[39]	Llewellyn MA; 2018	1/689 (0.1)
[17]	Alexander RE; 2013	0/27 (0)	[40]	Lopez-Beltran A; 1996	7/76 (9.2)
[18]	Alexander RE; 2014	24/36 (67)	[41]	Lopez-Beltran A; 1996	25/76 (32.9)
[19]	Badawi H; 2008	21/60 (35)	[42]	Mete UK; 2018	0/50 (0)
[20]	Barghi MR; 2005	21/59 (35.6)	[43]	Moghadam SO; 2020	24/106 (22.6)
[21]	Ben Selma W; 2010	0/125 (0)	[44]	Musangile FY; 2021	10/162 (6.2)
[22]	Berrada N; 2013	25/48 (52.1)	[45]	Pichler R; 2015	4/186 (2.2)
[23]	Chan KW; 1997	13/30 (43.3)	[46]	Samarska IV; 2019	19/38 (50)
[24]	Chapman-Fredricks JR; 2013	3/14 (21.43)	[47]	Sarier M; 2019	20/69 (29)
[25]	Collins K; 2020	7/33 (21.2)	[48]	Schmid SC; 2015	0/109 (0)
[26]	Cooper K; 1997	0/25 (0)	[49]	Shaker OG; 2013	58/70 (82.9)
[27]	De Gaetani C; 1999	17/43 (32.56)	[50]	Shigehara K; 2011	18/117 (15.38)
[28]	Fioriti D; 2003	1/32 (3.1)	[51]	Shigehara K; 2013	5/84 (5.95)
[29]	Gazzaniga P; 1998	11/35 (36.7)	[52]	Simoneau M; 1999	16/187 (8.5)
[30]	Golovina DA; 2016	38/101 (37.6)	[53]	Steinestel J; 2013	0/19 (0)
[31]	Gopalkrishna V; 1995	2/10 (20)	[54]	Tekin MI; 1999	2/42 (4.8)
[32]	Gould VE; 2010	6/23 (26.1)	[55]	Tenti P; 1996	26/79 (32.9)
[33]	Helal Tel A; 2006	1/114 (0.9)	[56]	Westenend PJ; 2001	0/16 (0)
[34]	Javanmard B; 2019	52/110 (47.3)	[57]	Yan Y; 2021	42/146 (28.8)
[35]	Kamel D; 1995	27/47 (57)	[58]	Yavuzer D; 2011	0/70 (0)
[36]	Kim KH; 1995	8/23 (34.7)	[59]	Youshya S; 2005	0/98 (0)

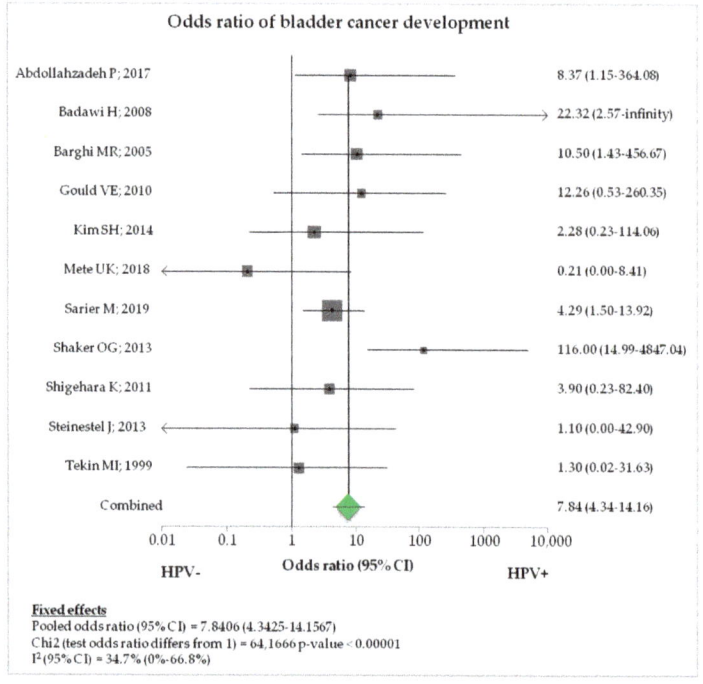

Figure 3. Forest plot of overall odds ratio in case-control studies. Adapted from [14,19,20,32,37,42,47,49,50,53,54].

Also, 69/479 (6.9%) were multiple infections [15,19,20,27,32,35,36,44,50,52,55,57].

The most prevalent genotype was HPV-16 (216/479; 45.1%), followed by HPV-18 (153/479; 31.9%), HPV-6 (25/479; 5.2%), and HPV-11 (17/479; 3.5%). Moreover, 68 (14.2%) infections were caused by other HR-HPV genotypes (Table S5).

3.6. Case-Control Studies

The studies with a case-control design numbered 11/46 (23.9%) in the selection, with a total of 611 cases vs. 227 controls [14,19,20,32,37,42,47,49,50,53,54]. The overall prevalence was 27.3% (167/611) and 4.4% (10/227) in cases and controls, respectively. The pooled odds ratio (OR) was 7.8406 (95% CI, 4.3425–14.1567; p-value < 0.00001; I2: 34.7%) for the association between HPV infection and occurrence of BCa (Table 5; Figure 3).

Table 5. HPV prevalence stratified by the presence (case) or absence (control) of any type of bladder tumor (case-control studies).

Ref.	First Author	HPV Positivity (n/N, %)	
		Cases	Controls
[14]	Abdollahzadeh P; 2017	15/67 (22.4)	1/30 (3.3)
[19]	Badawi H; 2008	21/60 (35)	0/20 (0)
[20]	Barghi MR; 2005	21/59 (35.6)	1/20 (5)
[32]	Gould VE; 2010	6/23 (26.1)	0/10 (0)
[37]	Kim SH; 2014	6/35 (17.1)	1/12 (8.3)
[42]	Mete UK; 2018	0/50 (0)	0/10 (0)
[47]	Sarier M; 2019	20/69 (28.9)	6/69 (8.7)
[49]	Shaker OG; 2013	58/70 (82.9)	1/25 (4)
[50]	Shigehara K; 2011	18/117 (15.4)	0/10 (0)
[53]	Steinestel J; 2013	0/19 (0)	0/21 (0)
[54]	Tekin MI; 1999	2/42 (4.8)	0/10 (0)

4. Discussion

This systematic review was performed to evaluate the prevalence of HPV infection in BCa, keeping into consideration confounding demographic, histological, and diagnostic variables.

An overall HPV prevalence of 19% was found in 46 studies, in line with previous meta-analyses which reported a prevalence of 16.88% [10] and 14.3% [61]. Despite the growing number of reported studies, the role of HPV in cancers other than genital, anal, head, and neck cancers is still debated, due to the heterogeneity in the study design, population enrolled, and HPV detection methods [6]. In fact, several systematic reviews, which evaluated the prevalence of infection of DNA-based vs. non-DNA-based methods confirmed the higher specificity and sensitivity of molecular-based methods [62,63]. Moreover, the use of genotype primers designed for shorter DNA sequences reduced the risk of "false negative" results in comparison with broad-spectrum primers (i.e., GP5+/6+), especially for FFPE specimens often undergoing DNA damage [10]. Therefore, the implementation of a standardized procedure for HPV detection could better clarify the impact of HPV in BCa pathogenesis.

A statistically significant difference in the prevalence of infection was found in different histological subtypes, with higher estimates in SCC than those in TCC and UC. The high affinity of HPV to differentiating squamous epithelium, previously demonstrated in cervical, head and neck, and anogenital carcinomas [64], as well as the ability of the virus to evade and inactivate the immune response, could explain the mechanism of carcinogenesis in the bladder epithelium. Since SCC has poor prognosis and is associated with worse outcomes in different sites [65], the confirmation of the role of HPV in SCC could improve the epidemiological burden and the prognosis of potential cases.

The assessment of the role of HPV as causative agent in different histological subtypes could have been affected by the adoption of the new WHO BCa classification [66]. This recent recommendation changed the traditional nomenclature of "transitional cell carcinoma" in "urothelial carcinoma", causing potential misinterpretations of the results. On this basis, the identification of standard accurate procedures for the detection and diagnosis of HPV infection could be helpful to estimate the burden of cancers associated with HPV. However, the available molecular techniques show a high diagnostic accuracy.

Although several studies suggested a relationship between advanced stage (i.e., $\geq$T2) and HPV prevalence [27,43,44], the poor information collected in the selected studies did not prove this association.

Similarly to other HPV-related cancers, HPV-16 was the most prevalent genotype in BCa, supporting previous findings on the increased risk of BCa in cases of infection caused by high-risk HPV genotypes, mainly by HPV-16 [10]. The high detection rate of HPV-16, together with HPV-18 and the low-risk HPV-6, strongly supports the administration of HPV vaccines to prevent HPV-related cancers in both sexes [67].

Finally, our study showed a significant association between HPV and BCa (OR: 7.84), confirming the findings of recent meta-analyses on the risk of BCa [10,62,65]. However, these results are in contrast with a previous study published by Khatami et al. [61], who described a non-significant association between infection and cancer and highlighted the scientific need of larger case-control studies. Although the majority of case-control studies were classified as "medium-quality", controls showed a prevalence of infection <10%, regardless of HPV detection methods, suggesting the etiological role of HPV in BCa.

Previous systematic reviews investigated the role of HPV infection in BCa and described a moderate association. Our study selection and analysis showed an important role of HPV infection in SCC BCa. However, some limitations should be acknowledged. More stratified analyses related to demographic (i.e., geographical area, behavioral factors, occupational exposures) and clinical (i.e., stage, HPV detection methods, prognosis of patients) confounders should be performed. The cross-sectional assessment does not help prove the temporal relationship between an exposure and the development of cancer.

5. Conclusions

The present systematic review highlights a potential role of HPV in the development of bladder cancer, indirectly supporting the adoption of primary preventive strategies in both sexes, as recommended by international authorities. Further epidemiological studies are needed to confirm those findings and assess the role of diagnostic and preventive strategies for HPV-related bladder cancer.

Supplementary Materials: The following supporting information can be downloaded at: https://www.mdpi.com/article/10.3390/diagnostics12071759/s1, Figures S1–S3, Tables S1–S5.

Author Contributions: Conceptualization, N.M., B.D.L., L.S. and G.S.; methodology, N.M., B.D.L., L.S., A.P. and G.S.; software, B.D.L., L.S. and G.S.; validation, N.M., B.D.L., L.S., I.S., A.P. and G.S.; formal analysis, B.D.L., L.S. and G.S.; investigation, N.M., B.D.L., G.S.; resources, N.M., B.D.L., L.S., I.S., A.D.R., A.P. and G.S.; data curation, N.M., B.D.L., L.S., A.P. and G.S.; writing—original draft preparation, N.M., B.D.L., I.S. and A.D.R.; writing—review and editing, N.M., B.D.L., A.P. and G.S.; visualization, N.M., B.D.L., L.S., I.S., A.D.R., A.P. and G.S.; supervision, A.P. and G.S. All authors have read and agreed to the published version of the manuscript.

Funding: Article Processing Charge was funded by Cariplo Foundation-Biomedical Research conducted by Young Researchers 2019.

Institutional Review Board Statement: Ethical review and approval were waived due to the design of the study.

Informed Consent Statement: Patient consent was waived due to the design of the study.

Data Availability Statement: The data is available in case it is requested for motivated reasons.

Conflicts of Interest: The authors declare no conflict of interest.

References

1. International Agency for Reasearch on Cancer (IARC). Global Cancer Observatory. Available online: https://gco.iarc.fr (accessed on 18 May 2022).
2. Sung, H.; Ferlay, J.; Siegel, R.L.; Laversanne, M.; Soerjomataram, I.; Jemal, A.; Bray, F. Global Cancer Statistics 2020: GLOBOCAN Estimates of Incidence and Mortality Worldwide for 36 Cancers in 185 Countries. *CA Cancer J. Clin.* **2021**, *71*, 209–249. [CrossRef] [PubMed]
3. Prout, G.R., Jr.; Wesley, M.N.; Greenberg, R.S.; Chen, V.W.; Brown, C.C.; Miller, A.W.; Weinstein, R.S.; Robboy, S.J.; Haynes, M.A.; Blacklow, R.S.; et al. Bladder cancer: Race differences in extent of disease at diagnosis. *Cancer* **2000**, *89*, 1349–1358. [CrossRef]
4. Di Meo, N.A.; Loizzo, D.; Pandolfo, S.D.; Autorino, R.; Ferro, M.; Porta, C.; Stella, A.; Bizzoca, C.; Vincenti, L.; Crocetto, F.; et al. Metabolomic Approaches for Detection and Identification of Biomarkers and Altered Pathways in Bladder Cancer. *Int. J. Mol. Sci.* **2022**, *23*, 4173. [CrossRef] [PubMed]
5. Saginala, K.; Barsouk, A.; Aluru, J.S.; Rawla, P.; Padala, S.A.; Barsouk, A. Epidemiology of Bladder Cancer. *Med. Sci.* **2020**, *8*, 15. [CrossRef]
6. Mushtaq, J.; Thurairaja, R.; Nair, R. Bladder Cancer. *Surgery* **2019**, *37*, 529–537. [CrossRef]
7. Muresu, N.; Sotgiu, G.; Saderi, L.; Sechi, I.; Cossu, A.; Marras, V.; Meloni, M.; Martinelli, M.; Cocuzza, C.; Tanda, F.; et al. Distribution of HPV Genotypes in Patients with a Diagnosis of Anal Cancer in an Italian Region. *Int. J. Environ. Res. Public Health* **2020**, *17*, 4516. [CrossRef]
8. Muresu, N.; Sotgiu, G.; Saderi, L.; Sechi, I.; Cossu, A.; Marras, V.; Meloni, M.; Martinelli, M.; Cocuzza, C.; Tanda, F.; et al. Italian observational study on HPV infection, E6, and p16 expression in men with penile cancer. *Virol. J.* **2020**, *17*, 161. [CrossRef]
9. Wu, J.; Xiao, F.; Zheng, Y.; Lin, Y.; Wang, H.L. Worldwide trend in human papillomavirus-attributable cancer incidence rates between 1990 and 2012 and Bayesian projection to 2030. *Cancer* **2021**, *127*, 3172–3182. [CrossRef]
10. Li, N.; Yang, L.; Zhang, Y.; Zhao, P.; Zheng, T.; Dai, M. Human papillomavirus infection and bladder cancer risk: A meta-analysis. *J. Infect. Dis.* **2011**, *204*, 217–223. [CrossRef]
11. Page, M.J.; McKenzie, J.E.; Bossuyt, P.M.; Boutron, I.; Hoffmann, T.C.; Mulrow, C.D.; Shamseer, L.; Tetzlaff, J.M.; Akl, E.A.; Brennan, S.E.; et al. The PRISMA 2020 statement: An updated guideline for reporting systematic reviews. *BMJ* **2021**, *372*, n71. [CrossRef]
12. Wells, G.A.; Shea, B.; O'Connell, D.; Pereson, J.; Welch, V.; Losos, M.; Tugwell, P. *The Newcastle-Ottawa Scale (NOS) for Assessing the Quality of Non Randomised Studies in Meta-Analyses*; Ottawa Hospital Research Institute: Ottawa, ON, Canada, 2011; Available online: http://www.ohri.ca/programs/clinical_epidemiology/oxford.asp (accessed on 10 May 2022).
13. Lockwood, C.; Porrit, K.; Munn, Z.; Rittenmeyer, L.; Salmond, S.; Bjerrum, M.; Loveday, H.; Carrier, J.; Stannard, D. Chapter 2: Systematic reviews of qualitative evidence. In *JBI Manual for Evidence Synthesis*; Aromataris, E., Munn, Z., Eds.; JBI: Adelaide, Australia, 2020; Available online: https://synthesismanual.jbi.global (accessed on 10 May 2022).
14. Abdollahzadeh, P.; Madani, S.H.; Khazaei, S.; Sajadimajd, S.; Izadi, B.; Najafi, F. Association Between Human Papillomavirus and Transitional Cell Carcinoma of the Bladder. *Urol. J.* **2017**, *14*, 5047–5050. [CrossRef] [PubMed]
15. Aggarwal, S.; Arora, V.K.; Gupta, S.; Singh, N.; Bhatia, A. Koilocytosis: Correlations with high-risk HPV and its comparison on tissue sections and cytology, urothelial carcinoma. *Diagn. Cytopathol.* **2009**, *37*, 174–177. [CrossRef] [PubMed]
16. Alexander, R.E.; Hu, Y.; Kum, J.B.; Montironi, R.; Lopez-Beltran, A.; Maclennan, G.T.; Idrees, M.T.; Emerson, R.E.; Ulbright, T.M.; Grignon, D.G.; et al. p16 expression is not associated with human papillomavirus in urinary bladder squamous cell carcinoma. *Mod. Pathol.* **2012**, *25*, 1526–1533. [CrossRef]
17. Alexander, R.E.; Davidson, D.D.; Lopez-Beltran, A.; Montironi, R.; MacLennan, G.T.; Compérat, E.; Idrees, M.T.; Emerson, R.E.; Cheng, L. Human papillomavirus is not an etiologic agent of urothelial inverted papillomas. *Am. J. Surg. Pathol.* **2013**, *37*, 1223–1228. [CrossRef] [PubMed]
18. Alexander, R.E.; Williamson, S.R.; Richey, J.; Lopez-Beltran, A.; Montironi, R.; Davidson, D.D.; Idrees, M.T.; Jones, C.L.; Zhang, S.; Wang, L.; et al. The expression patterns of p53 and p16 and an analysis of a possible role of HPV in primary adenocarcinoma of the urinary bladder. *PLoS ONE* **2014**, *9*, e95724. [CrossRef]
19. Badawi, H.; Ahmed, H.; Ismail, A.; Diab, M.; Moubarak, M.; Badawy, A.; Saber, M. Role of human papillomavirus types 16, 18, and 52 in recurrent cystitis and urinary bladder cancer among Egyptian patients. *Medscape J. Med.* **2008**, *10*, 232.
20. Barghi, M.R.; Hajimohammadmehdiarbab, A.; Moghaddam, S.M.; Kazemi, B. Correlation between human papillomavirus infection and bladder transitional cell carcinoma. *BMC Infect. Dis.* **2005**, *5*, 102. [CrossRef]
21. Ben Selma, W.; Ziadi, S.; Ben Gacem, R.; Amara, K.; Ksiaa, F.; Hachana, M.; Trimeche, M. Investigation of human papillomavirus in bladder cancer in a series of Tunisian patients. *Pathol. Res. Pract.* **2010**, *206*, 740–743. [CrossRef]
22. Berrada, N.; Al-Bouzidi, A.; Ameur, A.; Abbar, M.; El-Mzibri, M.; Ameziane-El-Hassani, R.; Benbacer, L.; Khyatti, M.; Qmichou, Z.; Amzazi, S.; et al. Human papillomavirus detection in Moroccan patients with bladder cancer. *J. Infect. Dev. Ctries* **2013**, *7*, 586–592. [CrossRef]
23. Chan, K.W.; Wong, K.Y.; Srivastava, G. Prevalence of six types of human papillomavirus in inverted papilloma and papillary transitional cell carcinoma of the bladder: An evaluation by polymerase chain reaction. *J Clin. Pathol.* **1997**, *50*, 1018–1021. [CrossRef]

24. Chapman-Fredricks, J.R.; Cioffi-Lavina, M.; Accola, M.A.; Rehrauer, W.M.; Garcia-Buitrago, M.T.; Gomez-Fernandez, C.; Ganjei-Azar, P.; Jordà, M. High-risk human papillomavirus DNA detected in primary squamous cell carcinoma of urinary bladder. *Arch. Pathol. Lab. Med.* **2013**, *137*, 1088–1093. [CrossRef]
25. Collins, K.; Hwang, M.; Hamza, A.; Rao, P. Prevalence of high-risk human papillomavirus in primary squamous cell carcinoma of urinary bladder. *Pathol. Res. Pract.* **2020**, *216*, 153084. [CrossRef] [PubMed]
26. Cooper, K.; Haffajee, Z.; Taylor, L. Human papillomavirus and schistosomiasis associated bladder cancer. *Mol. Pathol.* **1997**, *50*, 145–148. [CrossRef] [PubMed]
27. De Gaetani, C.; Ferrari, G.; Righi, E.; Bettelli, S.; Migaldi, M.; Ferrari, P.; Trentini, G.P. Detection of human papillomavirus DNA in urinary bladder carcinoma by in situ hybridisation. *J. Clin. Pathol.* **1999**, *52*, 103–106. [CrossRef] [PubMed]
28. Fioriti, D.; Pietropaolo, V.; Dal Forno, S.; Laurenti, C.; Chiarini, F.; Degener, A.M. Urothelial bladder carcinoma and viral infections: Different association with human polyomaviruses and papillomaviruses. *Int. J. Immunopathol. Pharmacol.* **2003**, *16*, 283–288. [CrossRef]
29. Gazzaniga, P.; Vercillo, R.; Gradilone, A.; Silvestri, I.; Gandini, O.; Napolitano, M.; Giuliani, L.; Fioravanti, A.; Gallucci, M.; Aglianò, A.M. Prevalence of papillomavirus, Epstein-Barr virus, cytomegalovirus, and herpes simplex virus type 2 in urinary bladder cancer. *J. Med. Virol.* **1998**, *55*, 262–267. [CrossRef]
30. Golovina, D.A.; Ermilova, V.D.; Zavalishina, L.E.; Andreeva, Y.Y.; Matveev, V.B.; Frank, G.A.; Volgareva, G.M. Loss of Cell Differentiation in HPV-Associated Bladder Cancer. *Bull. Exp. Biol. Med.* **2016**, *161*, 96–98. [CrossRef]
31. Gopalkrishna, V.; Srivastava, A.N.; Hedau, S.; Sharma, J.K.; Das, B.C. Detection of human papillomavirus DNA sequences in cancer of the urinary bladder by in situ hybridisation and polymerase chain reaction. *Sex. Transm. Infect.* **1995**, *71*, 231–233. [CrossRef]
32. Gould, V.E.; Schmitt, M.; Vinokurova, S.; Reddy, V.B.; Bitterman, P.; Alonso, A.; Gattuso, P. Human papillomavirus and p16 expression in inverted papillomas of the urinary bladder. *Cancer Lett.* **2010**, *292*, 171–175. [CrossRef]
33. Helal Tel, A.; Fadel, M.T.; El-Sayed, N.K. Human papilloma virus and p53 expression in bladder cancer in Egypt: Relationship to schistosomiasis and clinicopathologic factors. *Pathol. Oncol. Res.* **2006**, *12*, 173–178. [CrossRef]
34. Javanmard, B.; Barghi, M.R.; Amani, D.; Fallah Karkan, M.; Mazloomfard, M.M. Human Papilloma Virus DNA in Tumor Tissue and Urine in Different Stage of Bladder Cancer. *Urol. J.* **2019**, *16*, 352–356. [CrossRef] [PubMed]
35. Kamel, D.; Pääkkö, P.; Pöllänen, R.; Vähäkangas, K.; Lehto, V.P.; Soini, Y. Human papillomavirus DNA and abnormal p53 expression in carcinoma of the urinary bladder. *APMIS* **1995**, *103*, 331–338. [CrossRef] [PubMed]
36. Kim, K.H.; Kim, Y.S. Analysis of p53 tumor suppressor gene mutations and human papillomavirus infection in human bladder cancers. *Yonsei Med. J.* **1995**, *36*, 322–331. [CrossRef] [PubMed]
37. Kim, S.H.; Joung, J.Y.; Chung, J.; Park, W.S.; Lee, K.H.; Seo, H.K. Detection of human papillomavirus infection and p16 immunohistochemistry expression in bladder cancer with squamous differentiation. *PLoS ONE* **2014**, *9*, e93525. [CrossRef]
38. LaRue, H.; Simoneau, M.; Fradet, Y. Human papillomavirus in transitional cell carcinoma of the urinary bladder. *Clin. Cancer Res.* **1995**, *1*, 435–440.
39. Llewellyn, M.A.; Gordon, N.S.; Abbotts, B.; James, N.D.; Zeegers, M.P.; Cheng, K.K.; Macdonald, A.; Roberts, S.; Parish, J.L.; Ward, D.G.; et al. Defining the frequency of human papillomavirus and polyomavirus infection in urothelial bladder tumours. *Sci. Rep.* **2018**, *8*, 11290. [CrossRef]
40. Lopez-Beltran, A.; Escudero, A.L.; Vicioso, L.; Muñoz, E.; Carrasco, J.C. Human papillomavirus DNA as a factor determining the survival of bladder cancer patients. *Br. J. Cancer* **1996**, *73*, 124–127. [CrossRef]
41. López-Beltrán, A.; Escudero, A.L.; Carrasco-Aznar, J.C.; Vicioso-Recio, L. Human papillomavirus infection and transitional cell carcinoma of the bladder. Immunohistochemistry and in situ hybridization. *Pathol. Res. Pract.* **1996**, *192*, 154–159. [CrossRef]
42. Mete, U.K.; Shenvi, S.; Singh, M.P.; Chakraborti, A.; Kakkar, N.; Ratho, R.K.; Mandal, A.K. Human Papillomavirus in Urothelial Carcinoma of Bladder: An Indian study. *Int. J. Appl. Basic Med. Res.* **2018**, *8*, 217–219. [CrossRef]
43. Moghadam Ohadian, S.; Mansori, K.; Nowroozi, M.R.; Afshar, D.; Abbasi, B.; Nowroozi, A. Association of human papilloma virus (HPV) infection with oncological outcomes in urothelial bladder cancer. *Infect. Agents Cancer* **2020**, *15*, 52. [CrossRef]
44. Musangile, F.Y.; Matsuzaki, I.; Okodo, M.; Shirasaki, A.; Mikasa, Y.; Iwamoto, R.; Takahashi, Y.; Kojima, F.; Murata, S.I. Detection of HPV infection in urothelial carcinoma using RNAscope: Clinicopathological characterization. *Cancer Med.* **2021**, *10*, 5534–5544. [CrossRef] [PubMed]
45. Pichler, R.; Borena, W.; Schäfer, G.; Manzl, C.; Culig, Z.; List, S.; Neururer, S.; Von Laer, D.; Heidegger, I.; Klocker, H.; et al. Low prevalence of HPV detection and genotyping in non-muscle invasive bladder cancer using single-step PCR followed by reverse line blot. *World J. Urol.* **2015**, *33*, 2145–2151. [CrossRef] [PubMed]
46. Samarska, I.V.; Epstein, J.I. Condyloma Acuminatum of Urinary Bladder: Relation to Squamous Cell Carcinoma. *Am. J. Surg. Pathol.* **2019**, *43*, 1547–1553. [CrossRef]
47. Sarier, M.; Sepin, N.; Keles, Y.; Imir, L.; Emek, M.; Demir, M.; Kukul, E.; Soylu, A. Is There any Association between Urothelial Carcinoma of the Bladder and Human Papillomavirus? A Case-Control Study. *Urol. Int.* **2020**, *104*, 81–86. [CrossRef]
48. Schmid, S.C.; Thümer, L.; Schuster, T.; Horn, T.; Kurtz, F.; Slotta-Huspenina, J.; Seebach, J.; Straub, M.; Maurer, T.; Autenrieth, M.; et al. Human papilloma virus is not detectable in samples of urothelial bladder cancer in a central European population: A prospective translational study. *Infect. Agents Cancer* **2015**, *10*, 31. [CrossRef]

49. Shaker, O.G.; Hammam, O.A.; Wishahi, M.M. Is there a correlation between HPV and urinary bladder carcinoma? *Biomed. Pharmacother.* **2013**, *67*, 183–191. [CrossRef] [PubMed]
50. Shigehara, K.; Sasagawa, T.; Kawaguchi, S.; Nakashima, T.; Shimamura, M.; Maeda, Y.; Konaka, H.; Mizokami, A.; Koh, E.; Namiki, M. Etiologic role of human papillomavirus infection in bladder carcinoma. *Cancer* **2011**, *117*, 2067–2076. [CrossRef]
51. Shigehara, K.; Kawaguchi, S.; Sasagawa, T.; Nakashima, K.; Nakashima, T.; Shimamura, M.; Namiki, M. Etiological correlation of human papillomavirus infection in the development of female bladder tumor. *APMIS* **2013**, *121*, 1169–1176. [CrossRef]
52. Simoneau, M.; LaRue, H.; Fradet, Y. Low frequency of human papillomavirus infection in initial papillary bladder tumors. *Urol. Res.* **1999**, *27*, 180–184. [CrossRef]
53. Steinestel, J.; Cronauer, M.V.; Müller, J.; Al Ghazal, A.; Skowronek, P.; Arndt, A.; Kraft, K.; Schrader, M.; Schrader, A.J.; Steinestel, K. Overexpression of p16(INK4a) in urothelial carcinoma in situ is a marker for MAPK-mediated epithelial-mesenchymal transition but is not related to human papillomavirus infection. *PLoS ONE* **2013**, *8*, e65189. [CrossRef]
54. Tekin, M.I.; Tuncer, S.; Aki, F.T.; Bilen, C.Y.; Aygün, C.; Ozen, H. Human papillomavirus associated with bladder carcinoma? Analysis by polymerase chain reaction. *Int. J. Urol.* **1999**, *6*, 184–186. [CrossRef] [PubMed]
55. Tenti, P.; Zappatore, R.; Romagnoli, S.; Civardi, E.; Giunta, P.; Scelsi, R.; Stella, G.; Carnevali, L. p53 overexpression and human papillomavirus infection in transitional cell carcinoma of the urinary bladder: Correlation with histological parameters. *J. Pathol.* **1996**, *178*, 65–70. [CrossRef]
56. Westenend, P.J.; Stoop, J.A.; Hendriks, J.G. Human papillomaviruses 6/11, 16/18 and 31/33/51 are not associated with squamous cell carcinoma of the urinary bladder. *BJU Int.* **2001**, *88*, 198–201. [CrossRef] [PubMed]
57. Yan, Y.; Zhang, H.; Jiang, C.; Ma, X.; Zhou, X.; Tian, X.; Song, Y.; Chen, X.; Yu, L.; Li, R.; et al. Human Papillomavirus Prevalence and Integration Status in Tissue Samples of Bladder Cancer in the Chinese Population. *J. Infect. Dis.* **2021**, *224*, 114–122. [CrossRef] [PubMed]
58. Yavuzer, D.; Karadayi, N.; Salepci, T.; Baloglu, H.; Bilici, A.; Sakirahmet, D. Role of human papillomavirus in the development of urothelial carcinoma. *Med. Oncol.* **2011**, *28*, 919–923. [CrossRef]
59. Youshya, S.; Purdie, K.; Breuer, J.; Proby, C.; Sheaf, M.T.; Oliver, R.T.; Baithun, S. Does human papillomavirus play a role in the development of bladder transitional cell carcinoma? A comparison of PCR and immunohistochemical analysis. *J. Clin. Pathol.* **2005**, *58*, 207–210. [CrossRef]
60. Soukup, V.; Čapoun, O.; Cohen, D.; Hernández, V.; Babjuk, M.; Burger, M.; Compérat, E.; Gontero, P.; Lam, T.; MacLennan, S.; et al. Prognostic Performance and Reproducibility of the 1973 and 2004/2016 World Health Organization Grading Classification Systems in Non-muscle-invasive Bladder Cancer: A European Association of Urology Non-muscle Invasive Bladder Cancer Guidelines Panel Systematic Review. *Eur. Urol.* **2017**, *72*, 801–813. [CrossRef]
61. Khatami, A.; Salavatiha, Z.; Razizadeh, M.H. Bladder cancer and human papillomavirus association: A systematic review and meta-analysis. *Infect. Agents Cancer* **2022**, *17*, 3. [CrossRef]
62. Gutiérrez, J.; Jiménez, A.; de Dios Luna, J.; Soto, M.J.; Sorlózano, A. Meta-analysis of studies analyzing the relationship between bladder cancer and infection by human papillomavirus. *J. Urol.* **2006**, *176 Pt 1*, 2474–2481. [CrossRef]
63. Jimenez-Pacheco, A.; Exposito-Ruiz, M.; Arrabal-Polo, M.A.; Lopez-Luque, A.J. Meta-analysis of studies analyzing the role of human papillomavirus in the development of bladder carcinoma. *Korean J. Urol.* **2012**, *53*, 240–247. [CrossRef]
64. Chow, L.T.; Broker, T.R.; Steinberg, B.M. The natural history of human papillomavirus infections of the mucosal epithelia. *APMIS* **2010**, *118*, 422–449. [CrossRef] [PubMed]
65. Jørgensen, K.R.; Jensen, J.B. Human papillomavirus and urinary bladder cancer revisited. *APMIS* **2020**, *128*, 72–79. [CrossRef] [PubMed]
66. Humphrey, P.A.; Moch, H.; Cubilla, A.L.; Ulbright, T.M.; Reuter, V.E. The 2016 WHO Classification of Tumours of the Urinary System and Male Genital Organs—Part B: Prostate and Bladder Tumours. *Eur. Urol.* **2016**, *70*, 106–119. [CrossRef] [PubMed]
67. Human papillomavirus vaccines: WHO position paper, May 2017. *Wkly. Epidemiol. Rec.* **2017**, *92*, 241–268. (In English, French)

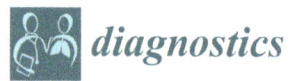

Article

Colposcopy Accuracy and Diagnostic Performance: A Quality Control and Quality Assurance Survey in Italian Tertiary-Level Teaching and Academic Institutions—The Italian Society of Colposcopy and Cervico-Vaginal Pathology (SICPCV)

Massimo Origoni [1,*], Francesco Cantatore [1], Francesco Sopracordevole [2], Nicolò Clemente [2], Arsenio Spinillo [3], Barbara Gardella [3], Rosa De Vincenzo [4,5], Caterina Ricci [5], Fabio Landoni [6], Maria Letizia Di Meo [6], Andrea Ciavattini [7], Jacopo Di Giuseppe [7], Eleonora Preti [8], Anna Daniela Iacobone [8,9], Carmine Carriero [10], Miriam Dellino [10], Massimo Capodanno [11], Antonino Perino [12], Cesare Miglioli [13], Luca Insolia [13], Maggiorino Barbero [14] and Massimo Candiani [1]

1. Department of Obstetrics & Gynecology, IRCCS Ospedale San Raffaele, Vita Salute San Raffaele University School of Medicine, 20132 Milan, Italy; francesco.cantatore@hsr.it (F.C.); massimo.candiani@hsr.it (M.C.)
2. Gynecological Oncology Unit, IRCCS Oncological Referral Center (CRO), National Cancer Institute, 33081 Aviano, Italy; fsopracordevole@cro.it (F.S.); nicolo.clemente@cro.it (N.C.)
3. Department of Obstetrics & Gynecology, IRCCS Policlinico San Matteo, University of Pavia, 27100 Pavia, Italy; a.spinillo@smatteo.pv.it (A.S.); barbara.gardella@gmail.com (B.G.)
4. Gynecological Oncology Unit, Department of Woman and Child Health and Public Health, IRCCS Policlinico Universitario A. Gemelli, 00168 Rome, Italy; rosa.devincenzo@unicatt.it
5. Department of Health Sciences and Public Health, Catholic University of the Sacred Hearth, 00168 Rome, Italy; caterina.ricci@policlinicogemelli.it
6. Department of Medicine and Surgery, University of Milano Bicocca, Clinic of Obstetrics and Gynecology, IRCCS San Gerardo dei Tintori, 20900 Monza, Italy; fabio.landoni@unimib.it (F.L.); marialetizia.dimeo@gmail.com (M.L.D.M.)
7. Gynecologic Section, Department of Odontostomatological and Specialized Clinical Sciences, Marche Polytechnic University, 60123 Ancona, Italy; a.ciavattini@staff.univpm.it (A.C.); jacopo.digiuseppe@ospedaliriuniti.marche.it (J.D.G.)
8. Preventive Gynecology Unit, IRCCS European Institute of Oncology (IEO), 20141 Milan, Italy; eleonora.preti@ieo.it (E.P.); annadaniela.iacobone@ieo.it (A.D.I.)
9. Department of Biomedical Sciences, University of Sassari, 07100 Sassari, Italy
10. Interdisciplinary Department of Medicine, University of Bari Aldo Moro, 70121 Bari, Italy; carmine.carriero@uniba.it (C.C.); miriam.dellino@uniba.it (M.D.)
11. Department of Obstetrics and Gynecology, University of Napoli, 80138 Naples, Italy; massimocapodanno@virgilio.it
12. Department of Obstetrics and Gynecology, University of Palermo, 90146 Palermo, Italy; antonio.perino@unipa.it
13. Research Center for Statistics, University of Geneva, 1201 Geneva, Switzerland; cesare.miglioli@unige.ch (C.M.); luca.insolia@unige.ch (L.I.)
14. Department of Obstetrics and Gynecology, Azienda Sanitaria Locale di Asti, 14100 Asti, Italy; barberom@tin.it
* Correspondence: massimo.origoni@hsr.it

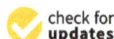

Citation: Origoni, M.; Cantatore, F.; Sopracordevole, F.; Clemente, N.; Spinillo, A.; Gardella, B.; De Vincenzo, R.; Ricci, C.; Landoni, F.; Di Meo, M.L.; et al. Colposcopy Accuracy and Diagnostic Performance: A Quality Control and Quality Assurance Survey in Italian Tertiary-Level Teaching and Academic Institutions—The Italian Society of Colposcopy and Cervico-Vaginal Pathology (SICPCV). *Diagnostics* 2023, 13, 1906. https://doi.org/10.3390/diagnostics13111906

Academic Editor: Gloria Calagna

Received: 5 May 2023
Revised: 17 May 2023
Accepted: 27 May 2023
Published: 29 May 2023

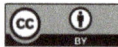

Copyright: © 2023 by the authors. Licensee MDPI, Basel, Switzerland. This article is an open access article distributed under the terms and conditions of the Creative Commons Attribution (CC BY) license (https://creativecommons.org/licenses/by/4.0/).

Abstract: Quality Control (QC) and Quality Assurance (QA) principles are essential for effective cervical cancer prevention. Being a crucial diagnostic step, colposcopy's sensitivity and specificity improvements are strongly advocated worldwide since inter- and intra-observer differences are the main limiting factors. The objective of the present study was the evaluation of colposcopy accuracy through the results of a QC/QA assessment from a survey in Italian tertiary-level academic and teaching hospitals. A web-based, user-friendly platform based on 100 colposcopic digital images was forwarded to colposcopists with different levels of experience. Seventy-three participants were asked to identify colposcopic patterns, provide personal impressions, and indicate the correct clinical practice. The data were correlated with a panel of experts' evaluation and with the clinical/pathological data of the cases. Overall sensitivity and specificity with the threshold of CIN2+ accounted for 73.7% and 87.7%, respectively, with minor differences between senior and junior candidates. Identification and interpretation of colposcopic patterns showed full agreement with the experts' panel, ranging from 50% to 82%, in some instances with better results from junior colposcopists. Colposcopic impressions correlated with a 20% underestimation of CIN2+ lesions, with no differences linked to level of experience. Our results demonstrate the good diagnostic performance of colposcopy and the need for improving accuracy through QC assessments and adhesion to standard requirements and recommendations.

Keywords: colposcopy; QC; QA; colposcopy sensitivity; diagnostic accuracy; cervical cancer prevention; CIN; SIL; colposcopy standards

1. Introduction

Colposcopy represents the recommended second-level procedure for the assessment of the uterine cervix as part of a cervical cancer screening program; it is indicated following the detection of primary test positivity according to specific guidelines, and its main objective is the early detection of high-grade cervical intraepithelial neoplasia (CIN2+) [1,2]. Colposcopic observation thus relies on the visual interpretation of macroscopic changes in color and morphology of the genital mucosae and on the correlation of specific patterns with different degrees of cervical disease. According to this intrinsic aspect of the procedure, colposcopy carries the cost of significant observer-dependent performance and thus the risk of lacking sensitivity and accuracy.

The performance of the exam is fundamental and mainly depends upon three steps: the identification of the squamocolumnar junction (SCJ), the correct assessment of the Transformation Zone (TZ) and the decision to take a biopsy/biopsies in the most appropriate cervical area.

Although colposcopy plays a fundamental role in the prevention of cervical cancer as it allows the identification, treatment, and/or follow-up of pre-cancer lesions, the accuracy of the procedure is largely influenced by a high degree of subjectivity and low reproducibility. This may lead to high rates of severe lesions under diagnosis or even cancer under detection. In this view, Artificial Intelligence (AI) may represent a promising option to overcome this limitation.

Colposcopy performance has been largely investigated and reported in different settings and different geographic areas [3–5]; almost all published data are consistent in reporting a large variability in terms of both sensitivity and specificity, with values ranging from 30% to 90% and from 40% to 95%, respectively. In this view, the colposcopic impression (CI), based on the detailed identification and interpretation of the different aspects of the TZ, represents the major issue, being closely correlated with the operator's decision to perform a targeted biopsy [6,7] and the success of the cervical cancer prevention strategy.

In the last few years, the application of Quality Control (QC) and Quality Assurance (QA) principles to assess the accuracy and performance of colposcopy has been advocated as of pivotal importance and is a strong recommendation worldwide [8–13].

The present study aims, through the multicentric involvement of major Italian teaching and academic gynecological institutions, to investigate the accuracy and quality assessment of colposcopy and, consequently, to determine the performance of operators with different levels of expertise in the field. In particular, the study was designed to assess the probability for a patient with a histologically confirmed cervical lesion of being incorrectly managed through the colposcopic workup (e.g., under detection of significant TZ alterations, not having a biopsy performed, or having a biopsy in an incorrect site). The secondary objective of the study was the development of a user-friendly online platform where Quality Control of colposcopy could be easily achieved and that could potentially be proposed and promoted for a nationwide QC and QA program.

2. Materials and Methods

One hundred (n. 100) colposcopic digital images were selected by a panel of experts among a large database of clinical cases with a comprehensive dataset of patients' demographic information, clinical history, cytological, virological (HPV-DNA detection), and pathological data. In particular, 35 were histologically negative (or without any type of lesion), 34 were low-grade lesions (HPV or CIN1), 24 were high-grade lesions (CIN2, CIN3, or in situ carcinoma), and 7 were pathologically proven invasive squamous or adenocarcinoma.

Images were deliberately identified when an objectively "difficult" colposcopic pattern was present. Nevertheless, the quality and resolution of all images, complete visibility of the entire cervix, absence of mucus/blood, and good representation of normal/abnormal colposcopic patterns were always identifiable; randomly selected images are illustrated as examples in Figures 1–3.

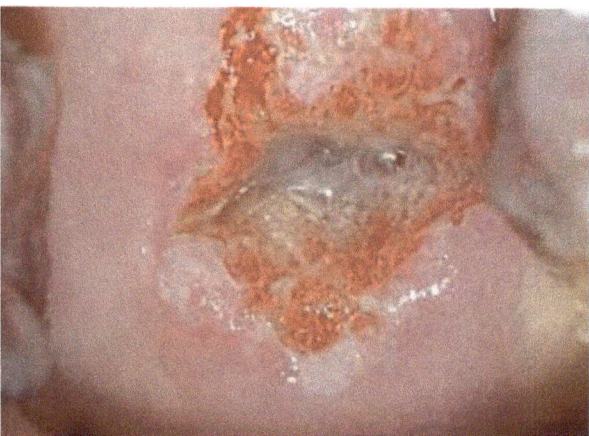

Figure 1. *Fully visible* SCJ—G2—biopsy indicated.

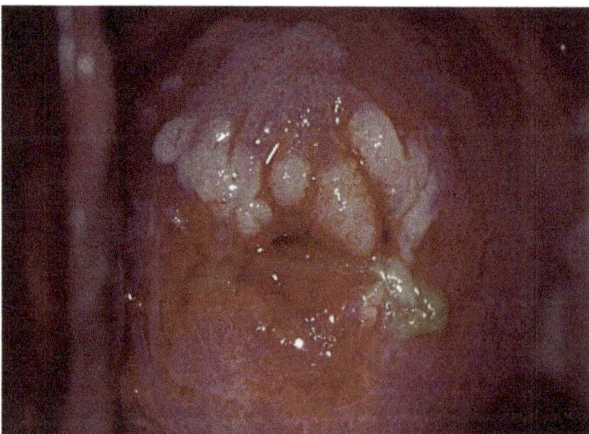

Figure 2. *Fully visible* SCJ—G2—biopsy indicated.

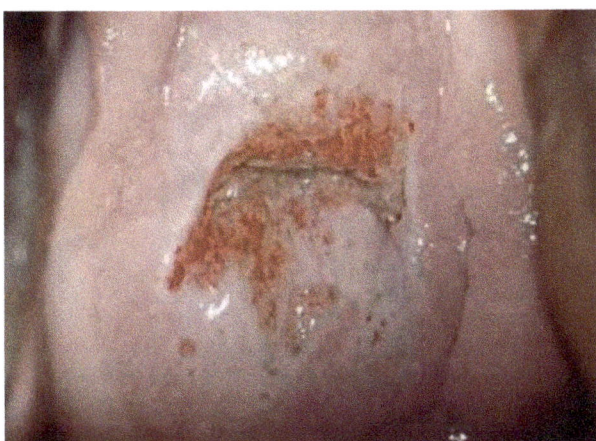

Figure 3. *Fully visible* SCJ—G2—biopsy indicated.

The experts' panel, for each single case, identified and recorded the following items: (1) assessment of colposcopic patterns according to the 2011 International Federation of Cervical Pathology and Colposcopy (IFCPC) nomenclature [14] and the 2017 American Society of Colposcopy and Cervical Pathology (ASCCP) terminology proposal [15]; (2) colposcopic impression, categorized as (2.1) negative, (2.2) favour low-grade lesion (Human Papillomavirus infection—Cervical Intraepithelial Neoplasia grade 1 CIN1), (2.3) favor high-grade lesion (Cervical Intraepithelial Neoplasia grade 2–3 CIN2+ or in situ squamous/adenocarcinoma), (2.4) favor malignant lesion (invasive squamous carcinoma or adenocarcinoma); (3) indication for taking a single biopsy or up to a maximum of 3 biopsies; and (4) the most appropriate area to be biopsied.

By the use of Qualtrix XM® software (2022 version) (www.qualtrics.com), an online platform was developed, either loggable via personal computers, tablets, or smartphones; following log-in, the application delivered the colposcopic digital high-resolution images integrated by a caption with details about the patient's age and primary screening results (cervical cytology and/or HPV-DNA detection), and a set of questions focused on: (1) squamo-columnar junction (SCJ) interpretation; (2) Transformation Zone (TZ) assessment; (3) biopsy indication; (4) areas suitable for performing biopsy; and (5) colposcopic impression.

The web link to the platform was forwarded to 10 academic and teaching Ob/Gyn Italian institutions, all having tertiary-level preventive oncological gynecology units, inviting colposcopy operators to anonymously attend the survey, detailing their respective level of expertise (<5 years vs. >5 years of colposcopy practice). Almost all juniors were residents/fellows of the participating institutions. The workload to complete the exam was anticipated to be at least 90 min according to the survey's characteristics, and it had to be finished in a single slot; at the end, each participant was provided with a final score but was not informed of the rate of correct/incorrect answers or the specification of the correct/incorrect ones. After completion of the test, the same could not be performed again because the platform credentials were no longer valid to log in to the application.

Data were collected, centralized, and recorded by the promoting investigators and analyzed using the R statistical software (www.r-project.org); participants responses to the test were compared with those of the committee and analyzed with those of variables treated as categorical. Pearson's chi-squared test (with Yates' continuity correction) and Cohen's *kappa* coefficient of agreement (95% CI intervals) were used to estimate the strength of associations; a *p* value < 0.05 was considered statistically significant, with *kappa* 0.60–0.80 indicating substantial agreement among observers [16,17]. The study design, methodology, and results were approved by the Scientific Committee of the Italian Society of Colposcopy and Cervico-Vaginal Pathology (SICPCV).

3. Results

The survey was conducted between January and April 2022 with the participation of 10 Italian centers: seventy-three (n. 73) colposcopists logged in to the web platform, 56 (76.7%) of them completing the whole test, and 17 (23.3%) only partially. The mean completion rate of the test for this latter subgroup of participants was 49%. The overall number of colposcopic observations/interpretations accounted for a total of 6155, upon which the survey has been performed. According to the level of colposcopic experience and practice, 27 (37%) participants reported a < 5 year practice in colposcopy (juniors) and 46 (63%) a personal experience > 5 years (seniors). No data were available regarding the number/year of colposcopies performed by participants.

The first part of the results analysis was primarily targeted at the identification of some intrinsic features of colposcopy, with the aim of evaluating the diagnostic accuracy and QC of the second-level colposcopy-based cervical cancer prevention workup. The overall analysis of the survey data in terms of colposcopy accuracy provided sensitivity and specificity rates of 61.6% and 77.1%, respectively; according to colposcopists' experience, sensitivity was 60.6% for seniors and 62.0% for juniors, while specificity was 76.7% and 77.4%, respectively. Considering the histology threshold of CIN2+, specificity increased to 87.7% (seniors 86.2% vs. juniors 88.6%).

In details, sensitivity increased from 60.9% in low-grade cases (HPV or CIN1) to 73.7% in high-grade cases (CIN2+); no statistically significant differences were obtained comparing seniors vs. juniors' rates of sensitivity (Table 1).

Table 1. Diagnostic accuracy of colposcopy.

	Histology	All	Experience in Colposcopy	
			Seniors	Juniors
sensitivity	HPV or CIN 1	60.9%	56.8%	63.4%
	CIN2-CIN 3	63.9%	64.9%	62.3%
	Cancer	47.9%	47.3%	48.3%
	CIN 2+	73.7%	73.5%	73.9%
	overall	61.6%	60.6%	62.0%
specificity	Negative	77.1%	76.7%	77.4%
	HPV or CIN 1	87.7%	86.2%	88.6%

Despite lacking statistical significance, senior colposcopists sensitivity was always inferior compared to juniors, with the only exception of CIN2-CIN3 cases (64.9% vs. 62.3%); when cancer cases were added to CIN2-CIN3 in a single analysis, the sensitivity rates of the two subgroups of colposcopists were closely comparable (73.5% vs. 73.9%). As for specificity, juniors' performance was again superior.

Table 2 shows the results according to the squamocolumnar junction (SCJ) evaluation, with the adoption of the 2011 IFCPC terminology [14]. Full agreement with the experts' panel was recorded in 81.2% when a *fully visible* SCJ was present, in 51.4% in *not fully visible* SCJ cases, and in 64.9% in *not visible* SCJ cases. Comparing seniors with juniors, a significant statistical difference was observed in *not visible* SCJ cases only (67.5% vs. 60.7%; $p = 0.011$). The Cohen's *kappa* correlation coefficient accounted for 0.49 (95% CI: 0.47–0.51) when the entire group of colposcopists was considered, for 0.49 (95% CI: 0.47–0.52) in the seniors group, and for 0.48 (95% CI: 0.45–0.51) in junior colposcopists. The highest rate of incorrect SCJ interpretation was recorded within the *not fully visible* SCJ group, where it accounted for 48.6%, with no statistical difference between seniors and juniors (48.1% vs. 49.5%).

Table 2. SCJ assessment (2011 IFCPC terminology [14]).

Experts Panel	Colposcopists	All	Experience in Colposcopy		
			Seniors	Juniors	
fully visibile	fully visibile [#]	81.2%	80.3%	82.6%	
	not fully visibile *	12.9%	13.4%	12.1%	p = NS
	not visibile	5.9%	6.3%	5.3%	
not fully visibile	fully visibile	29.3%	28.2%	31.2%	
	not fully visibile	51.4%	51.9%	50.5%	p = NS
	not visibile	19.3%	19.9%	18.3%	
not visibile	fully visibile	15.2%	12.5%	19.6%	
	not fully visibile	19.9%	20%	19.7%	p = 0.011
	not visibile	64.9%	67.5%	60.7%	

All colposcopists: $p < 2.2^{-16}$; Cohen's kappa correlation coefficient = 0.49 CI 95% [0.47–0.51]. Seniors: $p < 2.2^{-16}$; Cohen's kappa correlation coefficient = 0.49 CI 95% [0.47–0.52]. Juniors: $p < 2.2^{-16}$; Cohen's kappa correlation coefficient = 0.48 CI 95% [0.45–0.51]. [#] block letters = colposcopists vs. panel full agreement; * italics = incorrect SCJ judgment by colposcopists; SCJ = squamocolumnar junction; NS = not significant.

The same analysis was performed adopting the SCJ nomenclature proposal suggested by the American Society of Cervical Pathology and Colposcopy in 2017 [15], which divided the SCJ into two colposcopic categories only: *fully visible* and *not fully visible*. Full agreement with the experts increased to 75% in the *not fully visible* SCJ subgroup, with a statistically significant difference between seniors and juniors (77.1% vs. 72.8%, respectively; p = 0.011). The Cohen's *kappa* concordance coefficient also increased from 0.49 to 0.57 (95% CI: 0.54–0.59) for the whole set of participants, from 0.49 to 0.57 (95% CI: 0.55–0.60) for the seniors, and from 0.48 to 0.56 (95% CI: 0.52–0.59) for the juniors group. Table 3 summarizes these results.

Table 3. SCJ assessment (ASCCP 2017 Nomenclature [15]).

Experts Panel	Colposcopists	All	Experience in Colposcopy		
			Seniors	Juniors	
fully visible	fully visibile [#]	81.2%	80.3%	82.6%	p = NS
	not fully visibile *	18.8%	19.7%	17.4%	
not fully visible	fully visibile	24.6%	22.9%	27.2%	p = 0.011
	not fully visibile	75.4%	77.1%	72.8%	

All colposcopists: $p < 2.2^{-16}$; Cohen's kappa correlation coefficient = 0.57 CI 95% [0.54–0.59]. Seniors: $p < 2.2^{-16}$; Cohen's kappa correlation coefficient = 0.57 CI 95% [0.55–0.60]. Juniors: $p < 2.2^{-16}$; Cohen's kappa correlation coefficient = 0.56 CI 95% [0.52–0.59]. [#] block letters = colposcopists vs. panel full agreement; * italics = incorrect SCJ judgment by colposcopists; SCJ = squamocolumnar junction; NS = not significant.

Table 4 shows the results regarding colposcopists' interpretation of the Transformation Zone (TZ) compared with the experts' panel.

Full agreement was observed in 73.2% of Type 1, 53.8% of Type 2, and 66.7% of Type 3 TZ cases; within each group of TZ, a statistically significant difference was demonstrated comparing seniors to juniors: in particular, Type 1 and Type 2 TZ were better identified by junior colposcopists (79% vs. 69.5% and 55.9% vs. 52.3%, respectively; $p < 0.05$), while Type 3 TZ was significantly better identified by seniors (71.7% vs. 58.3%; $p < 0.05$).

In this analysis, the highest rate of incorrect interpretation was identified in senior colposcopists evaluating Type 2 TZ cases (47.7%), while the lowest rate was recorded in juniors' evaluation of Type 1 TZ (21%).

Table 4. TZ assessment.

Experts Panel	Colposcopists	All	Experience in Colposcopy		
			Seniors	Juniors	
Type 1	Type 1 #	73.2%	69.5%	79%	$p = 1.029^{-8}$
	Type 2 *	20.1%	22.3%	16.7%	
	Type 3	6.7%	8.2%	4.3%	
Type 2	Type 1	26.2%	23.7%	30%	$p = 7.006^{-8}$
	Type 2	53.8%	52.3%	55.9%	
	Type 3	20%	24%	14.1%	
Type 3	Type 1	11.1%	9.1%	14.5%	$p = 7.58^{-7}$
	Type 2	22.2 %	19.2%	27.2%	
	Type 3	66.7%	71.7%	58.3%	

All colposcopists: $p < 2.2^{-16}$; Cohen's *kappa* correlation coefficient = 0.46 CI 95% [0.45–0.48]. Seniors: $p < 2.2^{-16}$; Cohen's *kappa* correlation coefficient = 0.46 CI 95% [0.44–0.48]. Juniors: $p < 2.2^{-16}$; Cohen's *kappa* correlation coefficient = 0.47 CI 95% [0.44–0.50]. # block letters = colposcopists vs. panel full agreement; * italics = incorrect SCJ judgment by colposcopists; TZ = Transformation Zone.

The second part of the survey results analysis was conversely targeted to investigate the accuracy of the colposcopic procedure through the assessment of colposcopic interpretation of cervical patterns and its influence on the operators' clinical decisions.

As far as it concerned the assessment of grade (G) of the colposcopic pattern compared to proven histology, the following results were obtained: full agreement with histology was achieved in 60.59% of cases with G1/low-grade lesions, in 59.11% of G2/high-grade lesions, and in 64.64% of colposcopic patterns suspicious for cancer and histologically confirmed cervical malignancy; these concordance rates can also be seen as PPV of colposcopy.

Interestingly, 5.05% and 19.26% of cases with a histologically proven CIN2+ were categorized as colposcopically negative or G1 by participants, respectively.

On the other hand, overestimation of the colposcopic pattern reached the highest rate in histologically proven low-grade lesions (HPV-CIN1), which were classified as G2 in 24.70% of cases (Table 5).

Table 5. Predictive value of colposcopic grade (G).

Colposcopic Grade	Histology			
	Negative	HPV or CIN 1	CIN2-CIN 3	Cancer
Negative	76.25% *	18.70%	4.21%	0.84%
G1	20.15%	60.59%	17.97%	1.29%
G2	4.70%	24.70%	59.11%	11.49%
Cancer	1.52%	3.05%	30.79%	64.64%

Pearson's chi-squared test: $p < 2.2^{-16}$; Cohen's *kappa* correlation coefficient = 0.49 CI 95% [0.47–0.51]. * NPV; block letters = colposcopists vs. panel full agreement and PPV. G1 = minor colposcopic.

A similar analysis was performed considering the colposcopic impression formulated by colposcopists compared to histology.

A negative colposcopic impression correlated with a negative histology in 77.9% of cases, allowing this figure to be seen as NPV. Taking into consideration histologically confirmed high-grade lesions (CIN2-CIN3), which represent the main objective of the cervical cancer prevention strategy, the colposcopic impression of a high-grade lesion was correctly formulated by colposcopists in 59.4% of cases.

When cancer cases were added to CIN2/CIN3, the PPV of a high-grade lesion colposcopic impression increased to 70.5%.

The PPV of a colposcopic impression suspicious for cancer was 64.4% ($p < 0.05$; Cohen's *kappa* correlation coefficient = 0.51; 95% CI: [0.50–0.53]) (Table 6).

Table 6. Predictive value of colposcopic impression (CI).

Colposcopic Impression	Histology			
	Negative	HPV or CIN1	CIN2-CIN3	Cancer
Negative	77.9% *	18.5%	3%	0.6%
LG	18.8%	60%	19.7%	1.5%
HG	4.5%	25%	59.4% #	11.1%
Cancer	1.2%	6.5%	27.9%	64.4% ≈

Pearson's chi-squared test: $p < 2.2^{-16}$; Cohen's *kappa* correlation coefficient = 0.51—CI 95% [0.50–0.53]. * NPV = Negative Predictive Value; # PPV = Positive Predictive for CIN2-CIN3; ≈ PPV = Positive Predictive Value for cancer; LG = low-grade lesion; HG = high-grade lesion.

Directly correlated with the colposcopic impression and the G assessments, colposcopists were asked to indicate the need for taking biopsy/biopsies and the cervical site they thought was the most appropriate for histological confirmation; biopsies were performed in 3404 cases out of 6155 in the case of the experts panel (55%), and in 3482 cases out of 6155 (56%) in the case of candidates. Figures 4–6 illustrate how the biopsy/biopsies sites were indicated by colposcopists.

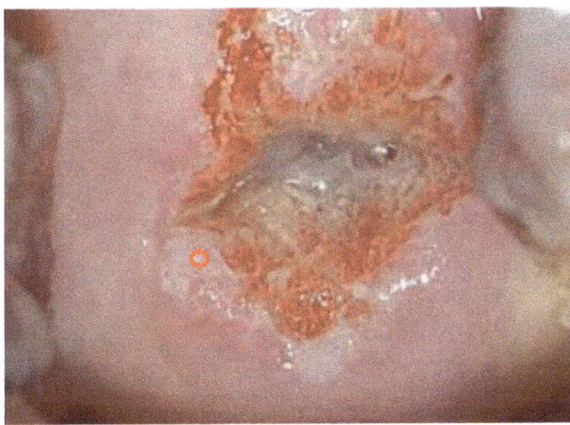

Figure 4. A single biopsy is indicated (correct site).

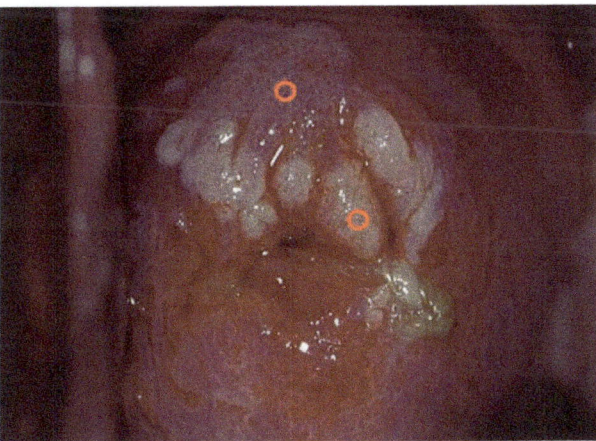

Figure 5. Multiple biopsies indicated (correct sites).

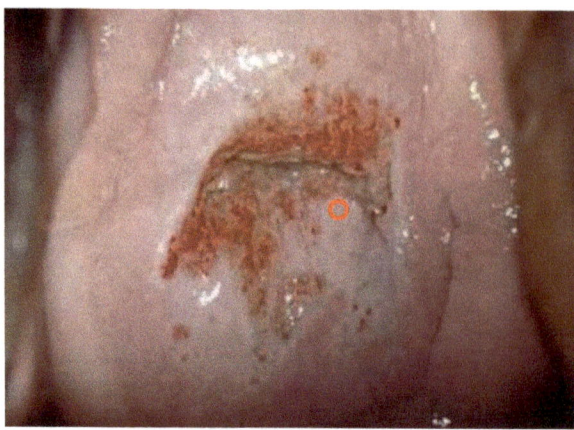

Figure 6. A single biopsy is indicated (correct site).

According to colposcopists experience, junior colposcopists performed biopsies in 52.7% of the whole set of cases, while more experienced operators performed them in 59%. Biopsies were omitted in 96.8% of cases evaluated by colposcopists as negative, in 30.4% of cases evaluated as LG lesion, in 2.1% of cases evaluated as HG lesion, and in 0.3% of cases evaluated as neoplasia. Furthermore, it was observed that as the degree of the lesion increased, the number of biopsies consistently increased; more than one single biopsy was reported in 12.6% of cases with a colposcopic impression of LG, in 52.5% of cases of HG, and in 82.5% of cases with a colposcopic impression of cancer.

The correct site for performing biopsies was recognized in 58.9%, 77.3%, and 91.7% of histologically proven LG lesions (HPV-CIN1), HG lesions (CIN2-CIN3), and cervical cancer, respectively, while an incorrect site was indicated in 16.8%, 13.6%, and 5.3%.

Noteworthy, non-biopsy rates accounted for 24.3% of HPV-CIN1 cases and for 12.1% of CIN2+ cases ($p < 0.05$) (Table 7).

Table 7. Biopsy decision.

		Histology			
		Negative	HPV or CIN 1	CIN2-CIN 3	Cancer
biopsy	not performed	58.6%	24.3%	9.1%	3.0%
	yes, wrong site	1.7%	16.8%	13.6%	5.3%
	yes, correct site	39.7%	58.9%	77.3%	91.7%

Pearson's chi-squared test: $p < 2.2^{-16}$.

Moreover, when the analysis focused on the subgroup of cases having a CIN2+ proven histology and a colposcopic impression of LG lesion expressed by colposcopists, the correctness of biopsy performance was significantly influenced by experience: junior colposcopists had a higher non-biopsy rate (20% vs. 10.1%), while seniors had a higher rate of correctly performed biopsies (73.9% vs. 66.9%) ($p < 0.05$) (Table 8).

Table 8. Underestimation of colposcopic impression vs. biopsy decision.

	Biopsy	Experience in Colposcopy		
		All	Seniors	Juniors
LG Colposcopic Impression with CIN2+ histology	not performed	13.6%	10.1%	20%
	yes, wrong site	15%	16%	13.1%
	yes, correct site	71.4%	73.9%	66.9%
			$p = 0.013$	

LG = low-grade lesion.

4. Discussion

As colposcopy is a fundamental step as part of screening programs for the detection of pre-cancer cervical lesions, the success of the preventive strategy entirely depends on the diagnostic accuracy of the procedure. The assessment of colposcopy accuracy, in other words, the QC and QA processes, requires figures of the highest reliability in order to correctly evaluate the performance and effectiveness of colposcopic practice or to promote changes in standard requirements for operators.

This practical need deals with the objective issue of the very wide range of colposcopy accuracy figures available in the literature; meta-analysis studies have been published with the aim of providing statistically credible data to be used as comparison or reference values, thus allowing effective QC and QA processes in clinical practice. As an example, the most recently published meta-analysis, based on 15 studies and 22,764 cases, reports a combined sensitivity and specificity of 92% and 51% for a LG-SIL+ threshold and of 68% and 93%, respectively, for a HG-SIL+ threshold [18].

Unfortunately, data obtained in this fashion suffers from the significant bias of including papers with different study designs that influence the outcome reported; widely different figures are in fact reported depending on how the outcome of colposcopy is evaluated. Some studies investigate colposcopy outcome based upon the Colposcopic Impression (CI) that a CIN2+ is present; others evaluate the outcome on taking a biopsy because there is thought to be a Disease Present (DP), with the threshold of DP usually being a CIN1+. For this reason, the outcome measures have a significant effect on accuracy evaluation [19], indicating wide differences in both sensitivity and specificity.

That said, the present study, due to its main object of investigating and analyzing the performance of colposcopy mostly in terms of the QC of colposcopists and of the procedure, has to be seen as CI-based. Thereafter, the reported results are mainly discussed and compared with similar literature data. Nevertheless, some DP-based outcome assessments have been possible and are similarly discussed and compared.

The combined CI sensitivity and specificity (CIN2+ threshold) values obtained from the survey were 73.7% and 87.7%, respectively (see Table 1), with no statistically significant differences between senior and junior colposcopists; in general, this can be seen as a favorable result of the teaching programs of the involved institutions. These figures, compared with previous reviews [7,20], may be placed above weighted mean values for sensitivity and fully comparable with weighted mean values for specificity. Being the QC of Italian colposcopy/colposcopists the major objective of the study, these figures, together with the absence of significant differences between juniors and seniors, in our opinion, allow a more than satisfactory general evaluation of the colposcopy/colposcopists performance. The strength of this impression may further be supported considering the difficulty of the survey and the workload required of attendants.

This is particularly interesting in consideration of the experience level of the participants: since junior colposcopists performance accounted for better accuracy in each subset of thresholds, though without statistical significance, this may either reflect the good quality of the teaching programs in the institutions surveyed or the need for senior colposcopists to consider some kind of self-improvement.

In terms of potential methodological biases, the use of static digital images of the cervix versus live colposcopy to assess the diagnostic accuracy and to perform QC evaluations, does not represent a limitation concerning the reliability of the sensitivity/specificity figures; as reported by Liu [21], recognitions of colposcopic patterns and colposcopic impression formulated on live colposcopy are reproducible on static digital images with high levels of agreement. Moreover, the use of a web-based program of digital colpophotographs, though with the different aim of assessing the accuracy of colposcopically directed biopsies, has already been proposed in Italy and demonstrated effective for QA purposes [9,22–24].

Regarding the results specifically directed to QC of colposcopists, we observed full agreement with the experts panel for the SCJ evaluation, following the 2011 IFCCP terminology [14], in 82.2% of *fully visible* SCJs, in 51.4% of *not fully visible* SCJs, and in 64.9% of *not visible* SCJs; in this analysis, a statistically significant difference was observed between seniors (67.5%) versus juniors (60.7%) for the *not visible* SCJ subgroup ($p = 0.01$).

When SCJ was categorized following the 2017 ASCCP proposal [15], grouping the *not fully visible* and the *not visible* SCJ into one single category named *not fully visible*, full agreement with the experts increased to 75.4%, still having a statistically significant difference between seniors (77.1%) and juniors (72.8%) ($p = 0.01$).

Comparable comments can be made as far as it concerns the Transformation Zone (TZ): full agreement with the expert panel was achieved in 73.2%, 53.8%, and 66.7% of Type 1, Type 2, and Type 3 (2011 IFCPC terminology) [14], respectively; statistically significant differences were present between seniors and juniors for all three categories (see Table 4). The lowest rate of agreement for both SCJ visibility and the type of the TZ was recorded in the intermediate category.

Several authors have addressed the issue and the practical implications of adopting uniform and standardized colposcopy terminology, underlining the importance and accuracy improvement of the procedure when precise definitions of cervical patterns are widely utilized in clinical practice. In this view, the 2011 IFCPC terminology has represented a significant step forward in terms of colposcopy accuracy, having demonstrated better correlation with histology compared to traditional methods [25]. Despite that, the SCJ/TZ parameters have been repeatedly identified as the weak side of the process, as the intermediate categories, namely the *not fully visible* SCJ and the *Type 2* TZ, were always associated with the lowest grade of accuracy and reproducibility [26,27].

Our results consistently confirm this analysis and support the 2017 ASCPC proposal, detailing a significant increase in accuracy when a two-tailed classification of the SCJ is adopted, as recently published articles report [15,28].

The analysis of the grade of the TZ (G) and of the colposcopic impression compared with histology allows some comments that, in our opinion, are particularly interesting in terms of providing accuracy figures having both QC and QA meanings.

In terms of minor/major acetic acid alterations, full agreement was achieved in 76.25% (negative), 60.59% (G1), 59.11% (G2), and 64.64% (cancer suspicious). It is noteworthy that a *negative* interpretation and a *G1* interpretation underestimated 5.05% and 19.26% of CIN2+ histologically proven lesions, respectively (Table 5).

As far as it concerned the colposcopic impression, a *negative* impression and a *LG lesion* impression underestimated 3.06% and 21.2% of CIN2+ histologically proven lesions, respectively (Table 6).

The analysis of these figures, performed consistently with the DP (CIN1+ threshold) principles of QA assessment, provided the following results: Overall, overrating the colposcopic impression was 1.5 times more common than underrating. However, when histologically proven HG lesions (CIN2-CIN3) were considered, overestimation and underestimation were fully comparable. It is in some way reassuring that only 3.06% of CIN2+ were considered colposcopically negative. Less reassuring is the detected 21% underestimation rate of CIN2+ lesions that were colposcopically interpreted as *LG lesions*. In terms of colposcopy principles, this should not represent a serious issue since an *LG lesion* colposcopic impression represents an indication for targeted biopsy, though the option of non-biopsy is acceptable [29]. Unfortunately, the balancing effect of the targeted biopsy in reducing the negative effect of colposcopic underestimation is largely influenced by real-life practice.

As shown in Table 7, our survey identified a 36.4% non-biopsy rate in histologically not-negative cases (24.3% of HPV-CIN1, 9.1% of CIN2-CIN3, and 3% of cancers, respectively). As reported, non-biopsy rates significantly decreased with increasing severity of histology ($p < 0.05$). These findings are interestingly consistent with several population-based studies on colposcopy QA [30,31]. Further, addressing the analysis specifically to cases with a *LG lesion* colposcopic impression and a CIN2+ histology, the non-biopsy rate accounted for 13.6%, with a statistically significant difference between seniors and juniors (10.1% vs. 20%) ($p = 0.01$) (Table 8). It clearly appears that experience in colposcopy plays an important role, significantly decreasing by 50% the risk of lower CI accuracy.

In parallel, together with the non-biopsy rates, our figures regarding the correctness of biopsy-taking deserve some comments; correctly performed biopsies accounted for 58.9% of HPV-CIN1, 77.3% of CIN2-CIN3, and 91.7% of cancers. In our data, the overall amount of incorrect-site biopsies performed accounted for 16.8% in HPV-CIN1, 13.6% in CIN2-CIN3, and 5.3% in cancers ($p < 0.05$%); in the subgroup with an *LG lesion* colposcopic impression and CIN2+ histology, a biopsy was correctly performed in 71.4% of cases (seniors 73.9% vs. juniors 66.9%) ($p < 0.05$).

As reported by Sideri [9], potential biases can be addressed when the accuracy of colposcopically targeted biopsy is investigated for QA purposes. Some may favor accuracy (e.g., the artificial conditions that may facilitate recognition of colposcopic features), while others may have the opposite effect (e.g., the impossibility of increasing the magnification and the single-shot chance given to participants). Nonetheless, the overall sensitivity does not appear to be significantly influenced by these factors.

Despite an overall good performance of the decision-making process for taking a colposcopically targeted biopsy, our results provide another confirmation that the sensitivity of biopsy for HG lesions is a justified concern; a large amount of data are available on the subject, consistently pointing to the need for improving options [5,32–35]. Colposcopists' experience, though with marginal differences, has consistently been identified as positively influencing colposcopy accuracy [36,37].

Being cervical pre-cancer lesions detection the primary objective of colposcopy within cervical cancer screening programs, results from the present QC and QA assessments of colposcopy in Italy suggest some final considerations: (a) the overall sensitivity/specificity figures are in agreement with, and in some aspects better than, the mean figures reported by meta-analysis; (b) underestimation of colposcopy is particularly relevant when a *LG lesion* colposcopic impression is formulated; (c) the recommendation of taking a colposcopically targeted biopsy in cases of *LG lesion* colposcopic impression is justified by the rate of missed CIN2+ cases; (d) the low rate of statistically significant differences between experienced and junior colposcopists allows a favorable judgment of teaching programs; and (e) the need for continuous update, improvement, and QC of colposcopists is recommendable. In conclusion, the authors of the present article strongly believe that the adoption of colposcopy standards and quality recommendations by scientific societies is a fundamental step for effective cervical cancer prevention [10–13,29].

Author Contributions: Conceptualization, M.O. and F.C.; methodology: M.O., F.C., C.M. and L.I.; data curation: M.O., F.C., C.M. and L.I.; formal analysis, M.O., F.C., C.M. and L.I.; investigation, F.C., F.S., N.C., A.S., B.G., R.D.V., C.R., F.L., M.L.D.M., A.C., J.D.G., E.P., A.D.I., C.C., M.D., M.C. (Massimo Capodanno) and A.P.; supervision, M.O. and M.C. (Massimo Candiani); validation, M.O., F.C., A.C., F.S. and M.B.; writing—original draft, M.O., F.C., A.C. and F.S.; writing—review and editing, M.O., F.C., A.C. and F.S. All authors have read and agreed to the published version of the manuscript.

Funding: This research received no external funding.

Institutional Review Board Statement: Due to the study design, no ethical approval was required.

Informed Consent Statement: Not applicable.

Data Availability Statement: Research data are available on request from the corresponding author.

Conflicts of Interest: The authors declare no conflict of interest.

References

1. Perkins, R.B.; Guido, R.S.; Castle, P.E.; Chelmow, D.; Einstein, M.H.; Garcia, F.; Huh, W.K.; Kim, J.J.; Moscicki, A.; Nayar, R.; et al. 2019 ASCCP Risk-Based Management Consensus Guidelines for Abnormal Cervical Cancer Screening Tests and Cancer Precursors. *J. Low Genit Tract Dis.* **2020**, *24*, 102–131. [CrossRef] [PubMed]
2. Perkins, R.B.; Guido, R.L.; Saraiya, M.; Sawaya, G.F.; Wentzensen, N.; Schiffman, M.; Feldman, S. Summary of Current Guidelines for Cervical Cancer Screening and Management of Abnormal Test Results: 2016–2020. *J. Womens Health. (Larchmt)* **2021**, *30*, 5–13. [CrossRef] [PubMed]
3. Cagle, A.J.; Hu, S.Y.; Sellors, J.W.; Bao, Y.P.; Lim, J.M.; Li, S.M.; Lewis, K.; Song, Y.; Ma, J.F.; Pan, Q.J.; et al. Use of an expanded gold standard to estimate the accuracy of colposcopy and visual inspection with acetic acid. *Int. J. Cancer* **2010**, *126*, 156–161. [CrossRef] [PubMed]
4. Massad, L.S.; Jeronimo, J.; Schiffman, M.; National Institutes of Health/American Society for Colposcopy and Cervical Pathology (NIH/ASCCP) Research Group. Interobserver agreement in the assessment of components of colposcopic grading. *Obstet. Gynecol.* **2008**, *111*, 1279–1284. [CrossRef] [PubMed]
5. Gage, J.C.; Hanson, V.W.; Abbey, K.; Dippery, S.; Gardner, S.; Kubota, J.; Schiffman, M.; Solomon, D.; Jeronimo, J.; ASCUS LSIL Triage Study (ALTS) Group. Number of cervical biopsies and sensitivity of colposcopy. *Obstet. Gynecol.* **2006**, *108*, 264–272. [CrossRef]
6. Zuchna, C.; Hager, M.; Tringler, B.; Georgoulopoulos, A.; Ciresa-Koenig, A.; Volgger, B.; Widschwendter, A.; Staudach, A. Diagnostic accuracy of guided cervical biopsies: A prospective multicenter study comparing the histopathology of simultaneous biopsy and cone specimen. *Am. J. Obstet. Gynecol.* **2010**, *203*, 321.e1–321.e6. [CrossRef]
7. Underwood, M.; Arbyn, M.; Parry-Smith, W.; De Bellis-Ayres, S.; Todd, R.; Redman, C.W.E.; Moss, E.L. Accuracy of colposcopy-directed punch biopsies: A systematic review and meta-analysis. *BJOG* **2012**, *119*, 1293–1301. [CrossRef]
8. Benedet, J.L.; Anderson, G.H.; Matisic, J.P.; Miller, D.M. A quality-control program for colposcopic practice. *Obstet. Gynecol.* **1991**, *78*, 872–875.
9. Sideri, M.; Garutti, P.; Costa, S.; Cristiani, P.; Schincaglia, P.; Sassoli de Bianchi, P.; Naldoni, C.; Bucchi, L. Accuracy of Colposcopically Directed Biopsy: Results from an Online Quality Assurance Programme for Colposcopy in a Population-Based Cervical Screening Setting in Italy. *Biomed. Res. Int.* **2015**, *2015*, 614035. [CrossRef]
10. Mayeaux, E.J.J.; Novetsky, A.P.; Chelmow, D.; Garcia, F.; Choma, K.; Liu, A.H.; Papasozomenos, T.; Einstein, M.H.; Massad, L.S.; Wentzensen, N.; et al. ASCCP Colposcopy Standards: Colposcopy Quality Improvement Recommendations for the United States. *J. Low Genit Tract Dis.* **2017**, *21*, 242–248. [CrossRef]
11. Waxman, A.G.; Conageski, C.; Silver, M.I.; Tedeschi, C.; Stier, E.A.; Apgar, B.; Huh, W.K.; Wentzensen, N.; Massad, L.S.; Khan, M.J.; et al. ASCCP Colposcopy Standards: How Do We Perform Colposcopy? Implications for Establishing Standards. *J. Low Genit Tract Dis.* **2017**, *21*, 235–241. [CrossRef]
12. Moss, E.L.; Redman, C.W.E.; Arbyn, M.; Dollery, E.; Petry, K.U.; Nieminen, P.; Myerson, N.; Leeson, S.C. Colposcopy training and assessment across the member countries of the European Federation for Colposcopy. *Eur. J. Obstet. Gynecol. Reprod. Biol.* **2015**, *188*, 124–128. [CrossRef]
13. Moss, E.L.; Arbyn, M.; Dollery, E.; Leeson, S.; Petry, K.U.; Nieminen, P.; Redman, C.W.E. European Federation of Colposcopy quality standards Delphi consultation. *Eur. J. Obstet. Gynecol. Reprod. Biol.* **2013**, *170*, 255–258. [CrossRef]
14. Bornstein, J.; Bentley, J.; Bosze, P.; Girardi, F.; Haefner, H.; Menton, M.; Perrotta, M.; Prendiville, W.; Russell, P.; Sideri, M.; et al. 2011 colposcopic terminology of the International Federation for Cervical Pathology and Colposcopy. *Obstet. Gynecol.* **2012**, *120*, 166–172. [CrossRef]
15. Khan, M.J.; Werner, C.L.; Darragh, T.M.; Guido, R.S.; Mathews, C.; Moscicki, A.; Mitchell, M.M.; Schiffman, M.; Wentzensen, N.; Massad, L.S.; et al. ASCCP Colposcopy Standards: Role of Colposcopy, Benefits, Potential Harms, and Terminology for Colposcopic Practice. *J. Low Genit Tract Dis.* **2017**, *21*, 223–229. [CrossRef]
16. Gardner, M.; Altman, D. *Statistics with Confidence. Confidence Intervals and Statistical Guidelines*; BMJ Books: London, UK, 1989.
17. Landis, J.R.; Koch, G.G. The measurement of observer agreement for categorical data. *Biometrics* **1977**, *33*, 159–174. [CrossRef]
18. Qin, D.; Bai, A.; Xue, P.; Seery, S.; Wang, J.; Mendez, M.J.G.; Li, Q.; Jiang, Y.; Qiao, Y. Colposcopic accuracy in diagnosing squamous intraepithelial lesions: A systematic review and meta-analysis of the International Federation of Cervical Pathology and Colposcopy 2011 terminology. *BMC Cancer* **2023**, *23*, 187. [CrossRef]
19. Brown, B.H.; Tidy, J.A. The diagnostic accuracy of colposcopy—A review of research methodology and impact on the outcomes of quality assurance. *Eur. J. Obstet. Gynecol. Reprod. Biol.* **2019**, *240*, 182–186. [CrossRef]
20. Mitchell, M.F.; Schottenfeld, D.; Tortolero-Luna, G.; Cantor, S.B.; Richards-Kortum, R. Colposcopy for the diagnosis of squamous intraepithelial lesions: A meta-analysis. *Obstet. Gynecol.* **1998**, *91*, 626–631. [CrossRef]
21. Liu, A.H.; Gold, M.A.; Schiffman, M.; Smith, K.M.; Zuna, R.E.; Dunn, S.T.; Gage, J.C.; Walker, J.L.; Wentzensen, N. Comparison of Colposcopic Impression Based on Live Colposcopy and Evaluation of Static Digital Images. *J. Low Genit Tract Dis.* **2016**, *20*, 154–161. [CrossRef]

22. Garutti, P.; Cristiani, P.; Fantin, G.P.; Sopracordevole, F.; Costa, S.; Schincaglia, P.; Ravaioli, A.; Sassoli de Bianchi, P.; Naldoni, C.; Ferretti, S.; et al. Interpretation of colposcopy in population-based cervical screening services in north-eastern Italy: An online interregional agreement study. *Eur. J. Obstet. Gynecol. Reprod. Biol.* **2016**, *206*, 64–69. [CrossRef] [PubMed]
23. Bucchi, L.; Cristiani, P.; Costa, S.; Schincaglia, P.; Garutti, P.; Sassoli de Bianchi, P.; Naldoni, C.; Olea, O.; Sideri, M. Rationale and development of an on-line quality assurance programme for colposcopy in a population-based cervical screening setting in Italy. *BMC Health Serv. Res.* **2013**, *13*, 237. [CrossRef] [PubMed]
24. Cristiani, P.; Costa, S.; Schincaglia, P.; Garutti, P.; de Bianchi, P.S.; Naldoni, C.; Sideri, M.; Bucchi, L. An online quality assurance program for colposcopy in a population-based cervical screening setting in Italy: Results on colposcopic impression. *J. Low Genit Tract Dis.* **2014**, *18*, 309–313. [CrossRef] [PubMed]
25. Rema, P.N.; Mathew, A.; Thomas, S. Performance of colposcopic scoring by modified International Federation of Cervical Pathology and Colposcopy terminology for diagnosing cervical intraepithelial neoplasia in a low-resource setting. *S. Asian J. Cancer* **2019**, *8*, 218–220. [CrossRef] [PubMed]
26. Fan, A.; Wang, C.; Zhang, L.; Yan, Y.; Han, C.; Xue, F. Diagnostic value of the 2011 International Federation for Cervical Pathology and Colposcopy Terminology in predicting cervical lesions. *Oncotarget* **2018**, *9*, 9166–9176. [CrossRef]
27. Li, Y.; Duan, X.; Sui, L.; Xu, F.; Xu, S.; Zhang, H.; Xu, C. Closer to a Uniform Language in Colposcopy: Study on the Potential Application of 2011 International Federation for Cervical Pathology and Colposcopy Terminology in Clinical Practice. *Biomed. Res. Int.* **2017**, *2017*, 8984516. [CrossRef]
28. Garutti, P.; Cristiani, P.; Ferretti, S.; Sassoli de Bianchi, P.; Ravaioli, A.; Bucchi, L. The Results of an Italian Quality Assurance Program Support the New American Society for Colposcopy and Cervical Pathology Recommendations for Colposcopy Practice. *J. Low Genit Tract Dis.* **2018**, *22*, 235–236. [CrossRef]
29. Redman, C.W.E.; Kesic, V.; Cruickshank, M.E.; Gultekin, M.; Carcopino, X.; Castro Sanchez, M.; Grigore, M.; Jakobsson, M.; Kuppers, V.; Pedro, A.; et al. European consensus statement on essential colposcopy. *Eur. J. Obstet. Gynecol. Reprod. Biol.* **2021**, *256*, 57–62. [CrossRef]
30. Benedet, J.L.; Matisic, J.P.; Bertrand, M.A. An analysis of 84,244 patients from the British Columbia cytology-colposcopy program. *Gynecol. Oncol.* **2004**, *92*, 127–134. [CrossRef]
31. Alfonzo, E.; Zhang, C.; Daneshpip, F.; Strander, B. Accuracy of colposcopy in the Swedish screening program. *Acta Obstet. Gynecol. Scand.* **2023**, *102*, 549–555. [CrossRef]
32. Buxton, E.J.; Luesley, D.M.; Shafi, M.I.; Rollason, M. Colposcopically directed punch biopsy: A potentially misleading investigation. *Br. J. Obstet. Gynaecol.* **1991**, *98*, 1273–1276. [CrossRef]
33. Chappatte, O.A.; Byrne, D.L.; Raju, K.S.; Nayagam, M.; Kenney, A. Histological differences between colposcopic-directed biopsy and loop excision of the transformation zone (LETZ): A cause for concern. *Gynecol. Oncol.* **1991**, *43*, 46–50. [CrossRef]
34. Moss, E.L.; Hadden, P.; Douce, G.; Jones, P.W.; Arbyn, M.; Redman, C.W.E. Is the colposcopically directed punch biopsy a reliable diagnostic test in women with minor cytological lesions? *J. Low Genit Tract Dis.* **2012**, *16*, 421–426. [CrossRef]
35. Costa, S.; Nuzzo, M.D.; Rubino, A.; Rambelli, V.; Marinelli, M.; Santini, D.; Cristiani, P.; Bucchi, L. Independent determinants of inaccuracy of colposcopically directed punch biopsy of the cervix. *Gynecol. Oncol.* **2003**, *90*, 57–63. [CrossRef]
36. Bifulco, G.; De Rosa, N.; Lavitola, G.; Piccoli, R.; Bertrando, A.; Natella, V.; Di Carlo, C.; Insabato, L.; Nappi, C. A prospective randomized study on limits of colposcopy and histology: The skill of colposcopist and colposcopy-guided biopsy in diagnosis of cervical intraepithelial lesions. *Infect. Agent Cancer* **2015**, *10*, 47–49. [CrossRef]
37. Stuebs, F.A.; Schulmeyer, C.E.; Mehlhorn, G.; Gass, P.; Kehl, S.; Renner, S.K.; Renner, S.P.; Geppert, C.; Adler, W.; Hartmann, A.; et al. Accuracy of colposcopy-directed biopsy in detecting early cervical neoplasia: A retrospective study. *Arch. Gynecol. Obstet.* **2019**, *299*, 525–532. [CrossRef]

Disclaimer/Publisher's Note: The statements, opinions and data contained in all publications are solely those of the individual author(s) and contributor(s) and not of MDPI and/or the editor(s). MDPI and/or the editor(s) disclaim responsibility for any injury to people or property resulting from any ideas, methods, instructions or products referred to in the content.

MDPI
St. Alban-Anlage 66
4052 Basel
Switzerland
www.mdpi.com

Diagnostics Editorial Office
E-mail: diagnostics@mdpi.com
www.mdpi.com/journal/diagnostics

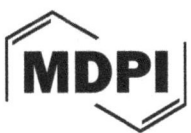

Disclaimer/Publisher's Note: The statements, opinions and data contained in all publications are solely those of the individual author(s) and contributor(s) and not of MDPI and/or the editor(s). MDPI and/or the editor(s) disclaim responsibility for any injury to people or property resulting from any ideas, methods, instructions or products referred to in the content.

www.ingramcontent.com/pod-product-compliance
Lightning Source LLC
LaVergne TN
LVHW070617100526
838202LV00012B/665